CITY OF PLAGUES

CITY OF PLAGUES

*Disease, Poverty, and Deviance
in San Francisco*

Susan Craddock

University of Minnesota Press

Minneapolis

London

The University of Minnesota Press gratefully acknowledges permission to reprint the following. An earlier version of chapter 1 appeared as "Tuberculosis, Tenements, and the Epistemology of Neglect: San Francisco in the Nineteenth Century," *Ecumene* 5, no. 1 (January 1998): 53–80; copyright 1998 by Arnold Publishers, used with permission. An earlier version of chapter 2 appeared as "Sewers and Scapegoats: Spatial Metaphors of Smallpox in Nineteenth-Century San Francisco," *Social Science and Medicine* 41, no. 7 (1995): 957–68; copyright 1995 by Elsevier Science Publications, used with permission from Elsevier Science. An earlier version of chapter 2 also appeared as "Embodying Place: Pathologizing Chinese and Chinatown in Nineteenth-Century San Francisco," *Antipode* 31, no. 4 (October 1999): 351–71; copyright 1999 by Blackwell Publishers, used with permission. An excerpt from the poem "Life in a Lung Resort," by Ruth Ashby, appears in chapter 5 and is reproduced with permission of the Bancroft Library, owners of the copyright in the Arequipa Sanatorium Records (92/894c, box 1:20).

Published by the University of Minnesota Press
111 Third Avenue South, Suite 290
Minneapolis, MN 55401–2520
http://www.upress.umn.edu

Printed in the United States of America on acid-free paper

The University of Minnesota is an equal-opportunity educator and employer.

Library of Congress Cataloging-in-Publication Data
Craddock, Susan.
    City of plagues : disease, poverty, and deviance in San Francisco / Susan Craddock.
        p.   cm.
    Includes bibliographical references and index.
    ISBN 0-8166-3047-X (hbk.) – ISBN 0-8166-3048-8 (pbk.)
    1. Epidemics–California–San Francisco–History.   2. Tuberculosis–California–San Francisco–History.   3. Communicable diseases–California–San Francisco–History.
    I. Title.
    RA650.5 .C73 2000
    614.4′9794′61 – dc21   99-057350

11 10 09 08 07 06 05 04 03 02 01 00   10 9 8 7 6 5 4 3 2 1

For Simon, whose smile is everything

CONTENTS

ACKNOWLEDGMENTS

Many debts accrue in the process of writing a book, most of which I am afraid cannot be repaid. This book would not have been possible without a Rockefeller / Social Science Research Council Grant on Poverty and the Urban Underclass, which allowed me the luxury of a year's archival research from 1992 to 1993. My thanks go to the staff of The Bancroft Library at the University of California, Berkeley, and especially to Dave Rez. Thanks also go to the staffs of the National Library of Medicine, the National Archives, the California State Archives, the San Francisco History Room at the public library, and the medical history library at the University of California, San Francisco. It would also not have been possible to finish this book without a semester's fellowship at the Udall Center for the Study of Public Policy at the University of Arizona. The wonderful office and other institutional support of the Udall Center made the final revisions much more enjoyable than they otherwise would have been. Many thanks go to Michael Watts, Richard Walker, Zak Sabry, Don Mitchell, and David Barnes for their wonderfully astute comments on the whole manuscript and to Chris Philo, Michael Brown, and anonymous reviewers for comments on various portions. Nayan Shah has inspired me with his own meticulous scholarship on San Francisco's Chinatown, and his enthusiasm concerning my endeavors has been more than appreciated. Mark Patterson and David Cantrell are responsible for the maps and graphs, and thanks especially to Mark for patience in doing and redoing even in the midst of finishing a dissertation. I will be forever grateful to Carrie Mullen, editor at the University of Minnesota Press, for believing in the project and providing support and advice at all stages. Hank Schlau's skillful editing made the book a better one and made the final stages of the process much easier for me. A Provost Author's Support Fund supported the costs involved in producing the book, enabling me to hire Adrienne Crump to do the index. Thanks to Adrienne for a great job on a tedious project. To my parents and sister I owe much for their continual support, but most of all I thank George for his unflagging patience and intellectual enrichment.

INTRODUCTION

Walking down the hallway of a homeless shelter in San Francisco, it is not hard to figure out why tuberculosis might have a significant presence among the residents. The hallway is long, narrow, and filled with smoke, and the few windows located near the ceiling look as if they have never been opened. In fact the hallway feels as if it has not been aired out for years, and cleaning is relatively perfunctory. Some shelters are organized by large wards, but the one I visited in 1991 was of the "honeycomb" architectural variety. In this type, a number of small rooms are located off a central hallway, each room containing six built-in bunk beds, three on each side with perhaps three feet separating each bed. None of the rooms has a window. Every evening each of these beds is filled with individuals needing a place to sleep that is not on the street or in a cramped doorway. Men and women occupy different halves of the building; the sexes after all should not be allowed to commingle even if germs are given every opportunity for promiscuous exchange.

It would seem that the homeless shelter was designed specifically with the transmission of tuberculosis in mind. The airless hallways, the cramped rooms, and the close configuration of bodies within them facilitate the transmission of a bacillus contained within dust particles and the microscopic sputum drops of infected individuals. It is not surprising to learn, then, that approximately one-third of San Francisco's homeless population were testing positive for the disease in the early 1990s.[1] A positive test does not necessarily indicate active disease, but the compromised diet, exposure, and general

1

physical debilitation of the long-term homeless individual suggest its greater likelihood.

Yet the homeless shelter alone cannot be blamed for the increase of tuberculosis among the poor and indigent. In the late 1980s and early 1990s, San Francisco implemented several small but significant structural changes designed to contain spatially an increasing — and increasingly annoying — homeless population. Bus stops were redesigned as narrow, metal-framed benches with rotating rubber seats to make them impossible to sleep on, much less sit on comfortably. Parks were patrolled more rigorously by police, and many acquired gates that were closed and locked after sunset. Parking lots and even vacant lots became noticeable for the chain-link fences surrounding them, and merchants increasingly took to locking steel-slatted gates across their storefronts at night to prevent the homeless from sleeping in their doorways. Ironically, measures intended to rid the city of an unwanted population may have inadvertently facilitated the rise of an even more unwanted disease because those measures left the homeless with fewer options to the homeless shelter. Park benches might not be optimal sleeping structures, but they are less conducive to the spread of tuberculosis than their municipally sanctioned alternative. From this perspective the homeless shelter becomes a trenchant symbol of society's tendency to make a marginalized population less visible rather than to implement policies of integration, job placement, and preventive health services. Though budget constraints serve as convenient rationales, it is difficult to overlook the punitive message behind the harsh architectures of indigence.

A century earlier, the San Francisco Board of Health formed a committee of physicians and businessmen to investigate Chinatown in the wake of a devastating epidemic of smallpox. After observing its inhabitants and surveying its stores, brothels, and lodging houses, the committee issued an 1885 report that was unequivocally damning. The choices, as the committee saw them, were either to intervene severely into Chinatown's everyday functioning through repeated sanitary purges that would leave few structures or inhabitants left unscathed or to raze Chinatown entirely and relocate it well outside of city boundaries. Choosing to ignore these solutions would leave the city vulnerable to those diseases repeatedly emanating out of Chinatown's dank interior. The mission of the committee, in other words, was not one of mere observation and objective description, even though its members considered themselves participants in such an endeavor. With the advantage of hindsight, it becomes more obvious that the committee was involved in a complex process of mapping deviance in a particularly hated district and inscribing it with a pathology that made intervention not only commendable but imperative.

These scenarios illustrate the purposes of this book, which examines tuberculosis, smallpox, plague, and syphilis in nineteenth- and early-twentieth-century San Francisco. One purpose is to disrupt the implicit location of public health outside social politics. At one level this disruption targets the ways in which diseases gain signification through the process of medical elucidation and public perception. Whether in the nineteenth or late twentieth century, the process has often been characterized by a tendency to see infectious diseases at the social margins and subsequently to generate epidemiological explanation through the frontispiece of social pathology. Hovering in the epistemological backdrop of this tendency is an age-old association of disease with deviance — a desire to explain epidemic through the culpability of the sexually aberrant, the nationally suspect, or the economically derelict. The implications of this signifying process are enormous, namely, in rendering "disease definitions and hypothetical etiologies...as tools of social control, as labels for deviance, and as a rationale for the legitimation of status relationships" (Rosenberg 1992b, xvi).

That interpretations of disease are necessarily political and that medical discourse plays an important disciplinary social function are not new points, as evidenced by Foucault's work of more than twenty years ago (Foucault 1977) and by the proliferation of recent social analyses of disease.[2] Following Foucault's lead, this book examines tuberculosis, plague, smallpox, and syphilis as diseases whose devastations were derived in part from their use as political tools and disciplinary mechanisms. The departure from Foucault comes in finding limitations to a primary focus on discursive meanings and genealogical explanations. The point of this book is thus not to simply uncover disease as a mechanism of power but to trace the effects of this power on particular communities. Interpretations of disease, in other words, do not remain within boundaries of the discursive. In the form of public health policy, they translate into carceral or exclusionary tactics, punitive intrusions into everyday life, or equally punitive neglect of basic welfare. It is largely through institutions of public health that diseases as political tools have sustained social as well as physical damage. This is not to say that public health policies through the years have not been responsible for much that is beneficial, but it is to say that there is a sustained failure within medicine and public health to recognize the effect institutional practice has upon those suffering real or ascribed burdens of disease (Rosenberg and Golden 1992). The other level of failure comes in the constrained disciplinary parameters of public health, a point that will be taken up again after a further discussion of signifying processes of disease.

Disease is by no means the only social force defining boundaries of the normal through a signification of the pathological (Canguilhem 1991). In her book *Purity and Danger,* Mary Douglas brings attention to the social need to erect boundaries against defilement, focusing her analysis on dirt as "matter out of place," a disruption of an ordered system (Douglas 1966, 36). Drawing from Julia Kristeva's notion of abjection, David Sibley broadens Douglas's analysis by extending associations of "dirt as a signifier of imperfection and inferiority" to the socially marginalized. Through both discursive and spatial tactics, the sexually, racially, economically, or mentally defiled are excluded from social visibility and confirmed as "low ranking in a hierarchy of being" (Sibley 1995, 14; see Kristeva 1982). A growing number of scholars are unpacking the variously assigned meanings of deviance and the mechanisms utilized to exclude, oppress, appropriate, or normalize the subjects of deviant discourse (Urla and Terry 1995; Philo 1989; Valentine 1993; Epstein 1995).

Disease is a particularly effective mechanism, however, because it does not just mark deviance. Used as accusation toward the already deviant (Douglas 1991), disease intensifies the rhetoric of hatred, fear, and blame utilized against undesirable populations. It shifts the quality of this rhetoric from the socially construed to the medically legitimated, from a vaguely if forcefully defined rationale of difference to a rational basis for surveillance, control, and exclusion. In short, it pathologizes, and with pathologization comes a more ominous set of meanings and a consequent imperative to intervene. The interpretation of smallpox in nineteenth-century San Francisco as a Chinese disease, for example, did not just deepen political enmity of a largely white society against a Chinese community. In shifting the status of the Chinese and Chinatown from different to pathological, it legitimated numerous public health intrusions into the community and, as evidenced in the 1885 committee report cited above, attempted to exclude it physically from the rest of the city. Important only as markers of discursive meaning are the facts that smallpox originated outside Chinatown (i.e., from within the white community) in at least three of four epidemics and that the Chinese died from the disease in rates proportional to their numbers but never more so.

In the present era, discursive constructions of disease are most often hidden within the guise of biomedical objectivity, yet this means that resultant designations of vulnerability are far more influential. The most egregious example of this process in recent years is the interpretation of AIDS. When most of the first cases of AIDS were identified as homosexual males, the result was what Gerald Oppenheimer terms "an exercise in epidemiological imagination" (Oppenheimer 1992, 268), because the causal factors and social relations behind the disease were interpreted as having to do with homosexuality and, more specifically, homosexual sex. The gay male body was subsequently pathologized as both the site and the boundary of infection, a contradictory epidemiology spawning a similarly contradictory social mapping. On the one hand, all gays became feared for the deadly germs their bodies might harbor and also inadvertently pass on through even the most mundane practices.[3] They were the reservoirs of disease but also the vectors, and the gay body was held suspect by virtue of its social categorization and regardless of its infectious status. On the other hand, the delimitation of AIDS as a gay disease generated a perception that no other social group was at risk, despite mounting evidence to the contrary. Historically as well as currently, the articulation of epidemiological boundaries poses risks to those situated outside vulnerable categories, as evidenced in this case by the rapidly increasing HIV rates among women and ethnic minorities (Treichler 1992b; Hammonds 1997).

In the steady evolution of epidemiological investigations, ascriptions of an HIV source did not end with gay men. The other three of the Center for Disease Control's "four Hs" of HIV infection — that is, Haitians, heroin users, and hemophiliacs — testify to the sustained tendency to see disease more quickly in groups already suspect for their marginal social locations as defined by the deviance of their bodies or social practices. As with the board of health's rendering of smallpox and the Chinese, the CDC and other public health institutions were quick to find the origins of an ominous new disease among, inter alia, an undesirable immigrant population rather than to acknowledge the possibility that Haitians became infected through their interactions with Americans (Farmer 1992). In the haste to construe a feared disease as lurking only on the margins, infectious status combined with social subordinance becomes more important than the actual tracing of transmission patterns. The subsequent attribution of HIV origins to Africa based on unsubstantiable evidence illustrates this very clearly. As Julia Epstein states, "AIDS stories are sedimented with the detritus of poverty, racism, and bigotry" (Epstein 1995, 5). Yet the authority of epidemiological determinations of source, especially when emerging from respected institutions such as the CDC, means that designated groups do not suffer their ignominy in the abstract. Rather, the impact of medical misinterpretation extends from health policies to legislation affecting new immigration reviews, insurance structures, the availability of drug rehabilitation programs, access to educational institutions, and employment.[4]

The pathologization of gays, Haitians, and Chinese points to the importance of recent theories of the body to a delineation of disease signification. Again Foucault's work has been instrumental in pointing to the importance of the body as the object of power relations and more specifically to the role of medicine in defining bodies and constructing both theoretical and institutional mechanisms for their control (Foucault 1975, 1977). Critiques by feminist theorists have subsequently expanded the social constructionist analysis to include the differential exercise of power upon particular kinds of bodies, emphasizing the tendency toward increased disciplinary action upon racialized and gendered bodies (Butler 1990; Grosz 1994, 1995; Bordo 1993). Not only do these actions inscribe bodies that are already marked as "Other" against the male white norm, but they work to produce them as sexualized, racialized, or gendered in particular ways according to a specific social lexicon of power. Elizabeth Grosz writes, "It is not simply that the body is represented in a variety of ways according to historical, social, and cultural exigencies while it remains basically the same; these factors actively produce the body as a body of a determinate type" (Grosz 1994, x).

Body types and their locations within relations of power raise questions informing much of this book, questions concerning the production of deviant bodies through the ascription of disease. Examining whose bodies are made deviant, how and by whom, and the consequences for targeted communities begins to unravel a politics of citizenship behind productions of deviance. As interwoven with race, sexuality, ability, class, and other social productions, disease becomes a means not only of demarcating social boundaries of acceptability but of erecting barriers between the acceptable and the deviant. Many scholars in cultural critiques of medicine have posed similar questions especially in regard to AIDS. Following the contention by Georges Canguilhem (1991) that the normal is known through the mobilization of its opposite, these scholars see the discursive deployment of AIDS, or more broadly of deviance, onto gendered and racialized bodies as serving to project the ideal healthy body as white, heterosexual, and male (Waldby 1996), as strengthening the advantageous socioeconomic location of the same (Waldby 1996; Wilton 1997; Treichler 1992b), or as mapping conflicting and complex social relations (Urla and Terry 1995). Conversely, the production of "Othered" bodies as dangerously infective through discourses of permeable body boundaries (Waldby 1996) and nonregulated bodily exchanges (Epstein 1995) contravenes political movements acting to shift undesirable groups' marginal social location toward the center.

The case studies contained in this book further exemplify but also extend the AIDS critique, adding depth through historical comparison to other discursive productions of diseased bodies and the political rationales underlying them.[5] It is clear in the examples of tuberculosis, smallpox, plague, and syphilis that the construction of bodies as diseased accomplished all of the above: it simultaneously marked the healthy body as white if not as male, mapped more definitively the hierarchical configurations of social subordination and dominance, rationalized relations of production, and precluded movement of marginal groups toward incorporation into the mainstream. But bodies were, and are, not randomly pathologized as if they were unmarked before medical inscription; particular bodies tend to be marked by particular types of disease. Examining the reasons for and outcomes of such differential epidemiological targeting reveals much about the interrelationships of medical theory, social relations, and public opinion.

Despite the preeminence of medical discourses in body production, the implication of unilateral action would be erroneous no matter how far reaching the signification of the disease. At any one time the discourses acting to produce bodies are multiple, some of them interdependent but others conflicting. In the case of AIDS, the pathologization deriving from medical discourses marked bodies already inscribed as deviant by the normalizing discourses of sexuality, ability, social function, and citizenship.[6] AIDS did not *make* gay men deviant any more than smallpox made the Chinese an undesirable community in San Francisco. Rather, both diseases articulated with already well-established political-social discourses, and in so doing they changed the nature of discursive production. In the case of AIDS, it changed the gay body from one reviled for multiple sexual transgressions[7] to one feared for its capacity to kill, a qualitative shift invoking intensified reactions. Gay male communities in cities such as San Francisco and New York have countered these productions through their own mobilization of political messages producing the gay male body as healthy, sexual, and demedicalized (Gilman 1995), yet the dominant negative imaging has not been entirely disarmed.

A focus on the body thus locates one important site of signification, illuminating the cultural values, boundaries of order, or normalizing imperatives of a particular place in time through reading the medical inscriptions of body types. Yet a discussion of the body is inadequate without an accompanying analysis of place. The body infected with HIV or other pathogens is not simply feared for its ability to spread disease to other bodies. It is feared because of its capacity to infect a whole community and from there to leak pathogens to an entire city, district, or region. Epidemiological responses to disease do not stop at the site of the body, nor even at relations between bodies. The cultural lexicon of any threatening disease always includes a set of meanings attached to those spaces inhabited either discursively or in reality by infected bodies. These meanings change the way places are understood just as the colonization of bodies by pathogens changes the way they are read. It is no consequence, then, that public health initiatives against disease have focused as much upon the appropriation and reproduction of space as upon the control over infectious bodies.

Social geographers not surprisingly have focused on theorizing how and under what conditions space is produced and on recognizing the multivalence of spatial form and function. According to Edward Soja, "Spatiality is socially produced and, like society itself, exists in both substantial forms (concrete spatialities) and as a set of relations between individuals and groups, an 'embodiment' and medium of social life itself" (Soja 1989, 120). Contained in the latter part of this statement is the central argument for reconceptualizing space as not simply a passive container for but a dynamic actor in the production of social relations (Soja 1989; Lefebvre 1991). Less represented in the literature but nevertheless important is the intervention of discursive representation (of inhabitants, buildings, signs, locations) inscribing space with symbolic meanings, a process that in turn shapes the parameters of social practice possible within that spatial arena (Lefebvre 1991).

Pervasive in much of social geographers' theorization of space is the centrality of power relations in its formation. Capitalist relations of production in particular form the basis in many studies for how space is produced and what form it takes, the imperatives of capitalist production creating landscapes embodying specific relations of power whose configurations in turn define what is possible in structuring subsequent hierarchies or their contestation (Harvey 1989; Henderson 1999; Lefebvre 1991; Mitchell 1996; Soja 1989). In recent years feminist geographers have argued successfully for the addition to class of gender, race, sexuality, ability, and other social categories in the analysis of power relations constituting and constitutive of space, recognizing that even within the framework of capitalism class is not always the preeminent factor structuring those actions productive of spatial formation and meaning (Bondi 1992; Pratt and Hanson 1994; Bell et al. 1994). Informed by this broadening of spatial theorizing, some geographers have turned their attention to uses of space in defining difference (Hubbard 1998; Cresswell 1996; Sibley 1995) as well as in containing it.

This book takes implicitly from the theoretical foundations established by social geographers, but it also redresses the absence in this corpus of literature of disease as a significant player in spatial formation. One of the central arguments of this book is that disease has played, and does play, a critical role in the production of place as lived, seen (built), and cognitively mapped. Understanding society and urban change at a given point in time thus necessitates the examination of disease and the formulation of responses to it. Diseases as they are socially interpreted take form primarily through spatial manifestations, either through their ascription onto particular structures, districts, or regions; through the real or symbolic mapping of contagion; or through the redeployment of social practices within particular spaces by association with or absence of disease. Conversely, spatial deployments inform subsequent perceptions of and responses to particular diseases. The embodiment of AIDS in inner cities, for example, has underscored the association of the disease with disorder, degradation, and a renewed sense of hopelessness. The spatial forms of medical intervention render a particular ordering of the urban body, too, through means of sanitary interventions, restricting movement of individuals or groups, reordering domestic spaces, purging diseased environments, and redesigning institutional structures.

A number of cultural analysts and medical historians have examined one or more of these angles in their analyses of disease, and many of their approaches have found resonance in this book. One salient discourse discussed by Epstein (1995) is the ability of disease to contest if not collapse boundaries largely through notions of leakage. Besides the permeability of body boundaries, diseases are feared for their ability to leak into any number of urban communities. Right now, HIV is largely contained within urban spaces such as inner cities and prisons, where it articulates with "poverty, street crime, injection drug use, welfare, teenage pregnancy, drive-by shootings, and other disasters of urban anomie" (Epstein 1995, 163) to create an insuperable marginality of these areas and to add the obloquy of a deviant disease to a long list of social pathologies. Preventing HIV and AIDS from leaking beyond the margins into the mainstream of middle-class neighborhoods, schools, and suburbs has been a central concern of communities and public health officials since the beginning of the syndrome.

Underlying this fear is the economic, political, and social interconnectedness of places, as well as the slipperiness of bodies as mobile entities or easily readable texts. The ascription of disease to particular bodies and places can only work as a containment measure, in other words, if bodies remain within their specified geographic locations and if they can be easily coded as to their sexual orientation, social practices, ethnic origin, or nationality. The possibility that an intravenous drug user could reside in an upper-class neighborhood, gay men could be in the military, Haitians or Africans could migrate to the United States, or peripatetic homeless populations could infiltrate shopping centers produces what has been called "border anxiety" (Young 1990; Epstein 1995), a collapsing of both social categories and spatial boundaries. The degree of border anxiety generated by HIV and resurgent tuberculosis is evident both in the discussion in medical literature and the media of threats to the mainstream and in attempts to represent risk as contained within the social margins. An increase in AIDS among women, for example, while appearing to be a leakage into the mainstream, was tied back into the social margins by CDC officials who focused attention on the women's sexual contacts with injection drug users and bisexual men (Wortley and Fleming 1998, 356).[8] Alternatively, when occasional cases of multi-drug-resistant tuberculosis leak out of the inner city into middle-class suburbs, the alarm is sounded over who and how many might really be at risk.[9]

The potential for diseases such as cholera, plague, or tuberculosis to break out of urban slums constituted similar anxieties for the public health constabulary of previous centuries (Barnes 1995; Calvi 1989; Kearns 1985, 1991; Wohl 1983). David Barnes notes that in nineteenth-century France tuberculosis was perceived as inseparable from the foul-smelling, ill-lit, overcrowded, and poorly ventilated housing of the urban poor, yet fear resided in the possibilities that this etiologic boundary would fail, leaking disease into upper-class neighborhoods through lower-class practices of spitting and the inevitable intermingling of lower- and upper-class bodies on city streets (Barnes 1995). Similar ascriptions of infectious disease to marginal districts and the resultant fear of leakage into mainstream communities constitute a major theme in this book: disease is ascribed to particular districts in part as a method of containment, yet in the very act of spatial delimitation the possibility is raised of diffusion, of the failure of containing boundaries and the dissemination of infection throughout an urban body.

The foundation for generating discourses of leakage rests, and rested, upon an underlying discourse of spatial pathology. Certain bodies are constructed as disease-ridden, but an equally important part of some framings is the concomitant pathologization of the spaces these bodies inhabit. Reiterating Barnes's statement, tuberculosis came to be synonymous with the specific material configurations of poverty in nineteenth-century Paris: disease did not just reside in the body; it resided in and was generated by slum housing. San Francisco's nineteenth- and early-twentieth-century construction of tuberculosis was similar. However, it is the case of San Francisco's Chinatown that begs an extension of the argument by Barnes and others of disease's association with particular spaces. Throughout the latter half of the nineteenth century, Chinatown was not simply associated with smallpox, plague, and syphilis; it was made metonymous with these diseases. That is, its labyrinthine alleyways, mysterious josshouses, and grimy brothels were construed not just as spawning these diseases or containing them but as actually becoming a part of them.

Spatial deployment tends, historically or currently, to be based in the reality of higher disease rates in particular districts. With the development of spot maps at the turn of the century came the ability to prove visually that poorer districts did in fact have higher rates of tuberculosis in nineteenth-century cities. Today geographic information systems display with ever greater technological detail similar patterns of disease burden among inner-city districts and gay neighborhoods. These differences of disease incidence deserve scrutiny in and of themselves, but especially significant is the way responses to them have been couched. The difference between epidemiological association and pathologization of place — that is, the difference between a physical map of disease and the social interpretation of it — warrants more attention for the contingent set of meanings generated and the types of interventions consequently implemented. Though the differences are not always predictable, they generally are founded upon either the nature of the disease itself or the groups and districts targeted in epidemiological interpretations.

Historically, for example, the association of tuberculosis with impoverished districts in San Francisco and elsewhere fostered policies of neglect or of more subtle spatial intervention such as the "hygienic gaze" (Barnes 1995; Armstrong 1983), that is, the institution of greater medical scrutiny over impoverished bodies and their environmental relations through the installation of public dispensaries. As will be seen in this book, neglect is its own form of violent action, and it is not to be underestimated how much suffering resulted from the unwillingness on the part of public health officials to intervene in a fatal disease and its material causes. But until its establishment as a contagious disease at the end of the century, tuberculosis did not generate the more overtly aggressive reactions that other epidemic diseases did. Nor were the poor populations who were characterized as tuberculous perceived to be as deviant as many other groups such as the insane, the criminal, or the nonwhite. Not until its association early in the twentieth century with more deviant groups such as hobos, and its association today with the homeless, were more strident spatial interventions initiated.

A more intense spatial pathologization occurs with diseases considered more threatening because of their greater virulence or because of their stronger association with deviance. As the spatial personification of epidemic infection, Chinatown was aggressively taken over by public health officials, cleansed, purged, and rebuilt very much like a physician attacking and cleansing the site of infection on a patient's body. With AIDS, gay urban spaces might have been utilized as sites of educational outreach. Instead they were characterized as embodiments of HIV transmission, and public health actions consequently focused on interrupting those practices seen in the new epidemiological imagination as potentially deadly. Bathhouses, nightclubs, beaches, and parks known to have largely gay patronage were either closed down, policed more closely, or intervened in with the intention of controlling how they could be defined and what actions could be performed within them (Brown 1997). Nonleisure spaces were affected as well, as gay men with AIDS were more likely to find themselves unwelcome in their places of work and habitation.[10] The lives of many gay men, in other words, changed significantly in part because of internally generated behavioral strictures (Brown 1997), but also in part because of such state and medical intervention into the spaces, resources, and configurations of male homosexual practice (Sullivan 1996; Gilman 1985).

For inner cites, AIDS has added the incubus of physical pathology to a long list of social pathologies including drug addiction, prostitution, gang warfare, and homelessness. Unlike the reaction to Chinatown a century previously or to gay neighborhoods more recently, the ascription of a feared disease to inner cities has not resulted in any significant measure in public health interventions. Declining tax bases if anything have resulted in further withdrawal from these areas of services such as subsidized housing, medical care, and drug rehabilitation programs. Ironically, these policies are probably contributing to rising levels of AIDS in these districts and its quicker diffusion into surrounding suburbs (Wallace 1990; Wallace and Wallace 1995). What programs and services are available for inner-city residents are confined to inner-city locations, however, thus keeping an unwanted population contained through locational politics of services rather than through other public health interventions.

Spatial association and pathologization are not always distinct processes, nor necessarily mutually exclusive. The point is to extend the argument beyond needing to understand disease as a product of a particular social context and level of medical understanding to recognizing that the same social context produces very different understandings and spatial deployments of diseases according to a complex array of factors including the nature of the disease (i.e., its symptoms), its interpreted epidemiology, the groups and districts to which it is ascribed, and the social ideologies and political economies of a given place in time. The point is also to question what purpose spatial pathologizations and their resulting interventions serve. The case studies that follow point to the need to scrutinize whether ideological and spatial entrenchment of difference, maintaining barriers between the healthy and the pathological, and normalization of deviant groups prove to be greater motivations for disease intervention than the prevention of disease itself.

Another purpose of this book is to show the folly of excluding broader social and economic factors from the parameters of public health. This is different from the first point in that it targets disciplinary boundaries rather than significatory practices. The ascendancy of germ theory at the turn of the century redefined the disciplinary parameters of public health to include a focus on the individual rather than the social and physical environment. How particular behaviors could place individuals at greater risk of disease became the modus operandi of public health practice, an operational shift that located the onus of responsibility for health onto the individual rather than environmental and institutional structures. The shifting focus of clinical medicine onto the isolated body and its internal mechanisms informed the parallel shift in public health policy and naturalized its separation from broader questions of social welfare.

Public health is still defined in these constrained terms, with consequences that are far-reaching and recurrent. As chapter 6 in particular shows, the refusal of a public health constabulary to apprehend the material deprivation underlying high tuberculosis rates in early-twentieth-century San Francisco meant a necessarily constrained capacity to deal effectively with this disease. Similar public health focus today upon tuberculosis case surveillance and contact-tracing may be responsible for stemming the rising tide of cases, but the refusal to see poverty, homelessness, or underemployment as significant causal factors will lead inevitably to new resurgences with every downturn in the economy or diminution in public spending.[11] Refusal to see rising HIV infectivity in inner cities as linked to poverty and sexual politics has led to relative inefficacy in preventive efforts, as steady rates of new cases attest.[12] If defined differently, public health could be a powerful force in social politics. An ontological turnaround could find livable wages, affordable housing, subsidized child care, and job training as a normalized part of what public health as an institution is about. One urban program for instance has health workers helping patients with job applications and interviews as part of a hypertension prevention program (*Economist,* September 12, 1998, 93–94).[13] Public health, in other words, has the capacity to address social inequities. Instead, as the following chapters show, it has often perpetuated them. The hope contained within this book is that the insights of historical analysis will eventually disrupt the status quo of public health practice and force a rethinking of institutional myopia.

Finally, this book tells a story that has not been told before. Most histories of disease in the United States focus upon the East Coast, the Midwest, and the South. Few have explored interpretations of disease in the West, and none has looked at the development of society and structures in San Francisco through the lens of epidemic.[14] Clearly other forces were important in shaping urban life in San Francisco during the last half of the nineteenth and first half of the twentieth centuries, but equally evident from archival materials is the degree to which disease, and public health responses to it, determined the quality and tenor of that life. It might seem that tuberculosis, smallpox, plague, and syphilis are especially morose optics for uncovering a local history of urban development and social injustice. But if Kierkegaard was right that "life can only be understood backwards" (cited in Thrift 1985, 377), then there is yet optimism in narrating a historical calculus of suffering.

Situating the Study

The purpose of conducting a regional study of disease lies in the value of illuminating those knowledge systems, ideologies, social structures, and economic patterns that are peculiar to a particular place in time and that determine the precise interpretations and utilizations of disease. Though such a study offers comparisons throughout, the primary engagement remains one of analyzing how diseases were interpreted and "spatialized" and why; this requires a narrow focus on one place and its particularity. Only then can the "beam of light" illuminate broader terrain (Tilly 1984).

I have not endeavored to write a microhistory, however, in that this book does not focus attention only or primarily on the subaltern. One of the purposes of the study is to suggest the disproportionate focus of disease constructs on the poor and marginalized, and one of the most effective ways to do this is by tracing those constructs back to their source, to those who participated in the dissemination of particular knowledges and their deployment in space. As such, this study focuses on the relationships between knowledge and power and on the social practices through which both are reproduced. Focusing on only lower-class populations would miss analysis of what group or groups were generating knowledge, of the conditions dictating the forms such knowledge took, and of the channels through which they were disseminated.

For example, the San Francisco Department of Public Health even in the mid–nineteenth century carried a significant degree of authority, but the policies and interpretations of diseases issued from this office originated primarily from one person, the city health officer. He, in turn, was influenced in his interpretations by the level of technical knowledge available to him, by social hegemonies spawned by the class of which he was a part, and by the frustration of a job whose horizons of unknowing were wide and whose liabilities were severe. His interpretations and the policies issued in consequence were in turn either embraced or contested as they filtered down through various levels of public attention — the news media, other physicians, school and hospital administrators, businessmen, and finally those (usually) poor or Chinese directly implicated. As is always the case with the dissemination of ideas, medical understanding was continually reshaped by these various factions through the filters of social location, political position, and location within the discourse itself. The overriding scenario is thus one in which medical discourses as articulated with sociopolitical ideologies of race, gender, and so on, formed the dominant regimes of truth, but always within a dynamic process that included the possibilities of contestation.

Finally, in producing a localized history, the question is raised of whether San Francisco was unique in its interpretations of and responses to disease. This question will be addressed at greater length throughout the text, but the answer in brief is both yes and no. San Francisco had an unusual beginning as a supply station for the Sierra Nevada gold rush of 1849 and after, meaning that its early social discourses focused on the capacity for every individual to succeed financially no matter what their previous economic background. Though this rhetoric was muted in later years of economic ups and downs, it nevertheless underlay relatively unsympathetic attitudes toward the impoverished in the latter part of the nineteenth century. With rapid population expansion and economic diversification in the latter decades of that century, San Francisco eventually was characterized by the same conditions fostering tuberculosis and epidemic diseases in all urban industrialized areas. Whether in Paris, London, Boston, or New York, sewers and other sanitation problems were largely the focus of public health authorities during this period, and San Francisco was no exception. One difference seems to show, however, in the degree to which the structural problems of the city, and more specifically of poverty, were effectively addressed. Health authorities in many cities such as London, Paris, Manchester, and New York focused attention by the mid–nineteenth century on the growing problems of poverty and implemented measures such as slum clearance and housing reform to ameliorate its impact (Barnes 1995; Duffy 1990; Hardy 1993; La Berge 1992; Woods and Woodward 1984). San Francisco showed few serious efforts in this direction, but it is difficult to say whether this was because of a struggle with its image or because it had simply not had as long a history of urbanism and its concomitant problems as had eastern U.S. and European cities.

Ascriptions of disease showed different patterns as well in San Francisco, a distinction residing in the social topography of the city. As one of the closer U.S. port cities to Asia, San Francisco had the largest Chinese population of any U.S. city until the Exclusion Act of 1882 barred further immigration. It also had a relatively high proportion of European immigrants, but its eastern European Jewish population in particular never approached that of New York or Chicago. The result was that the Chinese community received the brunt of disease scapegoating in San Francisco — the most "Other" of the non-Anglo populations was ascribed the most feared and deviant diseases. For other cities, scapegoating focused upon Jews (Kraut 1994), African Americans

(McBride 1991), or other groups residing at the bottom of the social hierarchy. The point becomes not so much which groups are being targeted in disease interpretations but why and under what circumstances. San Francisco was different in *whom* it scapegoated only because it had different groups constituting its social hierarchy. It was not different from any other city in *why* it scapegoated or in inevitably prolonging epidemics because of misdirected public health actions deriving from the act of scapegoating.

A Note on Sources

The officers' reports contained within the annual Municipal Reports of San Francisco formed a significant proportion of the primary material utilized for this study. Especially before the rise of scientific medicine in the early twentieth century, there was little concern for the goals of detachment and objectivity in reporting the incidence of disease and its origins and impact upon the city. Public health officers of the nineteenth century, then, gave full vent in their reports to their prejudices not only in theorizing the origins of smallpox epidemics or the etiology of tuberculosis but also in passing judgment on the poor or positing the subhuman character of the Chinese. The reports of the California State Board of Health, based in Sacramento, provided further social and medical commentary upon San Francisco's disease landscape, including documentation of policies formulated at the state level.

Supplementing these annual reports were publications of special medical committees called upon occasionally to investigate the conditions of Chinatown or the sanitary conditions characterizing the rest of San Francisco. These provided insight again into the interrelationship of medical theory, race or class politics, and public opinion. They described as well the condition of living quarters, sewer and water systems, streets, and other public spaces in the nineteenth century and the early years of the twentieth century. Also gleaned were the articles and editorials written by San Francisco physicians for medical journals, as well as editorials written by women for journals aimed at educating housewives on proper sanitary and hygienic methods of home care and child-raising. Newspaper articles were helpful in reporting public reaction to disease epidemics, as well as the "common interest" stories of individual experience or collective contestation of public health policies. For tuberculosis, the newspapers published by most sanatoriums provided valuable insight into life within these institutions, the rules governing patient behavior, the physical layout of sanatorium buildings and grounds, and the programs for rehabilitation.

Included in the annual municipal reports were the numerical records of disease incidence and mortality, broken down by ward, ethnicity, and age. These were indispensable in the analysis of disease rates and patterns, yet their limitations must be noted. Statistics of mortality by cause were accumulated by the late 1850s and reported in the annual Municipal Reports by the 1860s, but there is no description of how they were acquired and thus of whether some populations might have been overrepresented while others were underrepresented.[15] This would be a problem especially for tuberculosis after it became a reportable disease in the early twentieth century, but when the stigma of having the disease might have prevented private physicians from reporting their patients to public health authorities. Tuberculosis, or consumption, in the nineteenth century provides another problem given the relative subtlety of consumption's symptoms and the subsequent difficulty in diagnosing it. It must be presumed that only those who had more evident signs of tuberculosis and no visible signs of other diseases were given a diagnosis of consumption at death. In this last problem there is at least consistency in our favor, since tuberculosis did not get much easier to diagnose until the turn of the century. These limitations notwithstanding, the steep ascent of tuberculosis deaths in the latter half of the century is apparent. The Municipal Report of San Francisco for 1880–81, for instance, notes that tuberculosis mortality climbed from 223 out of an estimated population of 135,000 in 1865, to 690 out of 233,700 in 1880 (Municipal Reports 1881, 263). The distinctive symptoms of syphilis, smallpox, and plague made those diseases much easier to diagnose, but the possibility still existed for physicians to hide cases of these diseases from public health authorities. As chapters 2 and 3 attest, a stricter surveillance of the poor and poorer districts by public health officials also ensured their greater representation in morbidity (case) statistics.

There are other limitations to the statistics that do not allow as thorough a discussion of disease patterns as would be desirable. Mortality rates, for instance, were subdivided not by economic class but by city ward. Although this obviously enables a determination of citywide patterns, it makes more provisional the conclusions drawn concerning social and economic status since most wards encompassed poor as well as wealthier districts. The ward containing Nob Hill, the wealthiest enclave in the city, also contained parts of Chinatown, one of the poorest. And though mortality rates for Chinese were separated from those of whites, reporting was inaccurate for the former because health inspectors did not enter Chinatown or see Chinese patients regularly. Blacks, a relatively small percentage of the total population of San Francisco, were simply included within the white classification.

Setting

This book begins at roughly 1860 because it was around this time that San Francisco began taking shape as a city, beyond a motley collection of tents and wooden shacks. No longer just a stopping-off point before heading for the gold mines, it had acquired those institutional trappings such as city councils, administrators, jails, and hospitals that designate something as more than a temporary frontier outpost. From the somewhat chaotic amorphism of rapid growth at this point came the establishment of class and ethnic boundaries, differentiated residential neighborhoods, and the gradual evolution of ideologies positing standards for everyday social practices.

This period from 1860 to the turn of the century serves as the underlying structure of the next three and a half chapters, first for tuberculosis and then for smallpox, syphilis, and the first plague epidemic. The reason for this initial periodization is that, though medical theories and public health policies shifted during this period, the state of medical knowledge remained relatively constant. Medical understanding or lack thereof by no means served as the only factor engendering disease interpretations and metaphors, but it was important in determining the parameters of those interpretations. Medical theory influenced the dominant discourses on poverty and ethnicity and was directly responsible for ascriptions of disease origin or heightened contagiousness to particular communities and urban spaces. By the turn of the century, however, the germ theory of disease and the increasing authority of bacteriological science changed the tenor of disease interpretations.

Examination of the second plague epidemic in the second half of chapter 4 traces the impact of better epidemiological understanding in redefining particular communities and spaces within San Francisco. Between the first epidemic in 1900 and the second in 1907, the role of the flea and the rat in transmitting plague to human populations was elucidated, making for an interesting comparison of the changes in language if not of underlying social discourses generated by this change. Chapters 5 and 6 then examine tuberculosis from the turn of the century until about 1940, at which point the disease had diminished sufficiently to have lost its urgency even before the advent of antibiotics. The revolutionary breakthroughs in medicine by the late 1890s, though not proffering a cure for tuberculosis, nonetheless altered the ways in which the disease was perceived and treated. The advances in medical knowledge influenced shifts in the discourses of poverty and gender as well as generating new ways of manipulating the environment for purposes of disease treatment and prevention.

Finally, though this study focuses primarily on interpretations of disease and their role in producing space, it does not overlook the fact that disease is also a biological phenomenon. It changed the lives of those it touched physically as well as socially and symbolically. It invariably brought suffering to the afflicted and their families. For the duration of the nineteenth century and into the twentieth, there were few remedies to relieve that suffering. Although only a few of the most prominent diseases are examined in this book, the poor suffered as well from countless other diseases including diphtheria, pneumonia, inadequate nutrition, and alcoholism. They suffered more not because they were morally or biologically disposed to disease but because the conditions in which they lived were insalutary and their social and economic resources were limited. To those on the margins, disease could only have added further burden to the blight of poverty and the ignominy of difference.

1

TUBERCULOSIS, TENEMENTS, AND THE EPISTEMOLOGY OF NEGLECT

A history of tuberculosis in a nineteenth-century western U.S. city is a difficult one to trace. The disease took a significant toll on urban populations in terms of death and disability, yet it was given relatively little notice by medical, public health, and lay constituencies. First, it was not considered contagious until the turn of the century, and, second, there were far more frightening and virulent epidemics of cholera, diphtheria, and smallpox to contend with. The question arises, then, of why a history of tuberculosis in nineteenth-century San Francisco is important to tell, especially since the more virulent epidemics of smallpox and plague brought to the forefront contentious questions of race and citizenship far more than did consumption.[1] Tuberculosis was seen as a much less virulent and frightening disease despite its death toll, and responses to it in the latter half of the nineteenth century were decidedly more subtle. Nevertheless, together with the more generalized discourses on health and hygiene in nineteenth-century San Francisco, discussions of tuberculosis during this period shed light upon how the city of San Francisco itself changed during this period, how it was perceived and eventually pathologized, and how the spatial relations of the individual body within the city were conceptualized.[2]

The etiology of tuberculosis for most of the nineteenth century was somewhat debated, but one theme dominant during this period was that of climatic influence on the consumptive individual. More specifically, the influence of the West in general was considered by many East Coast physicians as just the thing for curing consumption. Although the impact of this movement should not be exaggerated for San Francisco, it nevertheless shaped debates over representations and realities of the city's salubrity and over the population residing within its boundaries. Policies recommended by public health authorities also inevitably emerged out of the context of these debates.

Framing the other side of the debate was the corresponding theory of predisposition. The consideration of external influences in consumption's causation was only part of the picture; if an individual was not predisposed to being susceptible to the disease, such externalities had much less effect. The impact of predisposition, generally considered to be hereditary, was to place the focus of the disease to a significant extent upon the individual. The individual body that contained an inherited susceptibility to consumption could be manipulated to a certain extent to attenuate the risk of disease, but little else could be done. What Ann Hardy has pointed out for Britain thus holds true for San Francisco in the mid–nineteenth century: "For most of this period, and for most people, tuberculosis was seen as an individual concern, to be prevented and treated by the individual and his family, rather than as a social problem to be tackled by the state on behalf of society" (Hardy 1993, 253). Even so, the image of the individual predisposed to consumption was not exactly a positive one, and for some physicians, attracting such unhealthy people to the city was undesirable.

By the latter decades of the nineteenth century this discourse had changed to some extent with the inclusion of consumption in a more generalized rhetoric of urban sanitation. As the city grew in size and population in the last decades of the century and as structural problems concomitant with this growth grew more evident, discourses about disease in general and about consumption were linked to "problematic" (i.e., poor) areas of the city and to a lesser extent to problematic habits of less-generic individuals. Although climate and predisposition did not entirely disappear as factors, the influence of damp housing, faulty and inadequate sewers, and individuals who lived in damp and unventilated dwellings became more the focus. Policies within the city and the state correspondingly began addressing both of these components of a shifting etiology: they moved, on the one hand, to reform housing and rebuild sewer systems and, on the other hand, to reform the behavior of individuals now perceived as placing *themselves* at risk for a largely preventable disease. The pathologies of the individual and of the city were thus closely linked in this scenario.

Yet this association between consumption and poverty, and the degree to which each component was pathologized, must not be exaggerated. The beginnings of the association may be seen by the latter decades of the nineteenth century, but not until the turn of the century did it strengthen, and the degree and specificity of pathologization become more obvious. In the nineteenth century tuberculosis began, usually indirectly or by implication, to raise questions about class, slum conditions, and the pathology of poverty that would become predominant by the early years of the twentieth century. It had not to any significant extent taken on a strong "moral etiology," to borrow Barnes's phrase (Barnes 1995, 76).

Indeed there was something of a dialectic in the way that physicians and public health officers represented San Francisco in the late nineteenth century. On the one hand, with more focus in public health reports on sanitary problems affecting particular areas of the city, previous rhetoric about the salubrity of the city and its citizenry was undermined at the same time that attention was increasingly being paid to specific subsections of the city, rather than the city as a whole. On the other hand, the almost careful inattention to the growing problems of poverty and its correlates at this time suggests what Edward Soja, borrowing from Marshall Berman and Henri Lefebvre, discusses as tendencies during and after this period toward a veiled urban spatiality that hid the consequences of uneven capitalist development and exploitation (Soja 1989, 23, 26). San Francisco was a briskly growing city in the latter decades of the nineteenth century, but like many other cities of the time, such growth produced problems not dealt with before in the form of large pockets of poverty abutting pockets of vast wealth. It would seem that municipal administrators chose to deal with some of these problems by not focusing undue attention upon them.

San Francisco the Salubrious?

Having found no other therapeutic remedy for the symptoms of consumption, some nineteenth-century physicians recommended to their patients a dose of "pure air . . . and the enlivening influence of bright sunshine and agreeable scenery" (C. J. B. Williams 1869, 1). By the mid–nineteenth century the West was being seen by East Coast physicians and their consumptive patients as the place to receive this dose, an "El Dorado" (Rothman 1994, 133) where the deleterious influence of the city was absent and where the magnificent effects of sun, dry air, and altitude could rid the weary consumptive of disease. Numerous western towns including Colorado Springs, Albuquerque, and Tucson claimed superior climates for the consumptive, but California was one of the preeminent destinations for health seekers during the latter half of the nineteenth century. According to Sheila M. Rothman, by 1900 one-fourth of all migrants to California were tuberculars who had come for their health and settled permanently (Rothman 1994, 132).

The movement of health seekers was the result of what Rothman calls a "peculiarly western form of medicine" based not in scientific fact but on observation of the "life-giving nature" of the West (Rothman 1994, 139). An association had been established in Europe and the eastern United States by the 1840s between tuberculosis and living in close, damp quarters and breathing "prerespired" air, that is, air that recirculated in and out of the lungs of inhabitants of unventilated dwellings (Barnes 1995; Hardy 1993; Bates 1992; Fee and Porter 1992). At the same time, narratives began circulating about consumptives on their last legs traveling west and becoming healthy again despite the odds, a fact attributed to the revivifying qualities of particular western regions. Claims centered on which climates and topography were better: the warm and arid desert, the high mountains, or the coast. The point of each was fairly basic, though: the regions and their accompanying weather patterns maintained atmospheres free of impurities, optimal temperatures, plentiful sunlight, and expansive open spaces (Rothman 1994).

Backing up these stories were more scientifically couched discussions published in medical journals of discoveries that tuberculosis was virtually absent among American Indians and other groups, from the Bedouin to the African bushmen to Portuguese fishermen. The remarkable health of these groups was attributed to the fact that their occupations and their ways of life kept them almost continually outdoors (MacCormac 1869; Abrams 1886–87; Remondino 1893). In addition, the time they did spend inside was generally in healthier constructions such as the hut or tent, rather than the peculiarly unhealthy "modern house with its well constructed and protecting windows and doors" (Remondino 1893, 33). The implication of these discussions was that the consumptive should adopt those lifestyle components of the "primitive," such as long hours outdoors and in the sun, that would ensure the evolution of their own disease-free lungs.[3]

Southern California received the largest number of those migrants heading to the West Coast to seek their cure, with towns such as San Diego, Santa Barbara, Los Angeles, and Pasadena widely promoting their climate and their facilities as the most beneficial to the consumptive (Rothman 1994, 146). San Francisco also did its part to enter the competition as another healthier-than-average town of the West. Several early San Francisco physicians and municipal authorities, for example, extolled the incredible climatic and environmental qualities of California and San Francisco, implying if not directly claiming that the consumptive could find physical redemption there. The sun shone almost continually, the winters were mild, the breezes refreshing.

The healthfulness created by such purity of atmosphere takes on near-mythic proportions in a quote from an early physician who had migrated from St. Louis to San Francisco in 1848:

> Nor is sickness that scourge of humanity here to harass and hinder us in our pursuits. . . . [T]he general salubrity of California has justly become a proverb. The surgeons of San Francisco have remarked that wounds heal here with astonishing rapidity, owing, it is supposed, in a great measure, to the extreme purity of the atmosphere. (Saunders 1967, 296)

The San Francisco health officer I. Rowell, making his report of 1867, claimed that the "invigorating climate" of San Francisco kept down the mortality rates and largely prevented any "idiopathic" (of unknown cause) cases of tuberculosis — that is, cases not traceable to tuberculous migrants. In his conclusion, his rhetoric becomes more expansive in claiming that San Francisco's mortality rates are lower than any other American city because of the "salubrity of the climate, the abundance of food, and the absence of poverty" (Municipal Reports 1867, 281, 285). That much of his claim was easily enough refuted did not deter this physician or others from taking the opportunity to advertise the salutary virtues of San Francisco.

Why these physicians and others felt compelled to attract tuberculous migrants to the city is not easy to explain. Unlike Los Angeles, Santa Barbara, and other southern California towns, San Francisco's economy was not dependent upon consumptive migrants; nor did it seem to accommodate the phthisic patient with as many facilities and services as did the southern health resorts (Rothman 1994). One reason might lie in visions of pecuniary advantages to physicians, given that it was the wealthier consumptive who was encouraged to seek the cure in western health resorts (Rothman 1994, 146). Frequently, physicians at this time had to struggle to acquire enough patients to make a livable income; the influx of moneyed consumptives needing long-term care would help alleviate financial pressures.

But a strictly monetary explanation for the call to health seekers is too simplistic. The claims of an extraordinary salubrity in San Francisco and elsewhere might have been a "peculiarly western" phenomenon, but it emerged directly out of a prevailing belief in environmentalist medicine, or the notion that the body was affected by any number of environmental factors — for example, weather, diet, air, and occupational exposures. Consumption was thought to be especially prone to occur or to improve under particular environmental conditions, and from the 1830s studies were undertaken in Europe to determine more precisely the impact of specific factors. In both Britain and France observations were made through the 1860s regarding environmental exposures of various occupations and their correlation with consumption. Physiologically, certain of these environmental exposures such as damp or unventilated buildings worked to weaken the body and deplete it of its resources, resulting in tuberculous degeneration. In his 1890s tract on the etiology and prevention of tuberculosis, the physician George Martin Kober specified that besides heredity, susceptibility could be determined by faulty nutrition, other diseases, dust-producing occupations, and damp soils (Kober n.d., 4).[4]

For most proponents of medical environmentalism, this theory fit well with notions of hereditary predisposition. For the predisposed and the already consumptive, if closed surroundings, lack of air, and damp living conditions were associated with their malady, then the environmental opposite to these must be the key to prevention or amelioration. As will be discussed further below, the medically prescribed antidote of fresh air and sunshine was not the only solution propounded by the British or French public health constabulary, but it was one of them. The same therapy had been recommended by many American physicians since the 1840s, in this case, according to Georgina D. Feldberg, stemming as much from the recognition that medical therapies such as bloodletting did nothing for consumption, as from the observation that some regions of the country seemed less plagued by tuberculosis than others (Feldberg 1995).[5] San Francisco physicians thus had national and international medical backing in advocating the benefits of a salubrious climate for the consumptive.[6]

Whatever the rationale, the comments of contemporary observers and more than one public health officer suggest that the promotion of San Francisco as a haven for tuberculars met with some success. The early city health officer mentioned above, I. Rowell, commented by 1867 that San Francisco's death rate from tuberculosis was due primarily to patients who already had the disease and died after coming to San Francisco (Municipal Reports 1867, 266). The contemporary historian H. H. Bancroft also mentions in his history of late-nineteenth-century San Francisco that the high consumption mortality rate in the city was due "mostly from eastern health-seekers" (Bancroft n.d., 704). Indeed it was common throughout the rest of the century for health officers to blame San Francisco's tuberculosis death rates on foreign migrants whose attempts to seek a cure for their disease in the city had obviously failed.

Such comments raise a few interesting points. First, it is clear that some physicians and public health officers did not support the trend of tuberculars migrating to the city. Most of these opponents to tuberculous immigrants focused their attention on the predisposition component of the etiologic question. Predisposition to consumption did not necessarily mean that the individual would come down with the disease, but it did mean that he or she had a much greater likelihood of acquiring it. Rather than focusing on the symbol of San Francisco as a salubrious space to which consumptives should come and cure themselves, the opponents of tuberculous immigrants focused on the consumptives themselves and their polluting effect on an otherwise exemplary city. Emphasis here was placed not on economic class but on the weak and flawed constitutions ascribed to consumptives and the undesirability of having such individuals swelling the ranks of the citizenry. The problem did not remain, however, with the phthisic individual. Since predisposition was considered largely hereditary, the public health officer concerned about having too many consumptives in the city had to worry as well about those consumptives marrying and reproducing more defective individuals.

Here again these San Francisco physicians were not alone. Taking a phrase coined by Jacques Lacan and discussed further by Catherine Waldby, the nineteenth-century consumptive in much of the United States and Europe possessed "imaginary anatomies," that is, anatomies that "are the products of the biomedical imagination, arrived at through processes of selectivity, idealization, utopian speculation and analogy" (Waldby 1996, 42–43). In other words, the imaginary anatomy is a socially constructed body based upon what is considered ideal at a particular moment in history and what is considered its opposite. Imbricating with Georges Canguilhem, it is also a strategy within medical discourse for demarcating the normal through creating undesirable and thus pathological bodies that require medical observation (Canguilhem 1991).

Thus the nineteenth-century consumptive, according to prevalent medical discourse, possessed a set of physical traits that included a narrow chest, "delicate physique and general vulnerability of the tissues" (Kober n.d., 4). As indicated by the term and the traits, the phthisic anatomy was as much a classificatory tactic and cultural embodiment as a scientific observation. It made a difficult-to-diagnose disease apparently visible; it marked the tuberculous off from the normative, healthy body; and it designated a set of characteristics increasingly suspect in an industrial milieu of productivity and the physical discipline of the worker. The body was at this time one of the most important spatial signifiers of a somewhat liminal disease, liminal in that it embodied, physically and symbolically, qualities antithetical to evolving imperatives of a capitalist society in need of healthy, robust laborers.[7]

Direct disdain for the consumptive individual was not the norm in medical or public health literature in San Francisco at this time, but the degeneration of the collective gene pool was obviously a fear of some. In the same tract on the etiology and prevention of tuberculosis, Kober makes an ardent plea for the discontinuation of consumptive migration:

> Would a stock raiser care to import diseased stock, however well bred?... Then, why should this glorious state be stocked with consumptives and their offsprings?... [I]t will never pay,... for instead of this state producing a people with mental and bodily vigor, courage, presence of mind, grace, and dignity, we shall have a race weak in mind and body, and deeply tainted with the predisposition to consumption. (Kober n.d., 4)

The mythology of a salubrious place could be sustained only if it was not marred by the taint of a disease afflicting the weak and undesirable. In this discourse, raised mortality levels from tuberculosis were of less concern to Kober than the more insidious damage wrought by defective gene pools.

The other interesting point indicated in this debate is the contradiction that it embodied. Even while espousing San Francisco or California as a healthier-than-average locale, public health officers also noted that tuberculosis mortality rates often were higher than for midwestern and eastern cities. The reason was usually attributed to the migrants who had come to San Francisco seeking health. With reasoning that rather defies logic, claims were then made that San Francisco *would* be healthier if it were not for the inflow of consumptives, even if it was the innate salubrity of the city that was supposed to cure these consumptives in the first place (Municipal Reports 1867, 1881).

Whichever side of the debate the physicians and city administrators took, their ultimate objective clearly was to sell an image of San Francisco as better than any city in the East or Midwest. In a scenario familiar to many western histories,[8] San Francisco was in a contradictory position in the early stages of its development. The degree to which it truly was healthier, more beautiful, and more bountiful in part was because of its location, but also because in the 1850s and early 1860s there were still insufficient people there to undermine those qualities. Yet in order to prove its claims of salubrity, to boost the economy, and to rival eastern cities as a hub of commerce and cosmopolitanism, individuals of all sorts including consumptives were invited to migrate. The thing necessary to fully realize the potential of San Francisco also undermined it considerably. Ultimately it did not matter whether the physicians of the city wanted consumptives moving there or not; the end result of their boosterism, together with national economic factors, was a large influx of population beginning in the late 1860s. Consequently, consumptives did not have to come from the outside; they were produced from within. That is the subject of the next section.

Before moving on, however, a word needs to be said about the way the consumptive was perceived in terms of municipal or state responsibility. As the last quote suggests, consumptives could be classed together and discussed as a delineated, anatomized, pathologized group. Yet in the first few decades of San Francisco's history, they were largely not considered to be the responsibility of the city or state. They might be undesirable, they might even raise the municipal mortality statistics, but they were not considered a direct threat to the public's health. To paraphrase Hardy's claim, consumptives were generally left to find medical care for themselves when they could afford it or to implement in their own lives a therapeutic regimen that might ameliorate their condition. If neither of these was possible, consumptives could find themselves eventually in the almshouse or City and County Hospital, or they might simply be left to die at home.

The assumption that consumptives were not the responsibility of the state did not go uncontested, however. A few physicians, writing in local medical journals, expressed the opinion that the state should fund an institution where consumptives coming to California or San Francisco seeking a cure could go. Such an institution would provide the kind of therapeutic regimen of rest, sunshine, and attractive scenery considered optimal for the consumptive and would be paid presumably through donations from each county. Such a plan, according to these physicians, was more cost-effective in the long run than not providing an institution for care, since many of the health seekers migrating into California ended up penniless and unable to get a job because of their debility. Maintaining these individuals within cities was more draining on municipal payrolls, given the potential for consumptives to be in and out of county hospitals or poorhouses for years. Better to fund one large state institution and share the costs toward a cure. As one anonymous writer put it, "keeping [consumptives] quarantined in the city only helps the work of decimation.... [T]here ought to be some place where such persons could be sent with another chance, at least, for life" ("About Hospitals" 1869, 214). Despite the humane logic of this plea, it went unanswered during the next decades.

Sanitation, Slums, and the City

The debate over environmental impact versus hereditary predisposition, and how each of these informed and was informed by perceptions of the city, continued until the turn of the century. In the meantime, however, another set of tuberculosis discourses focusing on housing, sanitation, and individual behavior gained ascendancy as San Francisco's growth accelerated after the completion of the railroad in 1869. Corresponding to these newer discourses was an ontology of place in San Francisco that changed from the capacity to heal to a dialectical and spatially delineated capacity for health *and* for disease. By the 1870s, the city harbored within its boundaries a growing underclass, a larger area of slums, and mounting sanitation problems. Responses to these factors shaped not only symbolic meanings of place but, through municipal policies, the physical characteristics of those areas the poor inhabited.

According to John S. Hittell, San Francisco grew an average of 8 percent per year in the late 1860s and early 1870s, and the growth accelerated in the next few years as families fled from a depression on the East Coast. The city's population thus grew from approximately 135,000 in 1867 to 178,276 in 1870 and 233,700 in 1880 (Hittell 1878, 397–99).[9] By 1875, San Francisco was also suffering its first major economic recession, caused, according to Olmstead et al., by the dumping of East Coast goods on the San Francisco market, a drought that impacted agricultural production, a fall in output from the gold and silver mines, and in 1875 the closing of the Bank of California, which caused a financial panic (Olmstead et al. 1979).[10]

The inevitable result of a rise in migration concomitant with economic recession was a proportionate increase in poverty, unemployment, and underemployment. As destitution and its correlates of crowding and squalor grew, what Soja calls a "greater social and spatial ordering of urban life" — that is, a closely contiguous yet spatially separate mapping of class — became apparent (Soja 1989, 176). The installation of first a steam rail in 1860 and then the cable car in 1873 allowed the wealthy to move to outlying areas, and later to ascend hilly areas such as Nob Hill, that were inaccessible to the poor. Poorer neighborhoods subsequently expanded over most of the South of Market area, Chinatown, downtown, and North Beach (see map 1.1).

Urban expansion and intensifying areas of poverty, on top of continued migration of consumptives, also caused an increase in tuberculosis rates. Indeed tuberculosis remained the leading cause of death in San Francisco for the remainder of the century — a fact only rarely commented upon. Even in an early mortuary report of 1860, consumption is listed as the chief cause of death and San Francisco is mentioned as having tuberculosis mortality rates comparable to New York or Boston (Municipal Report 1860, 11, 13). Although this comparison must be taken with extreme caution given the questionable reliability of statistics, it does indicate an early observation of significant tuberculosis rates that, according to the report's author, were not imported "as fully as common opinion warrants" (Municipal Report 1860, 13). By 1870, with 1,533 deaths, phthisis (consumption) headed the list of the most common causes of mortality in the previous four years, almost twice the number as the second leading cause, smallpox (Municipal Reports 1870, 229). Tubercu-

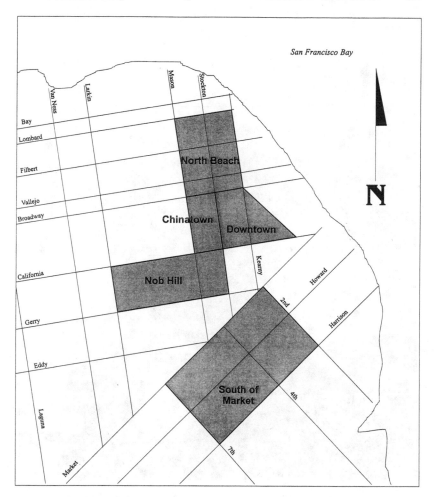

Map 1.1. San Francisco neighborhoods, 1870–90. Based on Issel and Cherny 1986; created by Mark Patterson.

losis mortality rates continued a steady climb through the next two decades, finally hitting a peak in 1894–95 of 1,165 deaths and 19.22 percent of all mortality in the city (Municipal Reports 1902, 499). Map 1.2 shows the tuberculosis rates by ward for the year 1890. The Tenth and Eleventh Wards, encompassing South of Market and Mission, contained the highest number of cases, with the Fourth Ward, encompassing parts of Chinatown and North Beach, showing a close second.

Not only were tuberculosis rates spatially defined at this time — they could also be mapped along gender and ethnic lines. For the duration of the

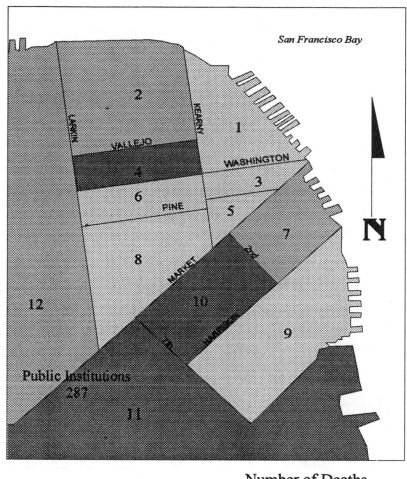

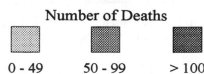

Map 1.2. San Francisco tuberculosis mortality by ward, 1890. Data from Municipal Reports 1889–90. Based on Issel and Cherny 1986; created by Mark Patterson.

nineteenth century in San Francisco, men died of tuberculosis at far higher rates than did women, a pattern that could easily be explained by the preponderance of men in San Francisco's early history, but which persisted even after the population evened out. In 1888, for example, a total of 643 men died of pulmonary phthisis while only 262 women did. For 1891, those numbers were very similar, at 674 and 285, respectively (Municipal Reports 1888, 483 and 1891, 537). The reasons behind this significant discrepancy are difficult to ascertain. One reason could stem from greater occupational exposure among men to dust and other substances that could compromise the lungs and the immune system.

Yet, as will be further discussed in chapter 4, women's employment at this time and for the decades to come was not necessarily any less hazardous in terms of exposure to tuberculosis. The employment options available to women in the latter part of the nineteenth century included domestic labor, nursing, and factory jobs. Domestic labor in the houses of the wealthy might have been the most salutary choice, but then the upper classes themselves were not immune to tuberculosis. The trend among all classes of keeping doors and windows shut against wind and fog also increased the likelihood that if tuberculosis existed within a household, it would be spread to others, including domestic servants.

Nursing at this time could be an extremely hazardous occupation given that contagion was not a widely embraced concept for most diseases other than smallpox. Even after the discovery of the tubercle bacillus, the contagiousness of tuberculosis was imperfectly understood and patients were not always isolated until after the turn of the century. Nurses acted more as domestic servants than medically trained personnel for most of the century, and their exposure to tubercle bacilli during the course of cleaning, feeding, and changing sheets would have been significant. Unfortunately there are no statistics to show the morbidity and mortality rates of nurses at this time, but it is likely that they were higher than the average population given the nature of nurses' occupational exposure. Factory work would have offered little reprieve. Even though factories at this time in San Francisco were relatively small operations,[11] they were largely unsanitary, dimly lit, and ill ventilated. Long hours and few breaks over time would have produced immunosuppressed bodies more vulnerable to tuberculosis and other infectious diseases.

The second liability of women's work was its wages. Poverty alone does not cause tuberculosis, but the spatial manifestations of poverty — that is, the suboptimal living environments, diets, and workplace conditions — increase the likelihood of exposure and immune system compromise. As Olmstead et al. point out, employment opportunities for women in this period not only were severely limited even in years of economic upturn but provided "little hope beyond the barest subsistence" (Olmstead et al. 1979, 197). According to Hittell, a contemporary historian of San Francisco, "Women who work at wages in industrial employment in California do not get more than half so much as men in similar jobs, and are excluded from most departments of labor in which pay is the highest, and the chances for advancement best" (quoted in Olmstead et al. 1979, 198). Whatever jobs women qualified for or were able to get, their remuneration was likely to be at the subsistence level, if even that. And though husbands sometimes supplemented these wages, the combination of suboptimal working and living conditions, long hours, and poor diet resulted in what Gerry Kearns has termed "the urban penalty," the price paid in physical deterioration by the poorest classes of industrial cities (Kearns 1991).

For those women who did not work, there were still the hazards of the home to contend with. Small houses, overcrowding, closed windows, and lack of sunlight were standard characteristics of underclass home environments, and these were also highly conducive to spreading tuberculosis. If women spent the better part of the day within the home, they stood a better chance of acquiring tuberculosis there than did men who left the home for several hours each day. One impoverished man in the late 1800s moved his family to San Francisco in hopes of a better life but found unemployment instead. As he summarized it,

> While I regret my circumstances I am aware others are a good deal worse off. I still keep house, of course in a poor fashion, but yet I manage to eat some and have enough of warmth and sleep, but my wife and children pent up from week to week without a sufficiency of warmth or of warm clothing, they feel the effects of this mode of living and it begins to tell upon them. (Cited in Olmstead et al. 1979, 137)

Whether this man was fed as part of his occasional jobs and found warmth through increased nutrition and active employment is unclear. Evident in his brief narrative, however, is the toll upon his family with what appears to be the beginnings of physical deterioration.

Given the above scenarios it is difficult to ascertain why men died at higher rates from tuberculosis throughout the nineteenth century in San Francisco. Absent well-paying jobs or salutary domestic environments, it would seem that women's mortality rates would have at least shown a less significant differential. Two reasons might be offered for the greater vulnerability of men. First, as hazardous as women's jobs were at this time, it is probable that many work sites for men were equally conducive to the spread of tuberculosis. Much employment for men was also seasonal or short-term, making erratic incomes, sparse meals, and sometimes even homelessness realities for many unskilled and semiskilled workers. According to Olmstead et al., winters saw an even greater number of unemployed in the South of Market district especially in the 1870s, as agricultural workers came in from the fields looking unsuccessfully for winter work in the city (Olmstead et al. 1979, 120). The greater number of men in, or looking for, employment would also mean a higher occupational vulnerability to tuberculosis overall.

A second reason for men's higher tuberculosis mortality rates might lie in the type of lodging common for single men. In what Paul Groth calls single laborer's zones, lodging houses of various sorts were built to accommodate large numbers of single men who came into the city searching for unskilled or semiskilled work, often on a day-by-day basis. San Francisco's single laborer's zones were located in South of Market and the waterfront districts, places "that mixed cheap work, cheap rooms, cheap liquor, and cheap clothes" (Groth 1994, 153; Olmstead et al. 1979). Lodging houses here were largely characterized by small, single rooms, many with only small windows allowing for insufficient light and air. The turnover rate would have been relatively high for these rooms, as men found employment for a few months and then moved on. Particularly with standards of hygiene of the time, it is doubtful that a thorough cleaning and even a changing of sheets always took place in between tenants.

Easier to explain are the higher rates of tuberculosis suffered by the Chinese and the small community of African Americans living in San Francisco in the nineteenth century. Statistics are spotty for both these groups, for the latter because they were incorporated into mortality rates for whites until later in the century, and for the former because of the "hands-off" nature of medical enumeration of Chinatown death rates, resulting in a majority of Chinese deaths being labeled as "unascertained" in cause. Nevertheless, a few insights are possible. In his report for 1881–82, Health Officer J. L. Meares states that 135 Chinese died of pulmonary phthisis out of a population of approximately 22,000. He adds that most of the 95 unascertained deaths were probably also from phthisis. In contrast, there were 495 deaths among the white population from tuberculosis, out of a population of 234,520 (Municipal Reports 1882, 360). Calculating the rates from these figures, this would mean that the Chinese died from tuberculosis in 1882 at a rate five times higher than the white population, or 1.05 percent of the population versus .21 percent, respectively.

Mortality rates for African Americans are more difficult to calculate because their population was not always differentiated from the white population, even when their disease rates were. In 1890, for example, only 9 African Americans died from pulmonary phthisis, versus 830 whites. But the African American community in San Francisco remained small throughout the nineteenth century; according to William Issel and Robert W. Cherny, they numbered approximately 2,000 in 1860, 1,176 of them living in the South of Market area according to the 1860 census. By 1880, there was no listing for African American residents in South of Market (Issel and Cherny 1986, 14; Olmstead et al. 1979, 182). Assuming a stable population, African Americans would have been dying of tuberculosis at rates over one and a half times the white population. Perhaps more telling is the statement by Thomas Logan, the president of the California State Board of Health in 1875, pointing out the higher mortality rates of blacks in California cities: though they constituted less than 1 percent of the population, they accounted for 1.5 percent of total deaths. His explanation for this is an interesting variant of the environment and predisposition theories. Blacks had higher tuberculosis mortality rates because of worse sanitary and housing conditions, but also because they were "more liable" to respiratory diseases and tuberculosis in particular — that is, they had an innate predisposition toward the disease, no matter what the external circumstances (California State Board of Health Reports 1875, 28).

The health officer's comment is one of the few at this period describing living conditions among the African American community. Although they apparently were not segregated within San Francisco as were the Chinese, discrimination in job opportunities and housing options meant that many lived in crowded underclass dwellings on meager incomes (Olmstead et al. 1979). The majority of Chinese, as will be seen further in the next chapter, lived in extraordinarily crowded housing, many living in basement apartments or rooms facing narrow streets or back alleys. Light and air would have been at a minimum in these habitations, and this makes it is easier to explain why the Chinese died of tuberculosis at significantly higher rates than did any other population group in nineteenth-century San Francisco.

Narratives of a Faulty City

The rhetoric of public health officers writing their yearly reports reflects the change in San Francisco from a small and relatively provincial town to a city with urban problems similar to many other U.S. or European cities experiencing rapid growth from industrialization. Rather than focusing on the attributes or disadvantages of the city as a whole, public health discourse began centering on specific problems of the city such as inadequate sanitation and sewers. The miasmatic theory of disease held that decomposing organic material emitted vapors that caused epidemic diseases and high death rates. Thus the structural problems of inadequate sewers and faulty garbage disposal were not just unsightly and odorous urban blights; in nineteenth-century medical currency, they were potentially deadly disease-producers, turning the unsanitary street into an epidemic corridor as vapors wafted out of backed-up sewers or uncollected waste. These problems, in turn, were ascribed to particular areas within the city, primarily poorer areas that by virtue of their economic status lacked the structural facilities serving the rest of the city.

The almost obsessive focus on sanitation in later nineteenth-century public health material was caused primarily by fear of diseases such as small-pox and cholera, but the inclusion of tuberculosis in the rhetoric of sanitary hygiene was occasionally made explicit. In an elaboration of the environmentalist theory of tuberculosis etiology, damp ground, poor soil drainage, foul air, and lack of ventilation were propounded as the causes of tuberculosis, or at least as exacerbating factors whose amelioration could prevent large numbers of cases of the disease. After a lengthy discussion of the city's inadequate sewers and his detailed plans to improve them, city health officer J. L. Meares in 1876 ended with the claim that in his plan he had "paid due attention to subsoil drainage, for it is well known that where the subsoil water has been removed from the foundations of buildings the result has always been to improve the health of the inhabitants by lessening the amount of consumption and all similar affections" (Municipal Reports 1876, 602). Similarly, the state board of health officer in 1879 claimed that consumption was one among many diseases with a close association to sewers and "whose death rate has been sensibly modified" by proper sewer facilities (California State Board of Health Reports 1879, 59).

In this and similar statements the association with poverty is veiled, leaving an otherwise uninformed reader no key as to where to map the faulty sanitation and undrained soil under discussion. Indeed a direct association between tuberculosis and poverty during the latter half of the century in San Francisco is rarely made. It is more evident at the state level, where disdain of poverty and poor habitats is revealed in more generalized discussions of ventilation and sanitation. Though tuberculosis is not overtly mentioned in these statements, it is implied in the discussion of ventilation, crowding, and filth, primary components of consumption's epidemiology. A moral etiology is also evident whereby the poor are implicitly blamed for their conditions and their disease, a blame stemming from a prevalent nineteenth-century association among immorality, poverty, and disease. The slums played a key role in this triumvirate, serving as active agents of vice and breeding grounds for the depraved — the filthy streets, crowded lodgings, and reeking sewers being concrete manifestations of the moral constitutions of the denizens within. In an elaboration of the association among depravity, poverty, and disease, slums are considered to directly influence the moral constitutions of their inhabitants, the key component in an otherwise tenuous etiology of poverty. The degraded, immoral slum body is thus a somatic by-product of the degraded structural surroundings. As the president of the California State Board of Health stated in 1870:

> To speak of overcrowding is suggestive at once of public lodging houses and tenements of the poor in filthy and narrow lanes, long a recognized and prolific source of disease, intemperance and vice. These haunts of the most depraved and abandoned characters serve as nurseries in which the young and yet uninitiated become familiar with every species of depravity, and their denizens... are among the first victims to epidemic. (California State Board of Health Reports 1870, 23)

Poverty in this statement is a highly spatialized phenomenon, a malignant blight on the urban landscape that in its "prolific" production threatens areas outside its own boundaries both in its capacity to spread and in its propensity to keep producing diseased slum bodies. It is thus a site even more troublesome in its capacity to reproduce itself. In this representational strategy of the state board of health officer, what Lefebvre terms the "marking" of space with symbolic meaning through discursive rhetoric is occurring, putting into place a clear rationale for poor neighborhoods to become loci of intervention by authorities of the state (Lefebvre 1991, 141). Even if the description of the officer was grounded in the realities of impoverished neighborhoods, the symbolic overlay of pathologic meanings operationalizes a struggle for spatial control in the name of epidemic containment.

Intervention as a solution to the spatial slur of poverty is suggested in a report four years later by the state board of health. In bemoaning the "multitudes" in the cities who were "so hemmed in by the barriers of foul air, filth and want" as to be unreachable through the more subtle means of education, the health officer suggests instead the tactic of structural modification of poor environments. To relieve the "unwholesome" burden of overcrowding, an "adequate supply of comfortable dwellings" is suggested, while the portent of preventable diseases and any "number of other evils" would be eliminated through proper drainage, ventilation, and a supply of good water (California State Board of Health Reports 1875, 4). Intervention by the state in the form of structural modification, combined with education, would thus contravene a cycle the poor themselves were unable to break (Duffy 1990; Fee and Acheson 1991; Poovey 1993; Leavitt and Numbers 1985).

This statement is more typical of nineteenth-century sanitarians whose concern with urban improvement stemmed less from humanitarian sentiments and more from a public health justification. If the slums spread disease, then intervention into those structural causes of disease was legitimated on medical grounds. Yet notwithstanding the suggestion of the state board of health officer and the widespread currency it enjoyed throughout the United States and Europe, little was done in the way of structural intervention into poor neighborhoods in San Francisco during the nineteenth century. Three ordinances, two passed in 1870 and the third in 1890, imposed regulations on space and structure that acted in theory as preventatives of consumption. The Cubic Air Law dictated a minimum of five hundred cubic feet of air per person in all residential dwellings, thus purportedly addressing the problem of overcrowding in poor areas and its association with increased consumption rates. This law was passed with little intention of improving overcrowded living conditions in poor neighborhoods, however. It was construed under the thin guise of a public health measure to legally enable health officers to monitor overcrowding in Chinatown as a way to jail the many individuals not adhering to the law. It was, in other words, a partial attempt at Chinese clearance. It was never enforced outside of the Chinese district, nor did it help to improve standards of living within Chinatown. Rather, the law was passed as a punitive measure against the Chinese community, a way to control and incarcerate foreign bodies perceived as far more inimical to public health than poor, white, tuberculous individuals.

The second ordinance enabled public health inspectors to serve notice to tenements observed to be too crowded or damp to be healthy. If after three days the problem had not been corrected, the inspector was empowered to evict the tenement residents until a level of occupancy was reached that was deemed safe for the health of the occupants. Further recalcitrance would be met with "total eviction and/or fines" (Act to Establish a Quarantine 1870, 24). The first problem with this ordinance was that it left the burden of amelioration on impoverished residents or indifferent landlords who would probably pass the cost of structural improvement on to tenants who could ill afford it. The second problem was that it was virtually never enforced.

The third act was passed at the state level and was aimed at improving workplace rather than domestic environments. The act provided for the sanitary condition of factories, workshops, and other business establishments and was to be managed by the commissioner of the Bureau of Labor Statistics. Given that the commissioner received no extra workers to implement this act, it was clearly never meant to be taken seriously (California State Board of Health Reports 1890, 6).

As the 1870 state board of health officer admitted after describing California slums, the board only had an advisory role and could not do anything about the buildings built for the poorer classes with lack of sanitation and ventilation. All they could do was make recommendations; in his view, the real agent for change was the public. "Public pressure only would make these changes" (California State Board of Health Reports 1870, 24), yet clearly this pressure was not forthcoming. Either the general population took a less bleak view of the slums described by the state health officer, or they were not versed enough in medical theory to understand the dangers embodied in South of Market and the waterfront. More likely, the delimited spaces of the slums also played a role. South of Market, the waterfront, and North Beach were all relatively easy to avoid if one did not want to trespass into dangerous zones of disease and depravity. The middle or upper classes could come in from the suburbs or descend from Nob Hill, spend the day at their workplaces, and return home without traversing the boundaries of lower-class slums. As long as these districts were contained, they were less feared, and the need for intervention into their public health nuisances remained at bay.

Class and Ethnic Contours

It is probable that some degree of racism lay at the root of the relative neglect displayed by public health authorities of tuberculosis and the slums in which it thrived. The poor in San Francisco in the latter part of the century, though relatively diverse and including Anglos of British descent, still tended to be predominantly Irish, Italians, and Chinese. Between 1860 and 1880 the numbers of Irish immigrating to San Francisco increased by 328 percent to a population of 30,720, while the Chinese population increased 780 percent to an approximate total of 21,200 (Olmstead et al. 1979). Although Italian immigration peaked at the turn of the century, the number of Italians was nonetheless significant by the 1880s (Cinel 1982). Many of these immigrants later improved their economic status in San Francisco, but the majority of them arrived in the city destitute, and a significant number of them stayed that way (Cinel 1982; Burchell 1980; Cather 1932). Consequently their only recourse upon arrival in San Francisco was to head for the lower-rent districts or to join relatives and family members already established in these areas.

That each of these groups was discriminated against during the latter half of the nineteenth century is without doubt, and the role of diseases such as smallpox in determining the nature and spatial deployment of social discrimination was salient (Trauner 1978; Craddock 1995). Yet tuberculosis, unlike many diseases, did not contain in its socially constructed form the myth of the foreigner as source of contagion. Even the Chinese, the perceived source of much that was wrong about the city, were rarely if ever blamed for the tuberculosis rates in San Francisco. One of the few passages during this period that discusses tuberculosis among the Chinese in essence describes an epidemiology commonly ascribed to the poor of any nationality:

> The Chinese did not contract tuberculosis due to climate, but because [of] their mode of life, in close, dark, diminutive habitations, with imperfect or no ventilation, in many cases in rooms partitioned off in cellars or beneath the street side-walks, where the fresh air of heaven never enters, and to which the pure sunlight is a stranger.... [T]hese would of themselves be supposed sufficient to induce disease. (Municipal Reports 1871, 28)

The source of tuberculosis is not attributed to the Chinese in this passage; rather, the degree to which the Chinese suffered from consumption is explained through the conditions of their structural environment. So were the poor of all nationalities blamed for their tuberculosis. In a more general epidemiological statement, for example, another San Francisco physician attributed a causal role to dank and crowded spaces in claiming that tuberculosis "may acquire more virulent infectious powers in the foul atmosphere of crowded rooms, and... the sporulation of the bacilli may be assisted by contact with the kind of organic matter found in such atmospheres" (Kober n.d., 2). This physician was obviously accurate in his presumption of an association between crowding, lack of ventilation, and tuberculosis, though his insight appears to be couched within a more clinical than social context of analysis.

With few exceptions, then, the ethnic contours of consumption's mythology were more subtle than for many diseases. High rates of tuberculosis among the poor imbricated with a racialized cartography of poverty to translate to some extent into a disease of the marginalized and a conscious marginalization of the spaces inhabited by the poor and tuberculous. A mapping of tuberculosis along racial lines, however, and even a mapping along class lines need to be undertaken with extreme caution. There is nowhere evident for San Francisco, for example, the type of racialized epidemiologies propounded by public health constabularies in other areas of the United States such as New York and Chicago. In these cities, a dominant discourse of tuberculosis targeted Jewish and eastern European immigrants not only as the focus of consumptive incidence but as public health menaces propagating the disease through their habits and lack of hygiene (Kraut 1994; Klein and Kantor 1976). Rhetoric in San Francisco and Sacramento (the seat of the state board of health) occasionally focused on the disease-breeding habits and habitations of the poor, but such discourse was neither pervasive nor dominant for the nineteenth century. Racialized constructions of tuberculosis were even rarer.

Overlaying any racial or class contours of tuberculosis epidemiology is the continuing discourse on tuberculosis as a disease of the defective and feeble-bodied. This framing did not disappear with the shift of focus to "foul air and damp housing" in the latter half of the century, but rather continued to exist alongside it. Within this discourse can be found the strongest statement of disdain concerning tuberculosis, a disdain that does not take on an overt class or racialized overtone. In 1883 the French physician Grancher published an article transcribed in the *Western Lancet* advocating tuberculosis as a "depurator" of those with "feeble natures, imperfectly endowed, and incapable of becoming the stock of a healthy race" (Grancher 1883, 550). Echoing his French colleague three years later, Albert Abrams of the California Medical Association stated in the *Transactions of the Medical Society of the State of California* that "it appears as if phthisis were the disease selected whereby disposition in obedience to the Malthusian doctrine is made of a surplus population" (Abrams 1886–87, 6).

Both Abrams and Grancher were writing in reaction to experiments being conducted to find a cure for tuberculosis, an undertaking they clearly objected to. Finding a cure for tuberculosis would only prolong the lives of those predisposed to the disease, a group defined by these physicians not necessarily by their social or ethnic standing but by their defective physiques. A tool in the services of "natural selection," tuberculosis, if left unchecked, could ultimately assist in the establishment of a "healthy race" by ridding it of its weaker components. How much support these eugenic viewpoints received in San Francisco is difficult to judge; the rarity of their appearance in medical literature suggests that it was a minority view. On the other hand, that the statements were published in major medical journals of the time suggests as well that they were not considered outside the boundaries of rational, expert medical opinion.[12] With a full third of mortality rates at the city hospital due to tuberculosis in 1890 (Municipal Reports 1890), these physicians were unfortunately accurate in their assessment of tuberculosis as an efficient depurator of the population.

Consumptive Spaces

The reasons for San Francisco's rising tuberculosis rates during the final decades of the century warrant scrutiny since this pattern was the opposite of what many cities were experiencing at this time. According to Feldberg, overall tuberculosis rates in America were on the decline in the last half of the century; even New York's high tuberculosis rates had begun to decline after the 1850s, and London's mortality rate began to fall approximately after the 1860s.[13] The precise reasons for the rise or fall of tuberculosis rates in any location are difficult to determine with accuracy, as is indicated by the continuing and prolific debate among medical historians.[14] Yet for San Francisco, increased crowding of poor neighborhoods, overburdened hospitals and poorhouses, and the subsequent lack of isolation of consumptives almost certainly played a significant role. The sustained institutional neglect of the poor by successive San Francisco administrations must also be scrutinized for the ways in which their inactions exacerbated those environmental factors contributing to higher disease rates among the poor.

One facet of this neglect was the dismal state of sanitation and water during the remainder of the century. Where many municipalities of the East Coast and elsewhere had managed to supply their residents with water by the latter part of the nineteenth century, potable water remained unavailable to some of South of Market and other poor areas throughout most of the century; similarly, refuse collection was haphazard and sewers faulty, inadequate, or nonexistent (Municipal Reports 1880, 1895). As public health officer Meares wrote about South of Market in 1876, "The house drainage in this district is exceedingly imperfect, consisting for the most part of small wooden sewers connecting with prolonged cesspools reeking with fermenting and putrefying animal and vegetable matter" (Municipal Reports 1876, 392).

Housing conditions worsened in poor neighborhoods during this period as well, a factor left unmitigated by the lack of tenement and housing reforms. The small wooden frame homes characterizing most of San Francisco's poor neighborhoods (figure 1.1) contained far more people than they were designed to accommodate, while their general state of repair declined over the years beyond the capacity of everyday upkeep. With characteristic fascination for lurid detail, a commission to inspect Chinatown in 1880 found that there were many underground dwellings reached by descending flights of steps into dank, crowded, and unsanitary apartments:

> Near the entrance to this underground den there are large waste pipes...which empty into open wooden boxes above the sewer.... Filth of...every description is everywhere patent to the senses both of sight and smell. Amidst all this smoke and stench and rottenness, in rooms 8x10 and 10x12 feet, 12 persons eat and sleep. (Committee to Investigate Chinatown 1880, 3)

Crowding was becoming more chronic and severe during the 1870s and into the 1880s outside of Chinatown as well. In excavating an area within South of Market, Roger Olmstead and his team found evidence that almost all of the households within their area of study increased their number of residents significantly during this period (Olmstead et al. 1979). Often this

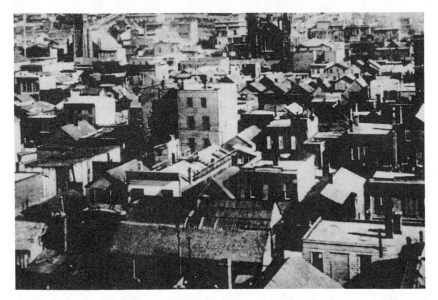

Figure 1.1. South of Market, circa 1860. Courtesy of The Bancroft Library, University of California, Berkeley.

was due to families taking in boarders, but in many cases relatives arrived who from lack of resources and income had no option but to move in with other family members. Whereas a modest house built for a single family in 1860 might house four to six people, that same house, according to Olmstead, would by the 1880s more likely house "a family of four with two additional roomers, perhaps with children, various aunts and brothers-in-law, or children with names totally different from the family name indicating perhaps the adoption of neighborhood children with no family left to care for them" (Olmstead et al. 1979, 183). For most of these dwellings, any yards that might have provided needed open space eventually were filled in with additions, storage areas, laundry spaces, or chicken coops.

The other primary structures of poverty influenced by municipal neglect were the city almshouse and the City and County Hospital. By 1867, an almshouse for paupers and the chronically ill was built well away from the core of the city, on eighty acres of land to the southwest. Unfortunately there is very little in the almshouse records about the percentage of inmates with tuberculosis. Yet high rates were inevitable given that there was no hospital specifically for consumptives at this point and given the inability of the City and County Hospital to provide long-term tuberculosis treatment; many of the poor and chronically ill ended up at the almshouse (Municipal Reports 1881). Evidence of high tuberculosis rates, at least for men, is given by Mary Smith, a Stanford sociologist writing about the almshouse in the late 1800s. She claims that more could be done "in providing especially for consumptive...cases. There are a considerable number of consumptives among the almshouse men, who not only suffer for want of careful attention, but who are a serious danger to the health of other inmates and employees" (M. R. Smith 1895, 42). In other words, even after the communicability of tuberculosis was established, tuberculous inmates were still being placed alongside other inmates of the almshouse with no special provisions for limiting contagion.

A further look into Smith's report gives a poignant character study of the women likely to find themselves in such a dismal institution, and why. Smith's tone in describing these women vacillates between condemnation of their penury and sympathy for the life they were forced to lead as a result of it. Most pathetic, according to Smith, were the women abandoned by their children because of financial difficulties or out of shame. As Smith comments,

> One of the commonest results of immigration seems to be that the children acquire a public-school education, become prosperous, and rise in social station; the old mother or father — foreign, uneducated, often vulgar, and unpresentable — becomes an unwelcome reminder of their common origin, and does not fit into the American life of the children. They are therefore quietly thrown back into the almshouse, where they will be...unknown to the children's friends. (M. R. Smith 1895, 20)

While not speaking directly to tuberculosis or how many women suffered from it, Smith's report nonetheless offers one of the few glimpses of poor women and the conditions in which they lived out their poverty. As with their male counterparts, it may be deduced that many almshouse women suffered from tuberculosis, an almost inevitable outcome of their poverty and their confinement in an institution indiscriminately housing the contagious and noncontagious poor together. The corridor in which the majority of women were forced to live was invariably cramped from overcrowding, a factor that not only made life less pleasant for the inmates but also facilitated the spread of tuberculosis.

In addition to overcrowding, physical conditions at the almshouse seem to have been substandard as well, based again on Smith's report and on successive claims by municipal health officers that the buildings and grounds of the institution were run down, inadequate, and in need of repair (M. R. Smith 1895, 20).[15] Staffing, too, was in short supply as evidenced both by Smith's claim above that the male tuberculous patients were ill cared for and by her subsequent observation that many times it was female inmates who bathed, fed, and cared for other inmates in the absence of qualified staff (M. R. Smith 1895, 9). This neglect evidences the very real, as well as symbolic, outcome of the distance between the almshouse and the city.

Apart from the almshouse, the City and County Hospital was the only option for those who could not afford private hospitals or private physicians. Built in 1872, the hospital was located on Potrero Street and was large enough to admit thousands over the course of a year. Unlike the almshouse, the records of the City and County Hospital are clear on the fact that from its opening, tuberculosis was the most common diagnosis among its patients (Municipal Reports 1870–90). But even more telling is the absence until the 1890s of a lengthy description of this hospital or the quality of care given to the indigent sick. Although careful reporting was done of the number of patients treated, their place of origin, their occupation, and their diagnosis, no account is given of the hospital itself.

When those accounts began to appear, they once again confirmed the city's patent refusal for more than three decades to deal adequately and humanely with the city's indigent sick and especially its indigent consumptives. The steward's report in 1890 states, for instance, that the grounds and buildings were "wornout, wretched and filthy," and Band-Aid repairs were subsequently done. Yet the main building, the steward continued, was still not sanitary since the plumbing was "so completely out of order" (Municipal Reports 1890, 406). By 1895 the former superintendent of the City and County Hospital reported that it was "notorious all over the English-speaking hospital world" for what a hospital should not be. "It has been censured as faultily constructed, wretchedly equipped, insufficiently manned and miserably sustained" (Municipal Reports 1895, 476).

The most thorough and thoroughly damning description came two years later from the superintendent physician of the hospital in his annual report to the board of supervisors. After citing the usual statistics on the number of patients admitted and discharged, the superintendent goes on to enumerate in descriptive and at times eloquent language every substandard aspect of the hospital. It would be difficult to discern from his report whether anything about the hospital was in decent working condition. And consumptives, according to the superintendent, were an especially neglected patient population. In order to get the clearest picture of the hospital and the conditions poor consumptives and other patients were forced to endure during the later 1800s, a lengthy quotation is warranted. The superintendent physician begins by mentioning the "unenviable public notoriety to which the hospital has been subject" and goes on to elucidate the particulars of that notoriety:

> The manner in which this hospital has been neglected in the past by the municipal authorities is a signal and standing reproach. The capacity of the hospital is the same as when erected twenty-five years ago. Since then the population of the city has doubled, but the annual appropriations have been progressively lessened. In every ward much of the bedding is in tatters and many of the windows uncurtained. The surgical appliances and instruments are...imperfect, of inferior quality, and many of them obsolete.... [T]he visiting surgeons are frequently compelled to bring to the hospital instruments from their own private collection in order that they may procure satisfactory results in their service. (Municipal Reports 1897, 11–12)

As the superintendent makes clear, the neglect he describes had been sustained over many years and several changes of the municipal guard. The egregious condition of the hospital thus was obviously not the result of one individual's or administration's parsimony, but instead was the manifestation of a long-standing social, medical, and administrative neglect of the poor. Most of the blame was owed more specifically, according to this superintendent, to the city government, an entity "which, at all times, has been apathetic, if not actually antagonistic, to any measures intended to reform the present imperfect and insufficient apology for a public hospital" (Municipal Reports 1897, 12).

In the final analysis, little was done in terms of structural intervention in San Francisco to ameliorate tuberculosis, except to offer the "imperfect and insufficient" apologies of a dismal almshouse and an even more dismal City and County Hospital for the indigent poor who sought medical care for their consumption. Addressing San Francisco's sanitary straits in 1875, a frustrated state board of health officer bemoaned that "we are scarcely dreaming of expanding our social garments, as our social body is outgrowing them." In other words, the same drainage and water supply systems adequate for a town of fifty thousand were still being used for a city five times that size twenty years later (California State Board of Health Reports 1875, 5). But where Mary Poovey suggests that using the metaphor of the body for urban problems enabled a strategy of institutional surveillance and control in early nineteenth-century Manchester (Poovey 1993, 6), a similar use of body metaphor here illuminated the consequences of institutional inaction. The prodigal city seemed determined to remain in its ill-fitting social garments, and there was nothing the state board of health officer could do — even though, as he laments, such a sanitary breach was tantamount to taking people out of their homes and forcibly putting them to death (California State Board of Health Reports 1875, 5).

It can only be assumed that given their options, many poor consumptives chose to remain at home to endure the course of their disease. Throughout the rest of the century and beyond, calls from within San Francisco and around California continued to be issued for the state to build an institution to house the consumptive poor. The number of poor dying from the disease in appalling institutional settings was clearly objectionable to these physicians, who out of humaneness and professional duty continued their attempts to offer the tubercular "another chance, at least, for life." The city and state administrations felt no such obligations toward their indigent populations.

The Body, the Healthy Home, and the Engendering of Health Reform

Slum intervention was not the only discourse being articulated (or ignored) concerning tuberculosis prevention at this time. Reform of the individual, bodily practices, and domestic spaces formed another common discourse voiced not as much by public health officers but by physicians in and outside San Francisco. The basic message contained in this discourse was that intervention could focus upon the individual rather than on environmental causes, shifting responsibility away from physicians or the more difficult prospect of structural change. More specifically, physicians addressing anti-tuberculosis tactics shifted responsibility for the regulation of health onto gendered bodies located in the domestic arena. The message targeted primarily middle-class housewives, but in invoking middle-class standards of domestic conduct as the antidote to tuberculosis, it implied that underclass women should emulate their higher-class counterparts. Hygiene and diet, for example, were two foci of class-coded bodily practice that could either hinder or help the onset of consumption. Both of these fell under the purview of the middle-class housewife as factors to regulate in herself as well as in her husband and children.[16]

With the sanitary emphasis on cleanliness, body hygiene took on greater importance and was to be fastidiously maintained at all times. Sanitary rhetoric suggested that dirt caused diseases of all sorts including consumption; a dirty body was a diseased body. Diet was also important, both because it was believed that good nutrition could improve the body's resistance to miasmas and other external causes of disease and because theories were batted around throughout the nineteenth century and beyond concerning the use of particular foods in connection with preventing or curing consumption. High-protein foods such as milk, eggs, and meat were sometimes considered the best dietary preventatives, while creams and other fatty foods were thought by some to combat the wasting tendencies of the tubercular. A good diet in general, however, was the most frequently articulated recommendation. As one physician stated, "every time nutrition is vitiated, tuberculization is possible" (*Western Lancet* 8, no. 11, 1880, 491).

The tone used by physicians was not suggestive but instructive; that is, individuals needed to be educated about everyday bodily practices because it was ignorance more than anything else that precipitated high rates of consumption. Discussion moved away from slum housing in the aggregate and the problems of crowding, filth, and cramped spaces. Instead, the home was discussed conceptually rather than structurally; it was the place in which the family resided, spent much of its time, learned bad habits or good, and constructed healthy or unhealthy lifestyles. It was the place, in the abstract, where the bodies within could maintain health or degenerate into disease. In this highly conceptualized medical discourse, homes were made healthy or insalutary not as much by their structural components as by the practices of those who dwelt inside them.

The key figure in this narrative was of course the woman. The "cult of true womanhood" of the nineteenth century had already construed the women of America as queens of the domestic sphere, arbiters of domestic harmony and moral development, doting mothers and selfless wives.[17] In a society highly gendered along spatial concepts of public and private, the woman became the real and symbolic sentinel of an increasingly sacred domestic concept, a place and an individual maintaining calm and order within an external world of capitalist anxiety. As Paula Baker puts it, home was not just the place *for* women and children; it became any place where women and children were (Baker 1984, 631). The domestic arena, then, was in part a symbolic space, a construct of feminine goodness and morality.

But the home was also a physical space, and it was here that medical discourse combined the moral and material in proposing that women were not just moral standard-bearers but domestic sanitary engineers. The combination of morality and cleanliness resulted in a healthy household; failure on one count or two would result in the degeneration of the family into disease and degradation. Women were pivotal figures in this equation because, in the words of one physician writing in the *Western Lancet,* "they are conversant with every nook of the dwelling from basement to roof." They needed more than maps of the house in their heads, however; they needed an awareness of its social cartography as well as innate feminine perception, for it was on "their knowledge and wisdom with regard to the conditions of the household necessary to health" that the physician relied. In fact, throwing moderation aside, this physician went so far as to state that "the future progress of the sanitary movement rests for permanent and executive support in greatest measure on the women of the country" (Richardon 1879, 15). A combination of medical prescription for domestic hygiene and maternal intuition would presumably preserve the health of the nation.

Besides keeping the house clean, women were also to teach their children how to love the outdoors and to instill in all family members the principle of fresh air and open windows. Bedrooms were particular targets because so much time was spent there where the air was motionless with inactivity. Unlike daytime rooms where activity in part kept air circulating, in the bedroom it was easy to "begin consuming narcotic poison as oxygen is used up" and fresh air was unable to seep in through closed windows and doors (*Medico-Literary Journal of San Francisco* 2, no. 7, March 1880, 7). The woman who did not properly monitor domestic apertures risked sending her family to early deaths through the breathing of vitiated air.

Though this discourse would gain momentum in the next century, the connection between immorality and disease also made the moral education of children a primary focus of physicians and sanitarians. As a prominent San Francisco physician questioned, "How many of the annual deaths [in San Francisco] can be prevented by proper sanitary regulations and a better understanding of the physical and moral training of children!" (McNutt 1879, 436). Such rhetoric was implicitly, if not explicitly, class- as well as race-based, relying upon the moral taxonomies of the white middle class as a guideline for lower-class efforts in preventing disease. Given the perceived influence of physical surroundings on moral constitution, for example, part of the process of moral training was the provision of a decent environment, such as middle-class housing. The methods by which the underclass were supposed to achieve this provision were not addressed — though the state board of health made recommendations for better provision of housing for the lower classes, the San Francisco city council chose not to act upon these (California State Board of Health Reports 1870). Apart from middle-class domestic surroundings, moral training also involved learning the manners, work ethics, and bodily hygiene of the middle class, and again the highly signified mother figure was to carefully instill these characteristics in her children if she wanted to ensure their survival into a healthy adulthood.

The construction of a gendered medical discourse centering on a highly conceptualized domestic space served several functions. First, physicians and sanitarians used an already existing discourse of true womanhood — one largely perpetuated by women themselves — in part to carve out a political space that did not impinge on male prerogative (Baker 1984). It was not a large leap to extend the perception that "home was anywhere women and children were" to "health in the home is health everywhere" (Richardson 1879, 15). If women were the (self-)appointed rulers of the home, then they also would be the domestic monitors of health. The nineteenth-century association between dirt, immorality, and disease made it inevitable that not just the house but the home would come to preeminence in preventive narratives. The home in this discourse became the symbolic umbrella of feminine fortitude, but it also became a structural opponent that women needed to know, to conquer, and to control if their duties as health providers were to be fulfilled. Medical science thus inscribed a slightly different gendered expectation onto and into the symbolic meanings and material structures of the home, giving both the home and women's roles added meaning in the nineteenth-century social lexicon.

The medical legitimation of women's roles was a second function of the domestic sanitation discourse. Women as domestic health providers might have seemed an empowering expansion of women's relatively limited social and political space, and in one sense it probably was. But this discourse also served to tie women more strongly to the home and rigidified through social and medical rationales the distinction between productive and reproductive spatial spheres. The social rationale was the strongly emotive argument that if women did not stay in the home and undertake the duties of moral and hygienic education of their families, then the rolls of the sick and degenerate would increase; hospitals would overflow with diseased individuals; urban crime would escalate; and society in general would display a precipitate and ugly decline. Quoting from another writer, the California State Board of Health officer in 1870 pontificated that

> specially should females be taught the responsible duties of maternity, in order that a race of better developed beings may bless the world; one of fewer excesses; one of more harmoniously developed natures; one of more healthy progenitive or hereditary influence. When women are thus taught, no fear need be had for the youth. (California State Board of Health Reports 1870, 70)

It would take a strong will indeed to ignore the sublime responsibility thus bestowed. Women were not just the custodians of health; they were responsible for the regeneration of the human race.

But it would take more than just will to ignore the call to maternal duty, because substantiating the soliloquy above was the medical theory that if women did not respond to the maternal prerogative, they themselves would sustain physical harm; most seriously, it could impair their ability to have children at all. A common nineteenth-century medical theory held the uterus to be something akin to the somatic duchy of the female anatomy, demanding preeminence in physical function and medical attention. But it was also considered extremely vulnerable to external and internal influences. Tuberculosis or other diseases impacted the uterus and weakened its ability to function, as did an overdeveloped sense of ambition or too much education. In his address to the graduating class of the University of California Medical School in 1879, W. F. McNutt railed against women in San Francisco who rather than obtaining knowledge that would "enable them to preserve their own health and save their offspring from misery, disease, and death" were instead "destroying their health and laying the foundation of disease in the acquisition of accomplishments" (McNutt 1879, 436). Straying outside the home sphere not only was a blatant shirking of social responsibility; it was physically incapacitating.

Hazarding a short stray from the subject of tuberculosis, it is important to note briefly that the medical rationalization for women's domestic confinement was embedded in part in pre-eugenic imperatives of social engineering. In the face of rising immigration rates, and more specifically an increase in non-European and non-British populations in the United States, some persons — physicians and nonphysicians alike — felt an urgency for Anglo women to increase their birth rates. This was a national phenomenon, but it was brought home to San Francisco as well. Embedded in the statement cited above by the state board of health officer is the necessity of race purity, the development not just of healthier humans but of better humans. The implications are clearer in the larger context of the report, which also discussed the problems of the Chinese community and, consequently, of miscegenation. Another report on female health and hygiene in San Francisco published in 1876 made the connection more explicit. After bemoaning the "uncommon amounts of reproductive difficulties" apparently suffered by women in San Francisco, the authors go on to discuss the statistics, which give "unmistakable evidence of the physical degeneration of the American race," a problem that would eventually result in the "occupation of the land by successive strangers" (Stallard et al. 1876, 6, 8). If there was a medical imperative for middle-class white women to fulfill their maternal duties, there was also an equally compelling social one. The precursors of a eugenic perspective invoking selective reproduction, middle-class gender values, and tuberculosis prevention in the service of a more "harmoniously developed" race are plainly evident in the opinions of these physicians.

A final function of the domestic sanitation discourse was a practical one. Focusing on women's capacity to make the domestic environment a healthy one meant shifting focus away from suboptimal structural environments.

Much like today's public health rhetoric, the discourse of health through lifestyle changes, hygiene, and other bodily practices relegated the onus of responsibility for a healthy body away from the urban blights of environmental pollutions, sanitary problems, and structural inadequacies. The implicit aim of this discourse toward the middle class was another unstated and subtle indication of the ability of physicians, and subsequently of municipal councils, to make the underclasses invisible. The behavioral discourse existed alongside that of sanitation, and though the two seem mutually contradictory, it is probable that the pervasive belief in education and individual responsibility influenced the decisions of successive municipal administrations to keep a deaf ear turned to the pleas for sanitary intervention. It was much less costly, after all, to reform the body and inculcate middle-class attitudes of hygiene than to redress social and structural antecedents to poor health.

San Francisco in Comparative Perspective

How unique San Francisco was in largely ignoring the problem of tuberculosis among its poor population is a question with no simple answer. Where the city stands most alone is probably in the relative silence of its public health constabulary on the association between tuberculosis and poverty. A formal institutional recognition and campaign targeting the tuberculous poor did not take place in the United States or Europe until the turn of the century, but well before that time public health officials and physicians in many cities had observed, if not systematically studied, the greater burden of diseases such as tuberculosis among poor populations. From Manchester to Paris, London to New York, medical administrators observed and studied associations of disease with occupation, degree of crowding, and poverty (Pooley and Pooley 1984; Ward 1989; Boyer 1978; Barnes 1995).

One of the best known of these observers was Louis Villermé, a French hygienist who observed the inequitable distribution of tuberculosis among classes and who in the 1830s and 1840s conducted systematic investigations of differential mortality among the arrondissements of Paris as well as among textile workers. His studies proved beyond a doubt that the poor in Paris sickened and died from tuberculosis and other diseases at higher rates than did the wealthy (Barnes 1995; Coleman 1982; La Berge 1992). Other hygienists in France conducted further studies elaborating the differential mortality of occupations and the impact of poverty on consumption (Barnes 1995). Numerous physicians' reports during the nineteenth century addressed the deleterious impact of crowded housing conditions and the general insalubrity of cities such as Manchester, London, and Paris, all of which were experiencing the increased poverty and pollution caused by industrialization (Povey 1993; Hardy 1993; Barnes 1995).

Such close investigation of the poor interfaced with a larger trend of fascination with poverty and its increased urban representation in the United States and Europe in the middle of the nineteenth century. This fascination resulted in countless characterizations of slums provided by reformers and medical officials whose verbal incisions into the interior environments of slums and bodily practices of slum-dwellers fell somewhere between clinical panopticism and tabloid sensationalism. Standard descriptions depicted slums as an urban wilderness out of control, breeding "incurable ills" and sanitary evils and threatening to take over the dwellings of the wealthy (Poovey 1993, 10). Fear of disease in particular generated the call to reform the environmental conditions propagating contagion in slum sectors, and in this sense the studies undertaken by physicians in the United States and Europe should not be interpreted as humanitarian gestures evolving out of an understanding of underclass exploitation and having the aim of reforming the structures of a capitalist society responsible for the degradation of the poor.

Rather, urban reform evolved first out of a fear that if action was not taken to intervene in the structural causes of disease in slum districts, upper-class areas would be endangered as well. It also evolved out of the medical theory that ameliorating the environmental conditions of the poor improved their moral constitutions and set them on the road to a more productive and upstanding life. In her history of public health in Boston, for example, Barbara Rosenkrantz notes that improving the physical environment of the poor was felt by public health authorities like Henry Bowditch to be the solution to their moral degradation. Improving housing and increasing the ability to buy food would "remedy the disharmony" of the cycle of poverty, disease, and degradation (Rosenkrantz 1972, 48). A similar attitude characterized the British sanitarian Edwin Chadwick, who reconciled a patronizing view of the poor with a belief in the efficacy of better housing to raise them out of their moral and physical turpitude (Eyler 1992, 280). As the president of the British Social Science Association declared more specifically in 1866, improving the "domiciliary conditions" of the poor would "destroy their appetite for spiritous liquors" (California State Board of Health Reports 1875, 4).

It is clear through these examples that the rhetoric used to describe the poor in most nineteenth-century urban areas pivoted around similar themes of disdain and unsympathetic interpretations of the etiology of poverty. To the degree that California or San Francisco physicians articulated this rhetoric, it was no different. In San Francisco and elsewhere in the United States and Europe, discourses about the poor also refracted along similar fault lines of the worthy and the unworthy. The worthy poor were generally perceived as industrious and moral individuals who met their penury through disease, a death in the family, or some other unfortunate external accident beyond their control. The unworthy poor were the aggregate mass whose poverty was a natural extension of their depravity and whose existence was nothing more than an open wound on the surface of the urban social body. Mary Smith's report on the San Francisco almshouse gives some indication of how the two categories were to be distinguished, but for all intents and purposes the classifications were a discursive strategy rather than a tool for policy implementation. The worthy poor rarely seemed to surface, leaving city administrations the rhetorical space to deal with the unworthy poor as they saw fit.

In the degree of rhetoric and of urban reform, however, San Francisco appears to stand opposed to most nineteenth-century U.S. and European cities with its comparative silence concerning the poor and their diseases. Probably the most important reason for this is that Chinatown was the district San Francisco demonized, though this occurred outside tuberculosis discourse. Tuberculosis played little part in a demonization of the Chinese because feared diseases such as smallpox made more effective tools for a racialized discourse of undesirability. As will be seen in the next chapter, diatribes against the contagiousness of Chinatown and its dangerous location in the middle of the city became pervasive by the 1870s and 1880s, with more than one attempt made to have the whole malignant "city within a city" excised. The body of the Chinese was made "Other" and vilified, and the type of poverty generated by these bodies was highly racialized. In Ann McClintock's words, "the geometry of the body mapped the psyche of the race" (McClintock 1995, 50), and body and psyche in turn were mapped onto a highly pathologized spatial arena that demanded constant scrutiny if not excavation. The problems of the non-Chinese slums were insignificant in comparison.

Another reason may stem from the relatively unique origins of San Francisco compared to older East Coast and European cities. The gold rush that spawned the growth of San Francisco in the late 1840s and 1850s generated for the decades to come an ideology of success, the ultimate manifestation of the American dream of financial reward for anyone who worked for it. Even if reality was different for many who tried it,[18] the cultural mystique surrounding this phenomenon was that anyone who came to California could get very rich very quickly, regardless of previous economic standing. As Neil Shumsky notes, this cultural (il)logic persisted in San Francisco well after the gold was exhausted and the economic disparities born of capitalist enterprise had long been established (Shumsky 1972). Of course other discourses existed contemporaneously with this one, and some contested the city's easy lifestyle, superiority complex, and facile way of ignoring those who could not make it. This will be discussed further later. Nevertheless, it is probable that gold rush mentality influenced to some degree the thinking of city administrators when they made successive decisions to withhold funding for urban reform.

Another factor in San Francisco's different responses to poverty and disease must lie in the context of longer histories of urbanization for East Coast and European cities and the sheer size of slums in cities like London, Manchester, New York, and Philadelphia. Population growth due to natural increase and migration was significant by the 1820s in these cities and continued over the course of decades; the volume of migrants entering port cities of the eastern U.S. seaboard in particular was unmatched in cities farther west. The intensity of crowding, the degree of pauperism, and the proportionate size of slums in large midwestern, East Coast, and European cities far outstripped what San Francisco would ever experience. The poor in San Francisco were a growing problem to comment upon occasionally; they were not the "urban wilderness" of larger cities to the east.

Yet the degree to which U.S. and European cities in the nineteenth century monitored, overhauled, or reconstructed their slums should not be exaggerated. Many of the calls for reform were issued by organizations such as the American Social Science Association, whose members thought that rigorous scientific investigation and enumeration of the poor would reveal quick solutions to social ills; or, in David Ward's words, "their faith was based upon the healing power of statistical facts" (Ward 1989, 40), not upon the desire for social change. Similarly, even the early French hygienists at the forefront of investigating links between poverty and disease stopped short of suggesting major urban reform; their interest, too, lay more in the enabling capacities of statistical investigation to illuminate heretofore uncharted slum interiors (La Berge 1992; Coleman 1982). The recommendations that were put forward often went unheeded by city or provincial administrations, and as such the experience of San Francisco on this front is typical. Although physicians and public health officials alike thought that the San Francisco city council and California legislature were especially parsimonious ("About Hospitals" 1869, 15; Municipal Reports 1870), other city administrations, balancing between social responsibility and "keeping public expenditures low and dependency at a minimum" (Bates 1992, 43), often sided with the latter.

It is difficult to ignore nevertheless the persistent claims of many living in or visiting San Francisco that the city and the state were particularly difficult to survive in under conditions of poverty. In her memoirs of traveling to San Francisco, Isabella Saxon in 1861 concluded after a five-year stay that "those who venture [to San Francisco] with a small capital may always have a good chance...of doing well.... Those who find themselves there without influence or capital...will be most unfortunate" (Saxon 1861, 24). A physician writing for the *California Medical Gazette* in 1869 claimed that "there is not, and never has been, a noble generosity in California." Absent a public institution for the destitute sick, these "languish in boarding houses and private families, often badly cared for...until death mercifully comes to their relief" ("About Hospitals" 1869, 15).

The comparative lack of funding put into sanitary repair and urban reform was also noted by a few public health authorities. The 1886 report of the California State Board of Health mentions that though California was one of the first states to establish a board of health (in 1870), "we have been forced to admit that California is now far behind some of her sister states in which state boards of health are maintained, in failing to have upon her statute books many needed sanitary laws, and having the same carried out by efficacious state aid" (California State Board of Health Reports 1886, 38). In his history of the California Medical Society, Roy Jones confirms that appropriations for health legislation in California were "miserly," but he goes further in claiming that "as years went on a parsimonious economy of the rulers increased rather than bettered." The funding appropriated for health legislation, in other words, decreased by one-fifth between the years 1870 and 1885, even though California's population doubled during that period (Jones 1964, 156). Though California and San Francisco legislatures were not alone in ignoring the stated needs of their public health boards, it would appear that they stood apart from many municipal and state legislatures in the degree of their concerted negligence.

The question remains to be answered, then, of whether the attempts at housing and workplace reform in London and other cities, however partial, played a role in the decline of tuberculosis rates in the last half of the century; or, conversely, whether San Francisco and California's lack of such reforms contributed to the increase in tuberculosis rates during the course of the century. Many cities provided more hospitals for phthisis patients (Bates 1992; Hardy 1993), a factor that would at least isolate the tuberculous individuals and prevent them from infecting others, even if it did not help cure their disease. San Francisco did not build a hospital for tuberculosis patients until the turn of the century, and the California legislature never did provide funds for a state institution. Elevated tuberculosis mortality rates from consumptive migrants was of course a factor, but this does not explain why tuberculosis rates continued to rise until the 1890s. The refusal of city officials to address the deleterious effects of unmitigated crowding, the delay in addressing serious sanitary deficiencies, and the inadequacy of institutional facilities for the indigent consumptive may very well have contributed significantly to tuberculosis rates that by the turn of the century were higher than those of the ten largest cities in the United States (Municipal Reports 1906). Contrary to the framing of the disease in other cities, tuberculosis never did become a social disease in nineteenth-century San Francisco.

Conclusion

As Sander Gilman points out, the infected individual is never value-neutral (Gilman 1988, 7). Tuberculosis and the tuberculous individual were interpreted in multiple and often complex ways, standing at the center of a debate by physicians and others about the therapeutic qualities of San Francisco's environment and about how the city should be advertised and developed. It was in part the solicitation of consumptives that contributed to the city's population growth and economy in the 1860s, though relative to other factors this influence declined in later decades. The presence of a significant number of consumptive migrants, and the discursive debates they generated, nevertheless leant meaning to the city as a cognitive space and an urban reality. It forced attention to the structural, climatic, and social qualities the city did or did not possess and at times spawned narratives enhancing the city's representation to distant audiences. Medical theories espousing, on the one hand, climatic capacity to alleviate consumption and, on the other hand, the hereditary predisposition toward the disease were the driving forces of this particular debate.

Contradicting the myth of urban salubrity, San Francisco harbored increasing numbers of poor and indigent with uncertain employment opportunities. Thousands arrived destitute from the East Coast hoping to find a better life in the West. Instead, many found limited or seasonal employment and a gradual intensification of their poverty as a survivable income continued to thwart them. An entry from one working man's diary during this bleak period in the 1870s and 1880s affirms this scenario:

> With this month ends a year I had hoped from its auspicious beginning to terminate in a far different manner, but while we hope still for the silver lining to the dark cloud of adversity; and as we think, we hope, and work and toil for it, yet as time revolves . . . our hopes become tinctured with despair. (Cited in Olmstead et al. 1979, 16)

Overcrowded conditions, inadequate diet, and lack of ventilation drove many of these more unfortunate individuals beyond despair and into tuberculosis.

Apathy toward the poor and toward slum districts in the nineteenth century, relative to rhetoric propagated elsewhere in the United States and Europe, might be explained by the continuing dialectic in San Francisco between the myth of salubrity and wealth and the increasing reality to the contrary. Following this line of thought, San Francisco may have been manifesting what Soja describes as a "complex and conflictful dialectic" caused by shifting modes of capitalist production and the social and political responses generated to make sense of these changes. The result is a "shifting and conflictful social context in which everything seems to be 'pregnant with its contrary'" (Soja 1989, 26). Economic growth produced much that was good in San Francisco, much that could affirm the boosterist claims of superiority; it also produced intense slum districts that the city administration did not seem to know what to do with. Perhaps embracing the cliché that if you ignore something it will go away, the city council largely decided to do nothing. The administration and city council concentrated their efforts on Chinatown instead.

Medical theories generated around the subject of tuberculosis and its larger epidemiological context also helped to inform gender roles in the nineteenth century and to keep well-delineated the spatial and social boundaries between productive and reproductive arenas. Underscoring the extant "cult of womanhood" ideology was the medical imperative for women not only to stay in the home but to produce it in specified ways. Key to the construction of a salutary domestic environment was the monitoring of cleanliness both in individuals and in architectural features as well as engendering proper bodily practices in all family members. As such, "home" became imbued with more complex meanings, both as a highly abstracted symbol of gendered order, hygiene, and middle-class morality and as a potent physical structure embodying the capacity to enable or constrain the health and social function of members residing within.

For the impoverished tubercular in nineteenth-century San Francisco, municipal inaction meant that few options were available other than the almshouse and City and County Hospital. As these became increasingly inadequate, many were left with no medical treatment at all. An anonymous editorial in the *California Medical Gazette* stated, "There probably never was a people so poorly provided with hospital accommodations, or one amongst whom they are so much needed" ("About Hospitals" 1869, 15). As Averbach and Shumsky both note, even public relief programs were largely lacking in San Francisco until the 1930s (Averbach 1973; Shumsky 1972). Only with shifting social ideologies at the turn of the twentieth century, and the recognition that tuberculosis was contagious, did San Francisco pay serious attention to its destitute, their disease, and the material conditions that linked them.

Responses to consumption in the latter half of the nineteenth century nevertheless serve important historiographic functions. As Allan Brandt states, "the manner in which a society responds [to disease] reveals its most fundamental cultural, social, and moral values" (Brandt 1991). Tuberculosis, then, more than many optics, illuminates more specifically for San Francisco the sometimes subtle struggles over class, social valuation of economic failure, and the physical shape and symbolic meanings of urban spaces during a time of rapid growth and economic uncertainty.

2

SEWERS AND SCAPEGOATS

Epidemic Diseases and Their Spatial Metaphors
in San Francisco, 1868–87

*There is no disease which in itself so impressively dejects the moral force
as small-pox, nor is there one from which the encouragement of hope, so
potent to cure, is more ruthlessly plucked away.*
— *California Medical Gazette,* August 1868

No disease in San Francisco's history produced more fear, and more reaction,
than smallpox. It remained relatively absent for years at a time before descending with little warning upon the city, killing hundreds within a matter
of weeks and causing a level of disruption of social activity that few other
diseases could have caused. The city suffered four major smallpox epidemics,
the first and most deadly in 1868, followed by subsequent episodes in 1876,
1881, and 1887. A vaccine provided some degree of hope, but its production
was so unreliable as to "pluck away" any convictions of preventive capability. In fact physicians and public health authorities were never completely
successful in nullifying the ravages of the disease or in preventing the next
epidemic, both because of their imprecise understanding of its etiology and
because they could not rely upon complete adherence to the rules they dictated. As one frustrated physician stated after the scourge of 1876, "Disease in
one of its most appalling forms held sway, and art stood helpless by" (*Western
Lancet* 7, no. 2, 1879, 534).

Yet ironically, it was this "appalling" form and the profound fear it engendered that shaped the social constructions and spatializations of the disease.

As may be predicted, these were vastly different from those of consumption. Whereas the social interpretations of tuberculosis were structured primarily along class lines, those for smallpox were overwhelmingly ethnic. In its most overt spatial manifestation, consumption was associated with the poor quarters and slums of the city, a disdainful disease associated with a disdained people. Smallpox, however, was not disdained but feared, and correspondingly its spatial association came eventually to focus almost exclusively on Chinatown, a place that in late-nineteenth-century San Francisco was increasingly feared and despised. As the century wore on, the "imaginative epidemiology" of smallpox focused on the Chinese as the sources of the disease, as well as its most efficient, if not exclusive, disseminators. By the late 1870s, Chinatown was almost synonymous with smallpox.

The framing of smallpox by public health officials and the public cannot be divorced from its larger material context. The 1870s and 1880s saw the rise of an anti-Chinese movement in San Francisco based most explicitly upon the perception that Chinese workers were taking jobs away from working-class whites. Smallpox served a strategic political role in this scenario, extending the boundaries of the debate from labor practices and the control of racially inscribed bodies to the control of a racialized area of the city. Few treatments of the anti-Chinese campaign take the political use of disease into account, and this begs for a broadening of standard explanations for why the anti-Chinese movement occurred and who its primary proponents were. Although economic recession and its predominantly Irish working-class victims were at the forefront of growing hostility toward the Chinese,[1] a purely economic explanation elucidates neither why disease was increasingly used to distinguish and vilify Chinatown nor why the primary proponents of this facet of the movement were from the ranks of professionals and the medical community, not from the South of Market working class.

In effect the anti-Chinese movement of the 1870s and 1880s was not simply a moment in the history of the city generated by a problematic configuration of labor supply and demand. It was part of a more complex ideology constructing the city as white and English-speaking, an ideology deployed spatially in the physical and social construction of Chinatown as a foreign and highly racialized district within an otherwise "American" city (Saxton 1971; Anderson 1987; Takaki 1989). Smallpox was a pivotal component of this construction, its race-based etiology serving to further map the degree and quality of otherness manifested in Chinatown inhabitants. The delimitation of disease origins to this district also changed political-medical perceptions toward it from an area to be shunned to an area needing intense scrutiny, intervention, and control.

Integral to this process was a political anatomy of the Chinese body that read disease and depravity into its fundamental structure. Following Foucault's statement that the body is an object and target of power (Foucault 1977), it is clear in the framing of smallpox in nineteenth-century San Francisco that inscribing the Chinese body with disease, in fact producing the entire body as diseased, functioned in part as a struggle for power over the microspaces of those bodies and the macrospaces between and surrounding them. Paraphrasing David Arnold, the Chinese body and the district they inhabited became cites of colonization *enabled* by smallpox; the inscription of disease, in other words, rationalized a degree of surveillance and control that would otherwise have been untenable (Arnold 1993). It was impossible to change the body's lexicon indicating racialized otherness, but it was possible to modify its reading through curtailing the degree to which disease comprised it. Curtailing disease among the Chinese, in short, would diminish their danger if not their foreignness.

Smallpox was not always interpreted through the nexus of Chinatown, however. As a generally feared and uncontrollable disease, it also galvanized support for scientific sanitation. Tuberculosis was a minor part of the movement for better hygiene of streets and sewers; the epidemic diseases of yellow fever, cholera, and smallpox were its primary driving force. Chinatown was targeted as the worst perpetrator of sanitary neglect, but the similar condition of many other areas of San Francisco was cause for alarm among public health authorities. Elaborating on the sanitary state of San Francisco from the last chapter, we can note here that garbage was ineffectually dealt with, sewers were inadequate, and privy contents were often dumped in the streets or in cesspools dotting the city. Horses, cows, and other animals frequently had free rein, and their bodies after death often rotted in the streets for days. Given these circumstances, the advent of an epidemic inside or out of the city boundaries was cause not only for panic but for better sanitation and improved conditions within the city. Although the role of smallpox was prominent, the threat of cholera and the Mississippi Valley yellow fever epidemic of 1878 considerably augmented the urgency with which these calls were made. Even if the mythology of Chinatown as the *source* of smallpox and other diseases remained relatively intact, it was increasingly impossible not to acknowledge that conditions pertaining in the rest of the city played a large role in spreading those diseases.

Devastating Diffusions

Experiences of yellow fever, smallpox, and cholera arrived in San Francisco via the immigrants coming from the Northeast and South. To have been born and raised in these areas meant to inherit a long history of infectious disease, since smallpox and yellow fever especially had plagued the eastern half of the country from the time of the first colonies. Cholera was added to the list in the 1830s when it finally straddled the barrier of the Atlantic Ocean. Epidemics were frequently devastating in their virulence and geographic breadth. Death tolls could be catastrophic; chaos reigned as municipal governments broke down; and roads and railways bogged down as the wealthy fled the area, leaving the poor to bear the brunt of disease. The scene in many of these cities during an epidemic must have somewhat resembled the European plague epidemics of centuries past, as this description of a yellow fever epidemic testifies:

> The plague has spread even to...northern cities, and terror has seized upon the inhabitants. Upon its approach, a regular panic took place. The town, situated in a low, marshy district, numbered four thousand, and within four days they had all fled except one hundred and twenty-five persons.... The streets were deserted, the only sounds heard in them were the shrieks of the delirious and the groans of the dying, as they came out on the hushed air from the chambers of the suffering. (*Medico-Literary Journal of San Francisco* 1, no. 1, September 1878, 13–14)

Beyond the social devastation wrought by these diseases, simply witnessing their physical manifestations and rapidity of onset could be terrifying. As one New Yorker stated during the 1832 cholera epidemic, "To see individuals well in the morning and buried before night...is something which is appalling to the boldest heart." The acute vomiting, cramps, and darkened extremities characterizing cholera could only have added to the horror (Rosenberg 1962, 3). Smallpox, however, was the most repugnant of all, a disease that progressed from fever and chills into a dense rash of blisters and pustules that turned "the miserable, aching victim...into a hideous, swollen monster." Not only was the body transformed, but its surroundings also became suffused with "a peculiarly sickening odor" (Hopkins 1983, 4). And if a victim survived the days of suffering, chances were that life would nonetheless be changed afterward since smallpox inscribed its indelible mark on the victim in the form of deep facial scarring, hair loss, frequent enlargement of the nose, and the potential for vision impairment.

Morbid Topographies

Seven years before San Francisco's first major outbreak, a smallpox epidemic broke out in 1861, during the early stages of the Civil War. Hitting the South first, the disease quickly spread northward and westward, facilitated by the wartime movement of people and troops and the greater social disruptions of war. It hit Washington, D.C., by the winter of 1861–62 and intensified the following year. Even President Lincoln was not spared the disease, although unlike thousands of others he obviously recovered. Although New England suffered as well, those states seemed somewhat better equipped to diminish the ravages by administering effective vaccines (Hopkins 1983). Indeed, the worst of the epidemic in the eastern United States seemed to focus in the South, where ravages of war, an economy in turmoil, and a number of newly freed slaves migrating to new locations served to further propagate the disease.

Blacks suffered considerably more than did whites in the 1860s epidemic. Donald R. Hopkins reports, for example, that black troops in the Union Army numbered 61,134, out of which 6,716 contracted smallpox. In comparison, white troops numbered approximately seven times as many (431,237) but suffered less than twice the number of cases (Hopkins 1983, 275). For some blacks it would appear that liberation from slavery was fleeting, as one report claimed that "delirious Negroes stumbled through the streets, and died on doorsteps and in police stations" in Washington, D.C. (cited in Hopkins 1983, 277).

Smallpox arrived in San Francisco when the rest of the country was finally breathing a sigh of relief at its subsidence. By the summer of 1868, four to five hundred people stood in line every day to receive the smallpox vaccination (*Alta of San Francisco,* August 1868, 1), and the smallpox hospital was already overcrowded (*California Medical Gazette,* August 1868). Nonetheless, the epidemic intensified the next year, and according to Health Officer Bates, at least 760 people died out of a population of approximately 150,000 (Municipal Reports 1870, 229). Possibly because the city had not seen a smallpox epidemic in many years, this was to be the worst epidemic in terms of mortality rates that San Francisco would endure.[2]

After the 1860s epidemic, the next major wave of smallpox arrived in the eastern states in the early 1870s — a timing that coincided with heavy immigration to the United States from Europe. According to Hopkins, it was this immigration that triggered epidemics in every major city on the Eastern Seaboard from 1871 to 1874, as well as in New Orleans, Cincinnati, Chicago, and other points westward. It reached San Francisco by 1876, where according to Health Officer Meares, 1,646 cases and 482 deaths occurred between May 19, 1876, and July 1, 1877. San Francisco in fact was also suffering under a simultaneous epidemic of diphtheria that killed 900 citizens, mostly children (Municipal Reports 1877, 392).

An interesting point concerning the dual epidemic in San Francisco is that, though diphtheria actually killed almost two times more people than smallpox, there was little mention of it in the health officer's report to the board of supervisors and correspondingly little coverage of it in the medical journals or media. Explanations for this are not definitive, but at least two factors probably contributed. First, diphtheria seems to fall somewhere in between the categories of subtle, endemic diseases, such as tuberculosis, and more spectacular epidemic diseases, such as smallpox. Although diphtheria acts relatively quickly, it is not as gruesome in its symptoms as smallpox or as rapid in its onset as cholera. And though some years brought especially heavy tolls from diphtheria, the disease was endemic to San Francisco, indeed to many cities in the United States at that time. As with tuberculosis, then, people were somewhat inured to the continual presence of the disease, a familiarity that engendered concern rather than fear or panic. Second, diphtheria struck primarily young children rather than adults, a fact that may have also dimmed the commotion over its presence. Infant mortality was extremely high during this period, in 1869 averaging two hundred out of every thousand births (*California Medical Gazette,* November 1869, 50). Diphtheria, then, was only one of many ailments felling young children during this period. For these and for perhaps other reasons, diphtheria's treatment and interpretation by the medical establishment and others in San Francisco were minimal.

Conversely, yellow fever never invaded the boundaries of San Francisco, yet the epidemic of 1878 in other areas of the United States brought a great deal of fear to the West Coast. Though perhaps not as mutilating as smallpox, yellow fever was another disease that produced frightening symptoms in its victims. Not only did chills, fever, and the jaundice giving it its name begin abruptly, but victims also hemorrhaged through the nose, gums, and stomach lining. Intense vomiting of this "digested" black blood ensued. Moreover, death rates could be appallingly high during severe epidemics, sometimes claiming as much as 60 percent of its victims (Humphreys 1992, 6). By the nineteenth century yellow fever was primarily a southern disease,[3] but the intensification of railroad use in the latter part of the century opened the way for yellow fever to break out of its previous geographic boundaries. Indeed, as the statement below testifies, the railroad was one of the primary factors in the spatial diffusion of the 1878 epidemic:

> The cars of the trains for several days went out literally packed to suffocation with people. Every station and town had shortly its quota of refugees from Memphis,... some of them carrying with them the seeds of the disease which, with time and conditions to propagate, afterward brought to their hospitable and generous hosts the misery and death which then plagued their relatives and friends. To the

cities of the far north and the far west they fled, too many of them to die on the way, . . . or, to reach the wished-for goal, only to die. (Keating 1879, 18)

In one of the worst epidemics to hit the United States, half of Memphis's population of 33,600 caught the disease and 5,000 people died; New Orleans lost a similar number (Humphreys 1992; Duffy 1990). In all, an estimated 20,000 deaths and 100,000 cases of yellow fever occurred within the Mississippi and Ohio Valleys during the course of the epidemic (Humphreys 1992; Ellis 1992). The report of the Tennessee Board of Health lamented that "1878 will be long remembered by the people of Tennessee as a year especially marked as one of disaster and death. The yellow fever . . . fastened its deadly fangs upon the Western Division of our State, carrying dismay and death into almost every household" (cited in Humphreys 1992, 60). Describing Memphis, the same eyewitness stated that "an appalling gloom hung over the doomed city. At night, it was silent as the grave, by day, it seemed desolate as the desert. There were hours, especially at night, when the solemn oppressions of universal death bore upon the human mind, as if the day of judgment was about to dawn. . . . Death prevailed everywhere" (Keating 1879, cited in Humphreys 1992, 61).

To the immense relief of San Franciscans, the yellow fever epidemic never made it to the West Coast. That relief was relatively short-lived, however, since the next wave of smallpox hit by 1880. Again it was a national epidemic, but this time San Francisco was at the forefront. Whether this indicates that the disease was brought in by ship from Asia and spread eastward by rail is not known for certain, although Hopkins attributes the California epidemic to a railway passenger from Chicago (Hopkins 1983, 285). As will be discussed later in this chapter, however, the Asian explanation was the one preferred by many in San Francisco. Perhaps because many had just been vaccinated during the previous smallpox episode, this wave at least proved to be milder, with 507 cases and 92 deaths reported for the city. By comparison, tuberculosis for the same year claimed 690 lives (Municipal Reports 1880–81, 254).

After a relatively brief respite, San Francisco experienced its last major smallpox epidemic in the fall of 1887. The disease again ravaged other parts of the United States first. One of the most devastated cities was Montreal, which suffered 10,000 cases and over 3,000 deaths out of a population of 168,000 (Hopkins 1983, 286). San Francisco fared better, with a total of 568 reported cases and 69 deaths, the vast majority of which occurred in the short span of time from December 1887 to February 1888 (Municipal Reports 1888, 471). By March, the city was declared out of the epidemic, notwithstanding the arrival in April of an infected steamer from Panama that sent a renewed wave of fear through the city. The steamer was quarantined in the bay, and no new cases were traced from it (Municipal Reports 1888, 469).

San Francisco was to have several more smallpox scares during the remainder of the century and on into the next, but the 1887–88 epidemic was to be the last significant episode of this disease. This trend pertained in the rest of the country as well, and while it would continue to be a topic of concern for public health officials until its eradication well into the twentieth century, its ability to incite terror in a population gradually diminished by the turn of the century.

Cholera was another disease, like yellow fever, that kept citizens concerned and public health officials on their toes trying to keep it from crossing city boundaries. Although cholera first swept through the United States in 1832, California did not get a major epidemic of it until 1850, when San Francisco lost 5 percent of its population and Sacramento 15 percent (Harris 1932).[4] Although there was another U.S. epidemic in 1866, and a milder one in 1873, San Francisco managed to remain unscathed. For inexplicable reasons, cholera did not hit San Francisco again with any vigor, despite occasional sweeps through the eastern United States, Asia, and Europe. Yet its existence on virtually all sides of San Francisco's borders, and the city's transportation links with Asia and the eastern United States, meant that cholera continued to hold emotional sway over the city. Unlike yellow fever, cholera had demonstrated once that California was not outside its geographic boundaries and hence could conceivably intrude again. As such, it made a political tool less utilized than smallpox, but it nevertheless was effective as a rationale for urban cleanup and sanitary reform.

Finally, leprosy was a disease that did not quite fit into the category of infectious epidemic diseases and therefore did not receive the attention that smallpox, yellow fever, and cholera did. Although it was known to be somehow communicable, it clearly did not spread with the ease and rapidity of other infectious diseases. Yet it was also, like smallpox, horrifying in its stigmatizing mutilation and for this reason inspired occasional diatribes against its presence in the city. It is difficult to ascertain what prompted these vituperative waves of "concern," but inevitably they culminated in a search for, and roundup of, leprosy victims residing within the city. Most were subsequently sent to the smallpox hospital on Twenty-Sixth Street, but, beginning in the 1870s, for many of the Chinese sufferers, leprosy was an automatic ticket back to China. Indeed, leprosy was another disease that became more strongly ascribed to the Chinese in the 1870s and 1880s, some going so far as to claim leprosy inherent among this community (Committee to Investigate Chinatown 1880, 12). Between 1876 and 1885, close to eighty Chinese lepers were shipped back to their home country (Municipal Reports 1885).

Productions: Race, Place, and Pathology

In her book *Vancouver's Chinatown,* Kay Anderson discusses the tendency of western cities to create a separate place or "landscape type" for those immigrants more distinctly different than others in the tide of primarily European immigration to North America in the nineteenth century. The Chinese were the furthest away from the European ideal; they were, more than any other immigrant group, the "Other" as distinct from the "us," a separate category requiring ascription to a particular space within the urban landscape (Anderson 1987).[5] More than just spaces encompassing the Chinese population of a city, though, these landscapes were social constructions with ascribed images and practices that in particular ways served the ideological needs of the larger urban arena. Although Anderson discusses disease as one of these socially constructed attributes of Chinatowns, it was perhaps the most developed and significant attribute of San Francisco's. More than economic arguments, the construction of Chinatown as the headquarters of disease became the most powerful tool to keep Chinatown not only a distinct but also a thoroughly undesirable part of San Francisco's landscape.

Yet the typical history of the Chinese in San Francisco focuses primarily on labor issues and the struggle between Chinese and white workers that began in the gold mines and continued throughout most of the century (Saxton 1971; Cross 1935). During the 1860s, demands for labor exceeded the supply in San Francisco (Issel and Cherny 1986; Shumsky 1972). The increasing number of Chinese immigrating into the city partially closed the gap, providing a significant percentage of the workforce completing the transcontinental railroad and later filling the needs of manufacturers short of labor (Cather 1932; Dicker 1979; Saxton 1971). According to Saxton, it was those manufacturers who produced items competitive nationally as opposed to locally — that is, the ready-made clothing, shoe, and cigar producers — who needed to hire the cheapest labor. Saxton argues that because these industries were new in the 1860s, there was no displacement of white male labor when women, children, and Chinese were hired (Saxton 1971, 70).[6] By the mid-1860s, 80 percent of the woolen mill workers and two thousand out of twenty-two hundred cigar-makers were Chinese; by the early 1870s, approximately half the factory workers were Chinese, with two thousand working in boot and shoe factories (Cross 1935, 315).

Friction between Chinese and white workers occurred nevertheless before 1870, but after 1870 tensions intensified. The influx of laborers after the completion of the railroad, coupled with the beginnings of an economic recession in 1870–71, led to the first serious bout of unemployment in San Francisco (Cross 1935). The worse depression of 1876–77 caused unemployment rates estimated to be as high as 20 percent, or fifteen thousand workers (Cross 1935). As noted by Cross, the scenes of destitution during this time were pervasive:

> Thousands of men tramped the city streets and the country roads in search of work.... At times the crowds that gathered at places of possible employment were so great that the police had to be called to clear the thoroughfare.... More than 4,000 applications for relief were made at the office of the San Francisco Benevolent Association in April, May, and June, 1877,... more numerous than at any time since its organization in 1865. (Cross 1935, 71)

The frustration of persistent fluctuations in job availability, lower wages caused by depression and the oversupply of labor, and a repeal of the eight-hour workday eventually found expression in the Workingman's Party of California, an organization formed to fight the causes of unemployment and to protect the jobs of white laborers. The WPC, in turn, vented its collective anger at the Chinese in response to a growing perception that Chinese laborers were taking jobs away from whites because they were willing to work for lower wages and longer hours (Cather 1932; Takaki 1989).[7]

By many accounts, the WPC *was* the anti-Chinese movement, a predominantly working-class Irish tide of bitterness directed at the industrial employers of the city and the Chinese workers they hired in preference to white laborers (Issel and Cherny 1986; Olmstead et al. 1979; Shumsky 1973). One of the WPC's most vocal advocates, Dennis Kearney, led a series of gatherings and riots beginning in 1877 that sometimes resulted in violence against the Chinese, their businesses, or the businesses of those who hired them. Figure 2.1 illustrates the perception, propagated by Kearney and his followers, of China and its emigrants as an overbearing tide of (sub)humanity usurping "American" businesses through shear force of numbers. Such representations, along with WPC agitations on popular and legislative fronts, fueled the passage of several ordinances barring Chinese from particular areas of employment. Chinese peddlers, for instance, were forbidden to sell their wares in the traditional way in baskets hanging from poles; a tax was levied in the 1870s on Chinese laundries; and by 1880 corporations were prohibited from hiring Chinese workers (Issel and Cherny 1986; Cather 1932; Takaki 1989). These ordinances were repeatedly ruled unconstitutional in court, but

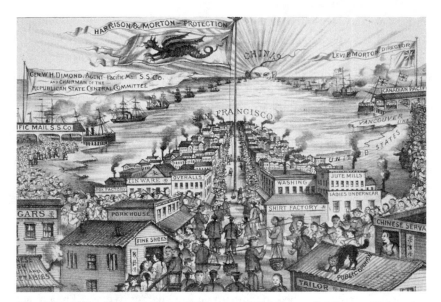

Figure 2.1. The Chinese threat. Courtesy of The Bancroft Library, University of California, Berkeley.

this did not stop the city legislature from persisting in their endeavors to undermine Chinese labor and business.

Yet the dismal economic situation affecting San Francisco did not fully explain the other significant but less-well-documented forms the anti-Chinese movement took. It was not only part of a broader-based movement within the city but part of a national movement ideologically reconstituting American cities as racially pure. Repercussions of this movement on Chinese communities is well summarized by Ronald Takaki's assertion that "historically, whites generally perceived America as a racially homogeneous society and Americans as white. Long before the Chinese arrived, they had already been predetermined for exclusion by this set of ideas" (Takaki 1989, 100). The Chinese were not "white," nor did they attempt assimilation into the dominant culture the way many other immigrant groups did. Continued difference in everything from appearance to language marked them as perpetual outsiders in a city and a country trying to meld a more singular paradigm of what an American should be. As Robert Burchell notes in his history of the Irish in San Francisco, "Politics and the economy, not to mention the language of officialdom and the level of civic aspiration, were all guided by Anglo-American norms.... [San Francisco was not] a society which had somehow managed to overcome the prevalent beliefs in racial superiority and inferiority and had admitted the Chinese to an equality with the whites" (Burchell 1980, 180).

Exclusionary mining policies in the 1850s attest to the presence of xeno-phobic sentiment ever since the arrival of Chinese in California (Cather 1932; Dicker 1979). It took severe strains on society, though, to force a "dejection of the moral force," and those strains came not just from the episodic depressions of the 1870s. The persistent threat of infectious diseases and realization of smallpox epidemics in the latter half of the century created a constant strain on San Francisco society. And though the temporal parallels between the economic and medical facets of the anti-Chinese movement point to an inter-relationship between the two, they also remained to a certain degree distinct in the causes they served and the effects they created.

First, the interpretation of smallpox as a predominantly Chinese disease did more lasting damage to the Chinese community than did the focus on labor practices. Whereas an improved economy and increasing jobs eventually eased the hostilities of the working class toward the Chinese, the stigmas of disease-breeding ascribed to Chinatown were harder to erase. The targeting of Chinese as the source of smallpox, in effect, was a more powerful political tool than accusations of job stealing. Second, it was a psychological tool. In the absence of medical elucidation, scapegoating remained not only a viable component of the framing of smallpox but a necessary strategy for placing boundaries around social disruption and fear (Gilman 1985). As these mounted with each subsequent episode of smallpox, perceptions that the Chinese were responsible grew more vehement.

The Intensification of a Racialized Spatialization

The most compelling difference among accounts of the four smallpox epidemics in San Francisco is the almost total lack of anti-Chinese rhetoric in descriptions of the 1868 incident. The city's health officer, for instance, made no attempt in his lengthy report to ascribe the source of the disease to the Chinese or to impute any special disease-breeding atmosphere to Chinatown. Even in laying partial blame for the wave of disease on the general sanitary condition of the city, he did not single out Chinatown as any more culpable than the rest of San Francisco (Municipal Reports 1868–69). Arguing for a better smallpox hospital, another physician pointed out that San Francisco was in a position to be invaded by the disease from Asia *or* from other countries, thereby acknowledging that smallpox could in fact arrive the long way from Europe (*California Medical Gazette*, August 1868, 39). An editorial on the epidemic written by a physician in one of the leading medical journals suggested that foreigners, "whether European or Asiatic," were generally better vaccinated than the native stock of lesser means (Morse 1869, 131). Although he does not give reasons for his assertion, it is nonetheless salient for its conviction that the Chinese were less responsible than others for the spread of smallpox.

One of the few times Chinatown is mentioned specifically regarding the 1868 epidemic was in an official resolution of the San Francisco Board of Health authorizing the health officer to have a medical inspector appointed for one month to "inspect those portions of the city inhabited by Chinese" (*California Medical Gazette,* July 1868, 16). Given the lack of anti-Chinese rhetoric in the rest of the epidemic accounts, a reasonable explanation for an extra inspector lay in the absence of any medical personnel in Chinatown during years between epidemics. For those Chinese falling victim to smallpox, as with non-Chinese, a medical inspector had to be available to authorize removal to the smallpox hospital or to determine the proper cause of death. The appointment of such an inspector, then, could simply signify the realization that official medical assistance was required for an area usually left to its own medical resources.

The more equitable attitude toward the Chinese changed rapidly within the next few years. By 1870, only one year after the end of the epidemic, the new health officer railed that the Chinese were a "moral leper in our community, . . . their habits and manner of life of such a character as to breed and engender disease wherever they reside" (Municipal Reports 1869–70, 233). This statement was not made in connection with an epidemic outbreak, but the officer's rhetoric struck a theme that was to be repeated with increasing vigor throughout the rest of the century. The Chinese from now on were blamed as the source of most diseases affecting the city.

Thus by the time smallpox appeared again in 1876, the social and spatial constructions had changed from a disease of arguable origin to a disease closely associated with Chinatown. Given the large volume of immigrants arriving in San Francisco by rail from the East Coast and Europe, it is more likely that the second wave of smallpox was introduced to the city via this trajectory. Yet there was no mention of this possibility by the city health officer or any other authorities of San Francisco. Instead, the blame for the 1876 epidemic was placed unequivocally on the Chinese, in particular the Chinese arriving on the steamship *Colorado* on May 19, 1876. "As if adding to the population of Celestials were not enough," wrote a newspaper reporter of the event, "that dreaded scourge, the smallpox, had manifested itself among the poor coolies during the voyage" (*San Francisco Chronicle,* May 20, 1876, 3).

More clearly evident in the framing of smallpox than of tuberculosis is the association of disease with the production of dirt, and the production of dirt with behavioral deviance. The epistemological moorings of this theory will be discussed in the next section; its practical manifestations, however, are clearly evidenced by the 1870s in the reactions by physicians and public health officials to smallpox. The 1870 municipal health officer, C. M. Bates, illustrates this triumvirate of dirt, disease, and deviance in his claim that "unless their style of life is changed, it is very much to be feared that some disease of a malignant form will be put among them and communicate itself to our Caucasian population" (Municipal Reports 1870, 233). "Style of life" is left unexplained in this instance, but the larger context of growing anti-Chinese rhetoric made it less oblique. It was a reference not just to the production of dirt but to the larger problem of un-American practices, physical characteristics, and language. An entire lifestyle, not just specific hygienic practices, here held the etiologic key to disease production. To stand out as un-American was quickly being pathologized as deadly and, worse, as infectious.

As if in fulfillment of his predecessor's prophecy, the succeeding health officer, J. L. Meares, attempted during the 1876 epidemic to explain why smallpox took hold so suddenly in San Francisco by blaming it on "the presence in our midst of 30,000 (as a class) of unscrupulous, lying and treacherous Chinamen, who have disregarded our sanitary laws" (Municipal Reports 1876–77, 397). The implication again in this statement is not just that lack of hygiene was dangerous but that lack of morals in this particular "class" accelerated the onset of disease and served as its effective conduit. The bias in Meares's view was so deeply entrenched as to be undeterred by mortality figures. When only sixty out of over sixteen hundred cases of smallpox during the 1876 epidemic were Chinese, he explained the discrepancy by claiming that over three hundred cases had been concealed within the labyrinthine spaces of Chinatown.

The conclusions were the same for the next two smallpox epidemics to visit San Francisco. On January 19, 1880, the *City of Peking* sailed into San Francisco's harbor flying the yellow flag because one of its Chinese steerage passengers had come down with smallpox on the way from Hong Kong and Yokohama. The ship was quarantined; the cabin passengers were kept on board for several days; and the Chinese passengers were transferred to the hull of an empty ship anchored in the harbor. Even if infection did begin with a Chinese passenger, one medical journal admitted that the captain had been allowed ashore during the quarantine period and that in fact "whilst at the wharf, there was a pretty free intercourse between the ship [where the white passengers were kept] and the shore" (*Western Lancet* 9, no. 1, 1880, 33). In other words, it was far more likely that this intermingling of potentially infected white passengers with wives and relatives on shore was the factor responsible for spreading the disease. Yet the epidemiological association of smallpox with Asian practices rendered impossible the idea of white infectivity. Meanwhile, the Chinese passengers, transformed into infectious agents dangerous to the urban populace, were left to suffer their disease imprisoned in the hull of a ship with no medical assistance.

Similarly, the 1887 epidemic was blamed on the *City of Sydney,* a ship that sailed to San Francisco from Hong Kong on May 3, 1887, purportedly carrying an infected Chinese passenger. While it was more likely that smallpox spread westward in an advancing wave of epidemic begun on the East Coast, this possibility was never considered by city authorities. Indeed the very potential for smallpox to arrive in San Francisco via other points in the United States seemed suddenly forgotten or discounted by the time of these later epidemics. Even though news of the 1885 epidemic hitting the rest of the United States and Canada must certainly have come to San Francisco, city authorities and others looked only westward to the shores of Asia for sources of infection.[8] Or, as Health Officer Meares's statement affirms, they looked inward to the heart of Chinatown. Indeed, Chinatown was considered an extension of the Asian "threat" into the boundaries of the city, and these shifting perspectives on smallpox were inextricably entwined with increasingly negative perceptions of this city within a city.

The Mapping of Myth

Henri Lefebvre asserts that "the dominant form of space, that of the centres of wealth and power, endeavors to mould the spaces it dominates (i.e., peripheral spaces) and it seeks, often by violent means, to reduce the obstacles and resistance it encounters there" (Lefebvre 1991, 49). Besides the violent tool of medical discourse, visual representations of Chinatown and its spatial organization were two more discursive tactics in the attempt to dominate the space of Chinatown and to reduce the resistance encountered there or encountered from individuals outside its boundaries. Descriptions of Chinatown circulating during this period combined reality and fiction, since spatial characteristics were sometimes exaggerated and invariably infused with ominous social meaning. Since few non-Chinese ever entered the boundaries of Chinatown beyond perhaps the restaurants on the main street, a certain degree of mythologization of the place could generally go undisputed by the white population. For these outsiders, the picture was of narrow and labyrinthine streets, with buildings so close together as to preclude the entrance of sunlight. Filth abounded; the stench was unbearable; and crammed into every basement, building, stairwell, and street were the huddling and disease-ridden bodies of Chinese.

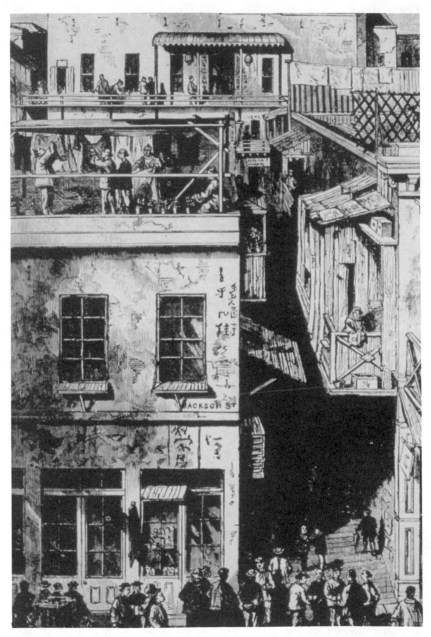

Figure 2.2. Artist's rendition of Chinatown, late nineteenth century. Courtesy of The Bancroft Library, University of California, Berkeley.

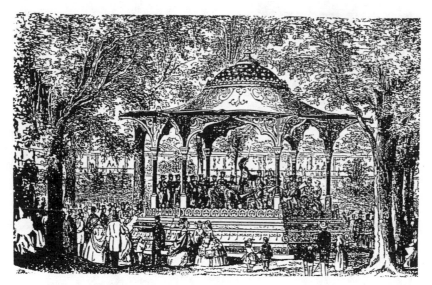

Figure 2.3. Park gazebo, San Francisco, late nineteenth century. From Olmstead et al., 1979.

In figures 2.2 and 2.3, this contrast between Chinatown and "white" San Francisco is represented. The image of Chinatown from 1873 shows more darkness than light; the buildings are so close together that balconies protruding from their sides are almost touching; and people are seen in almost every nook and corner of not only the sidewalk in front of the buildings but the alleyways, the balconies, and even the tops of the buildings. In addition to the crowding, there is dirt, neglect, and decrepitude evident in the way the buildings are shown: the front of the left building looks to be slowly flaking away while simultaneously being consumed by dirt and soot, while the balcony of the right building looks as if it could plunge to the ground below at any moment. The woman standing on this balcony also looks not just poor, but ill. A high proportion of Chinese women at this time were prostitutes, and given the corresponding agitation against them in connection with syphilis, this woman is possibly a personification of the sex-worker bringing death to her next unwitting customer.

In contrast is the wooded park and gazebo of the second picture. As a band plays from the stand, middle- and upper-class families are seen leisurely strolling in the light and airy (read: healthy) spaces of the park. The women are well dressed; the children are happy; and the men from their appearance are financially successful: everyone appears in the bloom of health, an im-

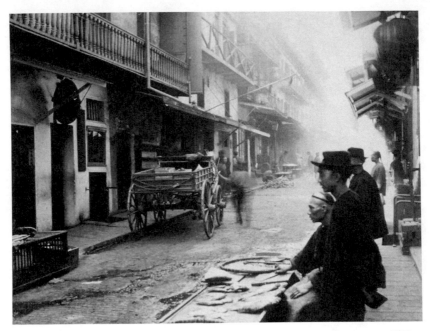

Figure 2.4. A street in Chinatown, late nineteenth century. Courtesy of The Bancroft Library, University of California, Berkeley.

plicit result of the middle-class "American" values to which they adhere. The park itself is an example of nineteenth-century innovations in city planning that consciously capitalized upon the equation of well-lit and open spaces with health and moral rectitude (Choay 1969; Ward 1989). Such innovations were in increasingly stark contrast to the intense crowding of poorer neighborhoods, and particularly of Chinatown.

Impressions of Chinatown were not left to the visual, however. Again and again descriptions of the spatial organization of Chinatown were verbally propagated, by physicians such as the health officer and later by others who took up the ideological tool of disease in the anti-Chinese campaign. In all of these descriptions, the numerous abrogations of social mores attributed to the Chinese are reflected in their degenerate use of space. In fact, it was above all in their use of space that the Chinese confirmed their subhumanness. In the Municipal Report of 1869–70, for instance, Health Officer Bates described Chinatown as a place where

> the great majority of them live crowded together in ricketty, filthy and dilapidated tenement houses like so many cattle or hogs.... In passing through that portion of the city occupied by them, the

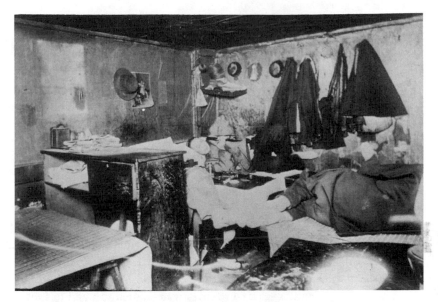

Figure 2.5. Accommodations in Chinatown, late nineteenth century. Courtesy of The Bancroft Library, University of California, Berkeley.

> most absolute squalidness and misery meets one at every turn.... Apartments that would be deemed small for the accommodation of a single American, are occupied by six, eight, or ten Mongolians. Nothing short of an ocular demonstration can convey an idea of Chinese poverty and depravity. (Municipal Reports 1869–70, 233)

Parts of the reports on Chinatown were probably true, as can be seen in figures 2.4 and 2.5. Streets were indeed crowded; buildings were built close together and were filled beyond capacity with Chinese residents and businesses. Long hours and low wages meant that most men survived at subsistence level, saving rent by rooming with as many other men as possible and buying only minimal belongings and food. Only then could enough money be saved to return to China.[9] Poor building and plumbing quality and the lack of regular sanitation services also meant that sanitary conditions inevitably were, indeed, quite abysmal. Rarely mentioned in the discourse of spatial use was the discrimination the Chinese faced in housing, both in the conditions they endured within Chinatown because of neglectful landlords and in attempting to go beyond the boundaries of Chinatown for housing. On the one hand, the borders of Chinatown could not expand because, given its location in the heart of downtown, there was little space for such expansion and because business and municipal interests would not allow it. On the other hand, the Chinese were not able to get housing anywhere outside the borders of Chinatown because of widespread discrimination; landlords would not rent to them, and neighborhood residents did not want them (Issel and Cherny 1986, 73). Rising Chinese populations until the 1880s, then, meant an exponential increase in crowding in the twelve-block area.

Yet the conditions under which most Chinese lived were clearly not viewed through humanitarian eyes. Like the inhabitants of South of Market slums, the Chinese were considered to live the way they did by cultural and genetic dictate rather than economic necessity. Their poverty was disdained, not pitied; as illustrated in the last sentence of Health Officer Bates's description, it was considered interdependent with their depravity. But unlike other impoverished and crowded areas of San Francisco, in Chinatown poverty and its physical manifestations took on a particularly sinister brand of depravity. They became not merely an annoyance but a threat and a subject of fear as they became more pathologized.

By 1880, a three-member team that included the city's mayor, its health officer, and a physician was selected to investigate Chinatown and to subsequently make recommendations for needed sanitary and other public health measures. In their report, entitled "Chinatown Declared a Nuisance," the authors called Chinatown a "cancer spot" endangering the otherwise (in this instance) healthy condition of the city; its buildings, sanitation, and inhabitants were described with ghoulish flair; and in the report's conclusion, Chinatown was designated a "laboratory of infection — situated in the very heart of our city, distilling its deadly poison by day and by night, and sending it forth to contaminate the atmosphere of the streets and houses of a populous, wealthy and intelligent community." The Chinese are construed in the report as living in their despicable conditions out of purposeful disregard of sanitary laws and out of malicious intent toward the well-being of the city's inhabitants. The injection of actual malice into the practices of the Chinese thus provided further rationale for action against them. Not surprisingly, the report recommended that the entirety of Chinatown be declared a nuisance, with concluding advice that "the Chinese cancer ... be cut out of the heart of our city, root and branch, if we have any regard for its future sanitary welfare" (Committee to Investigate Chinatown 1880, 2, 5, 6). The ambiguity of this statement seems consciously to leave open whether the authors were suggesting Chinatown's complete removal from the heart of the city or whether they were merely recommending a thorough sanitary purge.

In addition to Chinatown's highly pathologized space, there were two further differences between Chinatown and the poorer white quarters of the city that explain the greater threat posed by the former. The first was that

Chinatown was located in the heart of downtown San Francisco. Whereas middle- and upper-class residents of the city could choose to avoid South of Market and other poor enclaves, it was much more inconvenient to circum-ambulate an area in the middle of the city. Conversely, it was impossible for those Chinese exiting Chinatown on their way to jobs not to come in contact with white residents.

The second difference was the numerical preponderance of the Chinese, a persistent cause of concern and a factor that added force to the rendering of Chinatown into a locus of contagion. Between 1860 and 1880, the Chinese population increased 780 percent, from under three thousand to almost thirty thousand (Olmstead et al. 1979, 182). Fear of numbers played a significant role in the difference of interpretations between the 1868 and 1876 smallpox epidemics — that is, that the first was not framed as a specifically Chinese-originated phenomenon while the latter was. After completing work on the transcontinental railroad in 1869 and attracted by job opportunities in manufacturing, thousands of Chinese moved to San Francisco from other points in California in the early 1870s. As Saxton notes, Chinese residents in San Francisco as a percentage of California's Chinese population jumped from 8 percent in 1860 to 26 percent by 1870, and just under 30 percent by the end of the 1870s (Saxton 1971, 4). Meares's mention of the thirty thousand Chinese in the midst of San Francisco attests to the significance of their aggrandized population in determining the framing of epidemic disease.[10]

Given the first difference, it is not surprising that images of Chinatown increasingly focused on this potential for infecting the rest of San Francisco with myriad pestilences and disease-inducing miasmas. As can be seen from an 1882 cartoon in the *Wasp* (figure 2.6), the Butchertown, wharf, and South of Market areas are vaguely depicted under the three ghosts of malaria, small-pox, and leprosy. Chinatown, by contrast, is depicted more as a partner to the diseases rather than as their victim (*Wasp*, May 26, 1882). The less sanitary and more crowded areas of the city, in other words, were more susceptible to disease, but it was Chinatown that bred and disseminated it; it was the scythe in the metaphoric hands of Death.[11]

With smallpox epidemics, Chinatown was the one large pustule of contagion on an otherwise healthy body, a pustule that would inevitably spread to the untainted areas of the city. As Meares stated during the 1881 epidemic,

> Poisoned with the contagion of smallpox, coming in daily contact with our citizens, as servants, as laundrymen, and as ordinary labor-ers; manufacturing (as I have seen) clothing, slippers, etc. in the very house and in the very room in which a Chinaman was dying in the advanced stage of this disease; in short, coming in contact with our

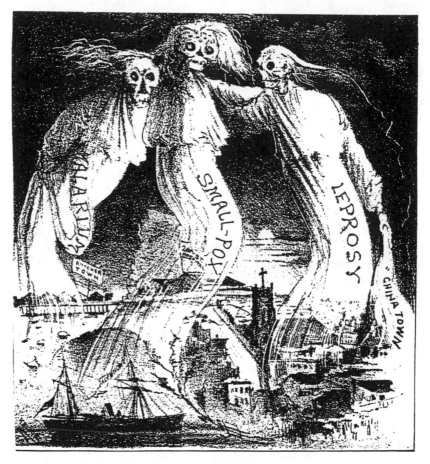

Figure 2.6. "Three Diseases over San Francisco," *The Wasp,* May 26, 1882. Courtesy of The Title Insurance and Trust Collection, California Historical Society.

people generally as no other class of our inhabitants do, they are a constant source of danger to the health and prosperity of the entire community. (Municipal Reports 1881, 253–54)

Evident in this statement is first an emphasis again on the indiscriminate use of space by the Chinese, this time objectionable because manufacturing activities were undertaken in the same room in which infectious disease was present. The implication, of course, is that smallpox germs were carried out on the surface of those manufactured items, to be sold to, and subsequently infect, healthy white Americans. Second, the daily trajectories of Chinese leaving Chinatown and going to jobs in factories and homes also posed a health problem to the general population, as these trajectories threatened to cause infection through the diseased bodies of Chinese to an unacceptable number of healthy white bodies.

An increasingly intrusive and hostile response was the result of these intensifying perceptions of contagion (Municipal Reports 1880). After the first smallpox epidemic, the previously mentioned Cubic Air Law was passed dictating at least five hundred cubic feet of air for each resident. The ordinance was almost exclusively aimed at decreasing the crowding within Chinatown, although it was eventually enforced with a fine and not with eviction and jail terms (Issel and Cherny 1986, 126). But by the second epidemic, such restraint by civic authorities on impingements of privacy had disappeared. Health Officer Meares ordered an extensive sanitary cleanup of Chinatown, hiring extra health inspectors and laborers to accomplish the task. For two months, this team invaded the community and the homes of the Chinese, fumigating and cleansing until "the whole of the Chinese quarter... [was] put in a sanitary condition that it had not enjoyed for ten years" (Municipal Reports 1877, 397).

Also during this second epidemic and for the next few years, Meares implored city authorities to build bigger prisons in order to enforce the Cubic Air Law "as the only possible means of correcting the sanitary evils of the Chinese quarter" (Municipal Reports 1880, 414). The same plea was made again during the 1880 epidemic. "It is to be feared, that only a repetition of virulent epidemics will awaken our people to the necessity of removing these constantly menacing causes of disease," he complained as city authorities continued to ignore his request for more prison space. This refusal almost certainly rested on financial and not philosophical grounds. While the board of supervisors agreed with Meares in his condemnation of Chinatown, their parsimony in funding municipal projects overruled their prejudice, as has already been established. Notwithstanding, it was the inability to carry out his plan that prompted Meares and the board of health to appoint a committee to investigate the sanitary conditions of Chinatown, this time having the backing of sound empirical "science" in declaring it a nuisance. Chinatown was given until March to clean itself up.

Here is evidence of a perception that the pathology of a district could be modified by a spatial and social reordering rendered through sanitary intervention. The behavioral deviance that fostered disease could be the key to prevention if it could be corrected. Conversely, as with the more limited rhetoric on slums, ameliorating the physical and structural environment could also induce behavioral reform. The degree of transformation necessary for satisfactory results was much greater among the Chinese than among the poor, but the assumption was that the same theory could be applied. For some, however, this approach was inadequate and flawed. The Chinese would not be reformed, because they were irretrievably foreign in their practices and physiognomies. Given the danger that Chinatown posed and would continue to pose, the only solution was to remove it entirely. The last level of extremity was reached with this constituency — that is, not just to purge Chinatown of its filth and disease but to purge Chinatown itself from the heart of San Francisco.

Although it was obviously never accomplished, calls for Chinatown's removal from the city came at several points during the last decades of the century, timed invariably with a terrorizing epidemic of smallpox or the threat of an epidemic of cholera or yellow fever. One member of the 1880 committee to investigate Chinatown, for example, went beyond the suggestions of his peers by stating that the Chinese were "unfit to have a dwelling place in the heart of a populous American city" and that "the city government should be empowered to assign them a location where their presence would be less obnoxious to the welfare and sanitary interests of the city" (Chipman 1880, 4).

During the last smallpox epidemic, a "People's Open Illustrated Letter" published in May 1886 confirmed that the desire to expel the Chinese on grounds of disease and sanitation had spread from the board of health to the general populace:

> As if the presence of these barbarians among us, depriving our workmen of employment, and causing our girls and boys to grow up in idleness,...was not a sufficient evil, they have been the cause of the pestilence which now "stalketh at noonday" through our streets, claiming as its victims our best and most enterprising citizens, and, entering our homes, lays low those who make home dear to us. Shall we stand supinely by and see Death triumphing over those we would so gladly save, and let this accursed race still hold their filthy and disease-breeding dens of infamy in the heart of our city?... Extraordinary cases of evil demand extraordinary means of prevention and removal of them.... Our citizens should organize and make these infamous wretches migrate outside of the city's limits. ("People's Open Illustrated Letter" 1886)

Much more than unemployment, it was disease that struck at the deepest fears of these residents, fears that had been primed by threats of yellow fever and cholera and by repeated visitations of smallpox. The temporary solution of cleaning up Chinatown was insufficient in their minds to expunge once and for all the existence of disease inside city borders and the threat of epidemics from without. Only expunging Chinatown itself would accomplish this. For these people, the synonymity of Chinatown and smallpox had become virtually complete. Getting rid of disease meant ridding the city of a racialized district and its inhabitants.

Dissenting Voices

The medical rhetoric focusing on Chinatown was widespread but not universally accepted. There were other physicians who contested the focus on Chinatown and questioned the board of health's actions taken against it and even the motives behind those actions. These dissenting voices seem to have been in the minority and did not evidently aggregate under a united oppositional banner, but they nevertheless made themselves heard through medical journals and, doubtless, other venues. The nature of dissent varied to a certain extent. One anonymous essay published in the *Medico-Literary Journal of San Francisco* in 1878 rebuffed the board of health for their disproportionate focus on Chinatown to the detriment of the rest of the city. This author did not disagree that Chinatown was a pesthole and a cancer spot that needed a thorough purging to make it less dangerous to the rest of the city. His quibble came over what he perceived as the highly political nature of the board of health's actions and the consequent neglect of their duties. "Certain politicians anxious to ride into power on the anti-Chinese hobby, have thought to strengthen their position by raising a great hue and cry over the sanitary condition of what is known as Chinatown, losing sight in their partisan zeal of the ten thousand other pest-holes that send up their mephitic effluvia to poison the air of the city" (*Medico-Literary Journal of San Francisco* 1, no. 2, October 1878, 19).

Contrary to affirming the metonymy of Chinatown and disease, this author admits the possibility that infectious diseases might have originated outside Chinatown. "Open sewers, sending forth their horrible stench, obstructed drains, defective privies and back-yards with years of accumulated garbage; all combine to keep alive if not to originate typhoid and scarlet fever, diphtheria and other scourges of the innocents" (*Medico-Literary Journal of San Francisco* 1, no. 2, October 1878, 19). Chinatown might be a blight on the city, but it did not stand alone. Neglecting the sanitary nuisances peppering the rest of the city only left the populace especially vulnerable to epidemic diseases. San Francisco *would* be a healthy city if the board of health could turn a blind eye to politics and instead do their jobs.

A stronger indictment of the board of health and their policies toward Chinatown came in another anonymous editorial published in 1880. Not surprisingly, the author addresses the recent appointment of the committee to investigate Chinatown and the results of their investigation. More surprising is his response. Like his colleague, the author finds in the actions of the public health constabulary a stronger regard for politics than medical evidence. The author begins by pointing out with thinly disguised disdain that the committee "thought" they had observed enough to justify their condemnation, even while never claiming to have thoroughly examined the whole district. "This hasty and wholesale denunciation of a section containing many hundreds of cleanly and respectable places does not look like the work of an honorable, distinguished body of officials... but rather like the party work of sandlot, Republican and Democratic politicians" (*Medico-Literary Journal of San Francisco* 2, no. 7, March 1880, 14). For this author, Chinatown is imagined not as a cancer spot plaguing the urban body but rather as a district like many others having its good qualities and its problem spots. To concentrate only on the latter was tantamount to unprofessional behavior and to the creation of an imagined space to supersede for purely political reasons a more varied and complex spatial reality.

A strong link between Chinatown and smallpox in the medical reports at the state level was also largely absent. This is interesting given that anti-Chinese rhetoric in general was present if not as pervasive as at the city level; it is also somewhat surprising given that San Francisco physicians often served stints on the state board of health. Nevertheless, Sacramento's distance from the locus of anti-Chinese agitation might explain why the discussion of smallpox in state board of health reports was further removed from political considerations and thus generally bereft of discursive ascriptions. In the 1882 report, the origins of the 1881 smallpox epidemic are discussed in more deductive epidemiological and geographical detail, focusing primarily on the role of the Central Pacific Railroad in bringing immigrants into California, some of whom were inevitably infected with the virus. "The great prevalence of smallpox in Chicago, and the constant communication with that city by rail, afford easy means for the conveyance of the specific poison to California" (California State Board of Health Reports 1882, 52). The board members claim, indeed, to have specific examples of infected individuals boarding trains in Chicago and proceeding to urban areas of California. Such evidence, it seems, escaped the notice of San Francisco public health officials.

Four years later, the secretary of the state board of health, Gerard Tyrrell, applied similar methods of epidemiological tracing in determining where the greatest threat from another smallpox epidemic lay. Concerned about the prevalence of smallpox in Canada, Tyrrell contacted members of state boards of health in the East to obtain information about the disease's progress. Having finished his inquiries, his deduction was that the greater threat came from

Japan, China, and Mexico rather than Canada, "as we found that the states bordering the Canadian frontier were strictly guarded by able and efficient quarantine officers.... [O]ur intercourse with Mexico being by rail as well as by sea, the liability of the conveyance of smallpox by immigrants is very great" (California State Board of Health 1886, 39). The focus on Chinese this time derives from the diminished capacity to monitor transborder transportation via ships, not from discursive strategies centered upon Chinese bodies, practices, and habitations.

Voices such as these physicians' are not abundant in the medical literature or popular media of the later nineteenth century, but it is nonetheless important to note that dissent did indeed exist even within the medical community. Not everyone sided politically or philosophically with the city board of health's attitude toward the Chinese and their way of life. Nor did they agree with the condemnation of Chinatown, or at least with the singling out of only one of many sanitary trouble spots in the city. Unfortunately, even the reports of the state board of health secretaries had negligible influence in matters of municipal policy; consequently, neither their more epidemiologically sound reports nor the more vehement protests of San Francisco physicians did much to contravene public health policy.

Comparative Perspectives

San Francisco's interpretation of smallpox was very much embedded in the broader social and political topography of the city. Had the Chinese been fewer in number, had their community been located on the outskirts of the city, or had racial politics not been in ascendancy at the time, public health officers undoubtedly would have framed the origins and epidemiology of the disease differently. So for other cities in North America or Europe, interpretations of smallpox in the nineteenth century differed from or paralleled San Francisco's according to their respective politics and social landscapes.

Anne Hardy's account of smallpox in London, for example, shows little evidence of a significant degree of scapegoating during the several smallpox epidemics that swept the city in the nineteenth century. This occurs in part because Hardy's agenda is to document why some epidemics were worse than others, which she does by focusing on public health responses, including vaccination campaigns. Notwithstanding, she does give evidence that the poor in London received a disproportionate degree of blame for disseminating smallpox through their habits and lifestyles. Descriptions of the poor and their epidemiological role in the epidemics indeed sometimes resemble the rhetoric used against the Chinese in San Francisco. As recorded by one London physician, the poor had been observed carrying on their everyday activities as if indifferent to the presence of the deadly disease, where "a small-pox patient lay in an adjoining room; and where dressmaking was going on in the same room"; where "a costermonger's barrow [was kept] under a bed upon which lay a small-pox patient"; or where a child was known to "go out to work in the day, and sleep at night with a sister suffering from small-pox" (cited in Hardy 1993, 135).

As with the rhetoric against the Chinese, the use of space is focused upon whereby out of ignorance or indifference the poor have endangered the rest of the city through their indiscriminate combination of sick space and economic space. Whether from an ill-advised use of space or whether from overcrowding, it was observed during London smallpox epidemics that the poorer districts did suffer disproportionately from the disease. Yet there is little sense in Hardy's account that the poor were targeted for extreme measures of intervention such as purgings of streets and razing of infested buildings or that there was any agitation for removing the poor to outly-ing areas of the city. One reason could be that the poor, despite the disdain held toward them, were nevertheless similar enough to the upper classes in physiognomy, language, and culture that actual scapegoating never became commonplace, even though "the minutiae of city-wide and cross-class in-fection through the medium of servants, laundries, dressmakers, and public contacts were repeatedly observed" (Hardy 1993, 136).

Milwaukee was another city hit by several smallpox outbreaks during the course of the nineteenth century and whose responses to each epidemic dif-fered considerably from San Francisco's. According to Judith Walzer Leavitt, the 1894 epidemic was particularly problematic in the tensions it engendered between immigrant districts and public health authorities. The tensions were of a different nature than San Francisco's, however. Polish and German immi-grants tended to be more resistant to vaccination, and in partial consequence their neighborhoods were hard hit during the epidemic. Friction crescen-doed when public health officials arrived in vans and attempted to take the infected away to the smallpox hospital (Leavitt 1985, 373–74). Despite higher disease rates prevailing in immigrant neighborhoods, there is again no evidence in Leavitt's account of scapegoating by public health officials or by other urban residents. One significant difference is that Polish and German immigrants had a degree of political and economic standing in Mil-waukee, as in many cities including San Francisco (Issel and Cherny 1983). Such standing obviated the kind of disdain or fear with which less success-ful, or more different, immigrants were frequently treated. Consequently, the armed blockade of Poles and Germans against health officers forced the latter to back down on more than one occasion. It did not incite extreme measures by the medical constabulary or antiethnic rhetoric by the rest of the community.

One city that did also pathologize its Chinese community to some extent was Vancouver. Interestingly, this process ran along similar lines as San Francisco's efforts to pathologize Chinatown, except in the case of Vancouver no particular infectious disease served as the catalyst. According to Kay Anderson, Californians advised Europeans in Vancouver about what to expect as significant numbers of Chinese began settling in Vancouver in the latter part of the nineteenth century. The parallels in descriptions of the two Chinatowns may derive in part from the influence of these Californians on how Vancouver saw its immigrant community. Equating Vancouver's Chinatown with disease and describing as contagious its dirt, culture, and values were effective ways to further isolate it and to mark it as undesirable within Vancouver's cognitive urban map. According to the city commissioner in the 1890s, Chinese settlement was an "ulcer lodged like a piece of wood in the tissues of the human body, which unless treated must cause disease in the places around it and ultimately to the whole body" (cited in Anderson 1992, 81).

Recalling Poovey, the metaphor of the social body served to visualize the city in a particular way, the aggregation of groups into spatial (bodily) components distancing the members of each group in the eyes of public health and municipal authorities (Poovey 1993). Introducing the metaphor of illness into that of the social body also, according to Waldby (1996), implies the necessity of reinscribing and reordering the diseased body part in order to mitigate the threat to the body as a whole. Acknowledging the common connection between the sociopolitical and the medical, Waldby suggests too that "if socio-political threat can be readily assimilated to infectious threat, so too can the spectre of literal infection, of infectious disease proper, be assimilated to socio-political threat" (Waldby 1996, 90–91). In the case of Vancouver's Chinatown, as in San Francisco's, the metaphor of the Chinese community as a disease helped galvanize sanitation campaigns to reinscribe the physical structures of the community as well as the cultural structures of the bodies inhabiting them. It also helped launch political campaigns to derail Chinese businesses such as laundries and to remove the community from the city (Anderson 1992, 81–89).

Sex, Shame, and Syphilis: Chinese Women

The framing of smallpox was not particularly gender-coded, but another disease ascribed disproportionately to Chinatown was. Syphilis was a disease not talked about as much as smallpox, but when it was, it was usually ascribed to

Chinese women. The framing of syphilis was necessarily different from that of smallpox because it was not a disease easily transmitted, nor was it ever epidemic. It was slower to manifest in the body, and though the symptoms in an untreated individual could become severe, they were not as physically transformative. But syphilis carried with it a larger degree of moral opprobrium. It was known to be transmitted sexually, and its social construction reflected this. Like most cities, San Francisco maintained a tension between its ability to support a flourishing sex trade and a deep-rooted moral condemnation of prostitution. Syphilis was both the symbolic representation and somatic manifestation of morally transgressive behavior, and the rhetoric surrounding it was proportionately vitriolic.

Syphilis was especially prevalent in a port city whose population inside and outside Chinatown was overwhelmingly male for most of the nineteenth century. In 1880, secondary syphilis was topped only by tuberculosis in number of admissions to the City and County Hospital (Municipal Reports 1881, 351). In the early years of the twentieth century, it was estimated that 10 percent of the population had syphilis, and 50 percent of men had gonorrhea (Commonwealth Club 1911, 2). Even if the incidence of disease was widespread, though, its origins were limited to a small area of the city.

San Francisco's zone of prostitution in the latter part of the nineteenth century was located in the heart of the city, bounded by Montgomery, Stockton, Broadway, and Market Streets (see map 2.1). As the map depicts, Chinatown constituted a relatively large proportion of this zone and contained one of the densest concentrations of brothels in the city (Shumsky and Springer 1981, 75). The reasons for this were several. First, Chinatown itself had an even higher imbalance between its male and female populations, registering over twenty-one males for every female in 1880 (U.S. Census 1960). The sexual needs of this primarily male population were quickly realized and capitalized upon by the Chinatown secret societies (U.S. Census 1960, 76). Chinese prostitutes were also patronized by white men, however, and this constituted the second reason for a higher number of Chinese brothels. It is possible that Chinatown's denigration enabled, ironically, a feeling of invisibility on the part of white men utilizing Chinese brothels since such denigration resulted in increased surveillance on some levels (e.g., sanitation) but conscious neglect in others. The contradictory appeal of the reviled "Other" might also have played a role (Stallybrass and White 1986), but a more certain answer lies in economics. Chinese prostitutes tended to be cheaper, sometimes charging half what a white prostitute outside Chinatown demanded for the same services (Shumsky and Springer 1981).

The existence of a flourishing sex trade within the boundaries of China-

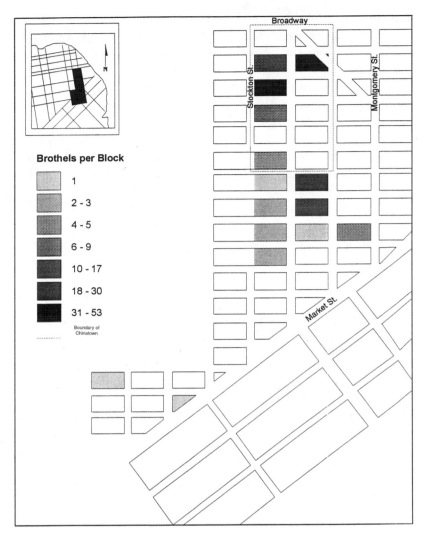

Map 2.1. Brothels in San Francisco, 1899. Based on Shumsky and Springer 1981; created by Mark Patterson.

town was thus not an invention of the board of health. In question is the degree to which they and other physicians held Chinese prostitutes responsible for the spread of syphilis. Like smallpox, it seems evident that syphilis held political importance disproportionate to its physical impact. Morbidity was significant, but mortality was negligible. In 1888, for example, a total of twenty-four people died from syphilis, accounting for only .4 percent of deaths in the city for that year. Many diseases—for example, typhoid fever, encephalitis, cancer, tuberculosis, and heart disease — each accounted for far more deaths, tuberculosis alone constituting 15 percent of the total (Municipal Reports 1888, 482). Nevertheless, syphilis played a strategic role in the anti-Chinese campaign. Smallpox inevitably affected more male Chinese than female given the population ratio within Chinatown. Its transformation into a Chinese disease, then, implicitly if not explicitly targeted the Chinese male. Syphilis was the female counterpart to smallpox, the disease that could be framed as a specifically female Chinese disease. The whole of Chinatown's population was thereby encompassed within a political vise enabled by medical discourse.

In the 1880 report written by the Committee to Investigate Chinatown, significant attention was brought to the problem of Chinese prostitution as further evidence of the vile character of Chinatown and its danger to the city. Representations of the trade, the individuals, and the disease they purportedly carried were bound up closely with representations of the infrastructure of Chinatown itself. Once again the use of space was an integral component of discursive medical tactics against the Chinese. Reports of sexual practices would have less emotional impact if descriptions were not embedded within the dank, dark, and ominous spaces of Chinatown. After elaborating on the baseness of Chinese lodging houses, then, the committee switched to the subject of Chinese courtesans by locating them in alleys described as "dark and narrow" and exhibiting "intolerable nastiness" (Committee to Investigate Chinatown 1880, 4). Though not explicitly stated, it was inferred that these courtesans plied their trade in the same type of rooms where every other sort of activity was discovered, from lace-washing to tripe-cleaning. These rooms invariably were not only small and cramped but remarkable for their odor and for walls "thick with dirt, slime, and sickening filth" (Committee to Investigate Chinatown 1880). The descriptions of stench, decay, and "oozing slime" virtually paralleled descriptions of late-stage syphilis. Place was again made metonymous with disease.

A second important component of the syphilis discourse centered around the bodies of the prostitutes themselves. A common framing of sexually transmitted diseases is the construction of affected women not as victims of disease but as propagators of it (Brandt 1987; Gilman 1988; Treichler 1992b). Danger in the infected female is thus "exogamous, the carrying of infection across specified borders" from female to low-risk male (Waldby 1996, 103). Whether in fifteenth-century Europe or in twentieth-century America, the image of the prostitute has been a potent one for symbolizing the pathological dangers of sexual transgression (Gilman 1988; Brandt

1987). Sexually transmitted diseases from syphilis to AIDS never seem to fell prostitutes; they instead become weapons of mass destruction against a collective male constituency made vulnerable by sexual need. In nineteenth-century San Francisco, however, the white prostitute largely was left out of this symbolic construction. Though white sex-workers were plentiful, it was the Chinese prostitute whose body was deadly. Citing Dr. H. H. Toland, the founder of Toland medical school in San Francisco and a member of the board of health, the committee claims that "in answer to the question to what extent these diseases [syphilis, sexually transmitted diseases] come from Chinese prostitutes, he says: 'I suppose nine-tenths'" (Committee to Investigate Chinatown 1880, 5).

The uncertainty implied by the word "suppose" is ignored by the committee, as is the highly unscientific basis of substantiation contained in the next sentence: "When these persons [syphilitics] come to me, I ask them where they got the disease, and they generally tell me from China women." Toland goes on to build his — and thus the committee's — case against the Chinese prostitute by recounting the number of syphilitics he has seen in his capacity as physician. He first strengthens the damning potential of this statement by focusing on the young age of many of the victims, some of the worst cases of which "occurred in children not more than 10 or 12 years old." Only a Chinese prostitute, its seems, would be immoral enough to seduce customers this young. He next focuses on the disease itself, bemoaning its potential to destroy life and to confront the infected male with a choice of a long course of treatment and the possibility of incomplete recovery. Allowing Chinese women to remain would only result in filling the hospitals with invalids. As such, according to Toland, "it would be a great relief to the younger portion of our community to get rid of them" (Committee to Investigate Chinatown 1880, 5). Further evidencing a political rationale to the committee's case is their neglect of an earlier report of physicians and board of health members constituted as a committee to investigate the presence of "social evil" in Chinatown. This committee, surprisingly, found "infrequent evidences of syphilitic disease" in either men or women (California State Board of Health Reports 1870, 46).

The 1880 committee was not the only locus of discontent against Chinese prostitutes, however. Other physicians also joined in the diatribe. One 1878 medical journal editorial entitled "How Chinese Women Are Infusing a Poison into the Anglo-Saxon Blood" extended the scale of the problem from one threatening San Francisco to one threatening the continuation of a white-dominated nation. The article began by questioning "the influence of the Chinese courtezans [sic] on the future of the American nation" and went on to claim that "if the future historian should ever be called upon to write the Conquest of America by the Chinese Government his opening chapter will be an account of the first batch of Chinese courtezans and the stream of deadly disease that followed." For this author, syphilis was a disease more destructive than any other, even smallpox, because it did not stop at one victim. Instead, it extended its symptoms over several succeeding generations, cursing a whole family line with disease and disability. For this author, syphilis was the "prime cause of human deterioration" (*Medico-Literary Journal of San Francisco* 1, no. 3, November 1878, 1, 8).

It was because of the nature of her disease that the Chinese prostitute held the capacity to derail an entire nation in practicing her profession. Where these prostitutes plied their trade is again significant, though, as the author brings his critique to bear on the location of Chinatown "in the very heart of San Francisco," a place where buildings had already been condemned by the board of health and whose stench continued to pervade the city. Much worse than the lepers hidden in Chinese basements were the "hundreds of Chinese women saturated with a far more loathsome disease" who were allowed "to spread the virus far and wide." To substantiate this latter claim, the author suddenly ascribes syphilis to half of the Chinese domestic servants in the city. The disease in this narrative has burst forth from the containing boundaries of Chinatown and invaded the homes of decent middle-class whites. Throwing aside the known etiology of the disease, the author further warns that allowing these servants to cook, launder, or raise children would result in syphilis breaking out of the containment of the Chinese body and into the spaces of the house itself, and its white inhabitants (*Medico-Literary Journal of San Francisco* 1, no. 3, November 1878, 4, 5).

In evidence again is Foucault's concept of political anatomy, whereby the body of the Chinese prostitute was the focus of fabrication and pathologization,[12] both of which in turn provided a rationale for increased control. As critics of Foucault's undifferentiated body have noted (Bordo 1993; Grosz 1994), however, the particular gendering and racialization of a body at times play a crucial role in determining whether and in what ways it is pathologized. Chinese men also may have suffered from syphilis, but their bodies were not inscribed with or by this disease to any significant extent, just as white men's and women's were not. As David Armstrong discusses, though, the medical gaze by the end of the nineteenth century had shifted to see disease not just in the space of the body but in the spaces in between them, that is, in the relations between bodies (Armstrong 1983). In this instance, syphilis was seen not so much in the relations between men and the prostitutes they encountered but in the spaces in between and surrounding Chinese women. It was seen as an extension of where and how they lived, in the rooms, lodgings, and alleys in which they practiced their trade, in the filth and odor evident around them. Body boundaries in this representation were almost porous with their surroundings; they contained a disease whose provenance was found equally within the body as within the spatial labyrinth of Chinatown.

Elizabeth Grosz states that "the ways in which space is perceived and represented depend on the kinds of objects positioned 'within' it" (Grosz 1995, 92). As with smallpox, the influence of the Chinese prostitute and syphilis on the ways in which Chinatown was perceived is significant; equally evident is the converse, however — that Chinese prostitutes were represented in a particularly negative light in part because they were Chinese and irretrievably Other, but in part because they occupied Chinatown, a place already pathologized.

One outcome informed in large measure by the discursive construction of syphilis was the immigration restriction in place by 1882 that, among other things, barred the entry of Chinese women of the laboring classes even if they were married to a Chinese laborer (Yung 1995). The rationale behind this ruling lay in the assumption that most if not all lower-class Chinese women migrating to California did so in order to engage in prostitution (Issel and Cherny 1986). Those prostitutes resident in San Francisco before this ruling nevertheless remained relatively unrestrained in their practices by outside authorities.[13] San Francisco, then, continued to maintain its dialectical relationship with sex. It demonstrated a need for the services of the Chinese prostitute, while at the same time it condemned her through a pathologization of her body, her trade, and its location.

Sanitation Narratives: The Coding of Cleanliness

To understand more clearly the anti-Chinese rhetoric and the associations of immorality, dirt, and disease, it helps to place these phenomena within the broader context of the sanitation movement. Taking shape in the 1860s and 1870s, the sanitation movement in San Francisco, as elsewhere, was the response of an increasingly concerned medical and professional constituency to the threats of epidemic diseases. More specifically, smallpox brought to an end upper-class complacency born of relative immunity to the increasing diseases of poverty such as tuberculosis, typhoid, and nutritional deficiencies. The epidemic of 1868 showed with terrifying clarity that no matter who disseminated smallpox, it spared no one its ravages and attacked the wealthy as much as the poor. Even at this time smallpox was generally considered contagious rather than the result of miasmas, yet it nonetheless galvanized concern over the sanitary status of the city.[14] As long as the city proper retained its faulty sewers and filthy streets, there was an implicit perception that it would remain susceptible to the emanation of smallpox from Chinatown. It would also remain vulnerable to possible incursions of yellow fever and cholera.

The focus on dirt and filth evidenced lighter and darker sides to the sanitation movement. Dirt, as seen in the previous chapter, was at this time a class-coded concept, produced by the poor and stigmatized by moral taint. And because dirt was both the by-product and the signifier of depravity, disease by association became increasingly overlaid with the same moral constructs (Nelkin and Gilman 1991; Fee and Fox 1988; Brandt 1991). The focus on dirt and disease thus became, through the interpolating channels of this ideology, attempts to reform social behavior and reorder personal and social spaces of the urban body as a whole, but particularly of the poor. Or as Peter Stallybrass and Allon White explain it, the upper classes began producing "new forms of regulation and prohibition governing their own bodies" and their own urban enclaves (Stallybrass and White 1986, 126). In the process, poor sectors became more disdained and, more importantly, more dangerous since epidemic disease had clearly shown that dirt had deadly repercussions across social and spatial boundaries.

Sewers: Cleaning the Underbelly of the Urban Body

Straightforward attempts at urban cleanup represented the more grounded and beneficial aspect of the sanitation movement, at least to the degree that these attempts were successful. Public memory was rather short, and the flurry of calls for sanitation frequently sputtered to a halt soon after the cessation of an epidemic. San Francisco's attempts at urban cleanup held such a pattern. Smallpox episodes and threats of cholera or yellow fever inevitably brought renewed demands for sanitary reform, but success was just as inevitably limited.

Bacteriology and germ theory made their way into mainstream medical theory slowly and in stages during the latter part of the nineteenth century.[15] Nor did these concepts upon acceptance necessarily supersede the miasmatic theory. An amalgamation of the two often was employed, whereby germs were imagined as the harmful component of noxious air. As one physician stated, "the most reasonable supposition seems to be, that the presence of decaying organic matter, or the gaseous emanations from putrefying dunghills, preserves, or may even revive the expiring vitality of germs brought by men, dogs, vermin, or perhaps the wind" (*California Medical Gazette*, November 1868, 110). The primary difference was that, in addition to causing disease by dissemination through the air, these "germ particles" could attach themselves to almost anything—clothing, hair, animals, or sidewalks (Stout 1868). The possibilities for infection were virtually limitless.

In addition to beliefs about the disease properties of malodorous air, most physicians and public health authorities by the later nineteenth century knew something about the connection between water and disease. This relationship was founded on observations that certain diseases seemed traceable not to germs wafting through the air but to water sources. The influence of the miasmatic theory on notions of water-born disease can be seen in a statement by two physicians writing in San Francisco in 1872 that water "polluted by fecal matter, [or] vegetable organic matter when derived from marshes, is injurious." Regardless of the details of this theory, the two physicians were accurate in their assessment of typhoid fever, cholera, and dysentery as being "caused by water contaminated by the evacuations passed in those diseases" (*Western Lancet,* January 4, 238).

The place that combined most perfectly these two main principles of nineteenth-century epidemiology was, of course, the sewer. Not only was the sewer the conduit for foul and contaminated water, but in the slow process of carrying this mephitic element away from the city, harmful gases were produced. Water and air of the vilest and most harmful sort found together in one topographical feature spelled out near obsession with the sewer for the nineteenth-century public health official.[16] As John Duffy discusses in his history of public health in the United States, sewers in East Coast cities were particularly problematic, having been built at a time when engineering was less advanced and cities were much smaller. Uncontrolled growth in the mid–nineteenth century quickly overwhelmed them, yet expense and logistics precluded their replacement in many cities (Duffy 1990).

San Francisco's sewers were newer than most, but similar problems were encountered when the city's population continued to explode through the later decades of the century. Beginning in the late 1860s, public health officials complained continually about the poor state of the sewers, their inefficiencies, and their dire inadequacy. Health Officer Bates in his 1870 report to the board of supervisors, for instance, bemoaned that

> there is a radical defect in our system of sewerage.... We have not only a bad system of sewerage in grade and size, but there is a deficiency in the amount necessary for the proper drainage of the city.... The grades of the streets being insufficient to afford proper drainage, there exists a very deleterious custom of permitting the debris and filth which accumulates in the sewers, to be taken out and placed in the open air, where it remains for hours, and sometimes for days. (Municipal Reports 1870, 231)

The result of this practice, according to Bates, was the production of "foul" and "poisonous" odors that, if not for the strong winds prevailing in the city, would cause yellow fever and cholera.

Even more ominous was an article written at the height of the 1868 small-pox epidemic by one of San Francisco's premier physicians, Arthur Stout, who stated more bluntly that wind or no wind, the sewers of San Francisco carried "many a strong man, many a fair woman, in the bloom of health, and still a larger proportion of young children, to a premature grave" (Stout 1868, 85). In addition to causing cholera and yellow fever, sewers were also the "most fertile sources" of smallpox, malaria, and epidemic fevers. But Stout faulted less the design of the sewers themselves than the way they were managed, confirming Bates's claim that when sewers clogged, the debris was shoveled out by one set of workers and left to rot for days on the streets. Stout adds cynically, however, that after being left for some time, the debris was then shoveled up by other workers into carts, thus "giving it a thorough ventilation, as though to sanify it, and again whirling its noxious effluvia into the air, and the noses of the faithful tax-payers, who pay so dearly and yet so cheerfully for the epicurean privilege" (Stout 1868, 85). What San Francisco needed to do, according to Stout, was to learn from London and Paris, cities that had taken the time and expense to build better sewers and to create more effective systems of managing them. Before they had accomplished this, these cities had been plagued by much higher rates of disease. Indeed London in particular was held by many in public health to be the sentinel in sanitary science because of the state of its sewers and the salutary urban order this denoted.[17]

San Francisco did not bring itself up to London's standards, however, because almost ten years later during the smallpox and diphtheria epidemics of 1876–77, Health Officer Meares was still complaining about the city's seriously defective sewers and their role in the spread of disease. With the exception of Chinatown, the problems were the worst in the South of Market area, but they were not limited to this district. Over a larger area of the city, defective sewers and house drains formed "an irrigating system which has already made a disease-breeding swamp of a considerable portion of the city, which is extending itself and becoming more and more polluted every year by the leakage from these pent-up sewers and wooden drains" (Municipal Reports 1877, 392). The problem was worse in localized areas, but the entire city was placed at risk because gases, after all, did not stick to delimited boundaries. As Health Officer Meares stated in 1876, "The diseases emanating from filth and pent-up sewerage are not confined to the districts in which these noxious and mephitic gases are generated, but these gases, being lighter than atmospheric air, ascend and penetrate dwellings far remote" (Municipal Reports 1876, 391). In other words, they migrated from lower-class to upper-class districts of the city.

To Meares's credit, he did make herculean efforts to improve San Francisco's sewers. Keeping abreast of the latest in sanitary engineering, he recommended the new perforated manhole covers to prevent harmful gases from being directed into homes or onto the streets (Municipal Reports 1877, 389). Several years previous to this, he had contracted with the city surveyor to draw a plan for replacing the city's outdated wooden sewers with the new and better designed metal pipes (Municipal Reports 1873, 596). These plans were not implemented for some time, a fact that distressed Meares each time a new epidemic hit the city. To him, inadequate sewers were the primary reason the city remained susceptible to Chinatown's diseases. Districts outside Chinatown, he acknowledged, produced their own quotient of "mephitic" gases that left them vulnerable.[18]

Sewer as Signifier

Turning back to the moral implications of the sanitation movement, sewers also in more symbolic ways straddled the tenuous boundaries between science and social reform. Stallybrass and White, in their highly provocative dissection of nineteenth-century mores, point out that the sewer became both the real and symbolic reminder to the upper classes that they could not completely disassociate themselves from the poor and their filth. The sewers transected and thus linked each section of a city whose topographical distinction by this point was a relative degree of class segregation. The upper classes had fastidiously removed themselves during the course of the century from what Stallybrass and White term the "metonymic chain of contagion which led back to the culture of the working classes" (Stallybrass and White 1986, 138). Upper-class residences, office buildings, theaters, and clubs became architectural enclaves of health within an increasingly dangerous city, enclaves whose cleanliness and respectability lay in stark opposition to the factories and slums and their ominous effluences.

But the sewer and the streets were those topographical features that precluded a complete separation, which insisted unyieldingly upon transgressing the boundaries of the more fortunate. Before the increase of epidemic diseases, this transgression was less a threat than an irritating reminder that the poor, by way of sewers, could still impart their ordure to the noses of the upper classes. But in the midst of epidemics, sewers suddenly became deadly conduits by which a marginal neighborhood's miasmas could be carried quite literally to the doors of the wealthy. The sewers, in essence, were symbolic of the " 'unutterable horrors of the city,' where there were no 'architectural barriers or protections of decency and propriety'" (Stallybrass and White 1986, 126). Even if the respectable classes via sanitary science could succeed in imposing order and cleanliness on themselves, the body of the city proved more difficult to purge (Stallybrass and White 1986, 125–48).

The most significant metonym in Stallybrass and White's analysis is that of the "Other" to signify the working classes. As reaffirmed in Anderson's theoretical genealogy of Chinatowns, the "Other" is a term symbolic of the emotional and cognitive space placed between mainstream sectors as the definitive embodiment of civilization and those perceived as distinctly antithetical to such a norm. Explicit in Stallybrass and White's argument is that sanitation helped expand that cognitive space, creating the "boundaries between high and low" that separated cleanliness from dirt. Perhaps more important, however, was how sanitary science rigidified those boundaries when epidemic diseases struck, turning the "Other" from an object of repulsion to a mortal enemy of the civic body. Abstract boundaries then became real through sanitary demarcation of poor neighborhoods and the attempts to screen upper-class districts from lower-class contagions. In their undifferentiated "Other" of nineteenth-century London, though, Stallybrass and White provide no comparative perspective to illuminate the proportional relationship between repulsion and degree of "Otherness." Nor is it their agenda to examine the role of disease in shaping this relationship.

For nineteenth-century San Francisco, the "Other" was bifurcated into the poor and the Chinese. The poor represent more directly the "Other" discussed by Stallybrass and White. The sewers and streets were indeed direct connections between upper-class enclaves and the slums of North Beach and South of Market, yet they were the only linkages to parts otherwise marginally located and easily avoided. And the poor themselves, though repugnant in their filth and "vicious immorality" (Ellis 1992), were deemed cognitively closer to the dominant class when seen relative to the Chinese. The tuberculosis associated with these areas, then, was a disdained but nonthreatening disease of like characterization to these "Others."

Chinatown, though, needed no sewers to remind the rest of the city of its presence. Imposing itself in the very heart of the city, it spewed its filth and effluvia sans mediating pipeline directly into the nerve center of town. It left no boundaries unassailed between clean and dirty, culpable and innocent. It was everything antithetical to the sanitation movement. Not only did it infect the city with its filth, but its inhabitants refused to subscribe to the self-righteous tenets of social and sanitary propriety: they refused, in other words, to live like whites. To purge the area, then, was merely to swab out a wound only to watch it fester again and reinfect itself, threatening once more to infect the rest of the urban body. The inevitable outcome could only be the vilest and most threatening of diseases — smallpox. The fear this disease inspired corresponded precisely to the fear undergirding much of the sanitary and public health movements: the fear of transgression. Just as Chinatown transgressed virtually every social and sanitary code, so did smallpox. It ignored all boundaries, striking down the wealthy as often as the poor and marginal; it gave no warning of its actions; and the very viciousness of its character only belied the baseness of its origin.

In an age when the construction of the "Other" was well developed, the Chinese and their habitat represented the most "Other" of all others. Even if sewers and filthy streets kept the rest of the city susceptible to disease, the worst diseases must invariably be attributed to the worst offender of sanitation, the strongest link in the "metonymic chain of contagion."

Conclusion

"Blaming," write Dorothy Nelkin and Sander Gilman, "has always been a means to make mysterious and devastating diseases comprehensible and therefore possibly controllable" (Nelkin and Gilman 1991, 40). At this level of generality, San Francisco's resort to scapegoating in reaction to smallpox epidemics was not unique in the history of responses to epidemic disease. Neither was the friction between municipal health mandates and individual negotiation of disease (Calvi 1989; R. J. Evans 1992), nor the systematic cleaning of city streets and sewers (Duffy 1990; Wohl 1983). All of these reactions have, throughout history, served a need to create boundaries where none was heeded, to impose order where chaos reigned, and to formulate meaning from senseless devastation and suffering. The distinct forms these reactions take come in the more detailed interfacing of a disease and the social, ideological, and political concerns of a particular time and place. To paraphrase the historian Giulia Calvi, the coded meanings inherent in responses to disease must be uncovered in the "density of the social fabric" (Calvi 1984, 2). For San Francisco, this meant a social fabric dominated by a drive for social order derived from a fluctuating economy and the perception of uncontrolled urban growth, and which found its greatest force in confronting what was perceived as the most disordered, uncontrollable constituency — the Chinese and their own "city within a city."

But these coded meanings must also be looked for in the disease itself, since responses are not to an abstracted concept but to a particular set of symptoms and intrinsic qualities. In contrast to tuberculosis, smallpox engendered reactions commensurate with its own violence and pervasive reach. Accordingly, it attracted in San Francisco the most powerful social and political meanings of any disease until the outbreak of plague at the turn of the century. Its metaphorical behavior was antithetical to a time and place focused on reinforcing cultural norms and rigidifying social boundaries. As such, it was perceived as paralleling a community equally impervious to these constructs. Beyond simply blaming the Chinese for smallpox, this association provoked a deeper fusing of disease and place as the characteristics of smallpox and syphilis were reified within the spaces of Chinatown. A despised urban space was reproduced in the image of a threatening disease, a metonymy serving both political and social purposes.

The absence of medical understanding enabled a more flexible interpretation of smallpox, but it was not solely responsible for it. As Allan Brandt writes, disease is never just a biological phenomenon (Brandt 1991, 93). Epidemiological understanding does not deprive a disease of its social context or prevent the ascription of social meanings. Nor does medical explication always denude a disease of the fear that drives a search for meaning, spatial limitation, and control. For smallpox, a "disinfecting" of its metaphors would only come with its virtual extinction in the next century, but even then the vestiges of meaning would remain.

3

NEGOTIATING THE BOUNDARIES, POLICING THE BORDERS OF DISEASE

Thus far in the examination of smallpox, those responses more collective and institutional in nature have been depicted. But underneath these more visible public reactions were the personal confrontations of a disease that was terrifying at the same time that it was constraining. It made the conduct of everyday life difficult by interjecting contagious space into everyday pathways or by disrupting those structural and social features constitutive of everyday practices. Sometimes even more constraining, however, were the public health measures invoked to combat smallpox. In their urgent attempts to mitigate the spread of disease, public health officials commonly disregarded the personal and economic needs of the individual. As Foucault stated in the context of a similarly disrupting disease, "discipline, the ordering of every detail of individual and collective life, was the correlative of the real and imaginary disorder of plague" (Foucault 1977, 198).

In his genealogy of the increasingly meticulous ordering of social and personal terrain in the midst of epidemics, however, Foucault overlooked individual contestation of imposed order and bodily surveillance. It is obvious from extant journal and newspaper accounts that San Franciscans did not simply acquiesce to the imposition of public health mandates. Like many before them,[1] they found ways, unorganized and individualistic, to negotiate those urban areas that were constitutive of their economic or social livelihood but that had been made dangerous by disease or inaccessible by public health dictate. As will be seen, such negotiations entailed a spatial dialectic between two overlaid topographies: that of office buildings, homes, and parks and that of contagious spaces, liminal areas, and demarcated zones of disease.

The rigidity of public health ordinances enacted during the San Francisco epidemics derived in part from the inability of physicians to elucidate the etiology of disease. Embracing both sides of the contemporary debate over contagion versus anticontagion, San Francisco public health authorities acknowledged that sanitary measures alone were insufficient to prevent the spread of smallpox. That is, while still believing in "mephitic" gases, they also observed that spatial diffusions of smallpox within the city indicated a person-to-person transmission. Thus did the board of health impose two primary measures: vaccination and quarantine. The latter deployed rules almost identical to those first implemented during plague outbreaks in Europe four centuries earlier (Cipolla 1979, 1981; Carmichael 1986). Beginning with the first smallpox epidemic in 1868, the health officer was authorized to remove anyone diagnosed with the disease to the new smallpox hospital on the grounds of the almshouse. This constituted the most important quarantine law (*California Medical Gazette,* July 1868). Because the new hospital could accommodate only a small fraction of cases during an epidemic, however, the second quarantine statute mandated placing a yellow placard on the door of the victim's residence (Municipal Reports 1870).

In addition to the two methods of quarantine, ordinances were written detailing every aspect of behavior on the parts of the victim, physician, community, and public health officer when confronted with a case of smallpox. The list was quite lengthy: every physician was ordered to report any observed cases of smallpox to the health officer; every householder was required to report anyone boarding in their home suspected of having smallpox; no one having come in contact with a smallpox victim was to go out into public or in any way come into contact with unaffected persons; special vehicles were to be used to remove the smallpox victim from the premises; the health officer was authorized to fumigate and disinfect any residence of a smallpox victim or one suspected of having the disease; and no smallpox victim was to be removed from the house except under authorization of the health officer (Municipal Reports 1872, 563–65).

Landscape of Exile

Both the smallpox hospital and the yellow placards were wrought with often conflicting symbolic meaning for the San Francisco resident living in the latter part of the nineteenth century. The smallpox hospital, for instance, was opened in the early spring of 1868 with a degree of pride on the part of civic administrators and public health officials. As reported in one newspaper, the city health officer proclaimed that the hospital "had an enchanting view of the bay, hills, and Precito Creek," a parlor in front, and the latest structural innovations for better ventilation (*Alta of San Francisco,* April 13, 1868, 1). In its design, too, the hospital made evident that its purpose was not just to isolate the sick from the normal but to police "transborder" exchanges between bodies. It did this by separating classes and ethnicities into different wards, thereby maintaining boundaries more effectively than could the city with its public spaces and promiscuous streets. One ward was allocated for women and two for "negroes"; the Chinese were housed in a separate building entirely; and the upper classes used private rooms (*Alta of San Francisco,* April 13, 1868, 1).

But by August of that same year, disparaging reports of the hospital were already beginning to circulate. The San Francisco Medical Society had sent a committee to investigate the hospital, with the rationale that "the most opportune moment to obtain reform in hygienic institutions is when the invasion of an alarming epidemic disturbs the public comfort... [and] relaxes the constriction of the public purse." The results of the committee's findings were revealing of how divergent the abstract design of an institution could be from the real exigencies of an epidemic. Spatial boundaries collapsed when only one woman occupied the entire female ward, while the other wards were crowded to the point of overflow even though the peak of the epidemic was months away. Used bed clothing and linens were found discarded near the building, and the "parlor" had already been converted into another ward because there was no space for convalescent patients. It was no wonder, the committee stated, that "the obloquy of the pest-house is as much dreaded as the fear of the pest" (*California Medical Gazette,* August 1868, 37, 38).

More than their direct observations, though, the committee provided a sympathetic analysis of what the smallpox hospital signified to those suffering within its walls. In their view, the hospital was for those outside it a necessary evil, a highly contagious place whose thick walls and distance from the city boundaries could contain smallpox within its circumference. For the victim trapped inside this overcrowded and ill-conceived structure, however, there was the "horrible and revolting" spectacle of "universal bathing... in each other's effluvia." Though the quarantine law mandating isolation in the smallpox hospital was designed to protect both the patient and the community, the committee found instead that "the law [was] one-sided, it protects the public, but sacrifices the subject, as though the diseased were the criminal, and the pest-house the punishment.... In the excitement of an epidemic, the contaminated are deserted in the general zeal of the uncontaminated to obtain immunity" (*California Medical Gazette,* August 1868, 38). In a clear illustration of "exercising power over men, of controlling their relations, of separating out their dangerous mixtures" (Foucault 1977, 198), the pesthouse served a carceral function, keeping a society placated through the separation of the diseased from the normal. It did not necessarily always fulfill the function of healing.

As poignant as the committee's observations were, other reports were even more revealing of hospital practices. Whereas the medical committee found the care at the hospital commendable in the circumstances, a series of articles in the *San Francisco Chronicle* claimed the opposite. An article dated late July claimed that patients "raving with fever" were placed in straight-jackets (*San Francisco Chronicle,* July 28, 1868, 2), while another article in August added that patients were sometimes locked in the dark or simply left to die of neglect (*San Francisco Chronicle,* August 5, 1868, 2). A third article derisively titled "Nursing a Smallpox Patient" claimed that when a patient delirious with fever escaped from the hospital, four nurses chased him down, beat him, and lashed him to a cot. On their return to the hospital, they carried the unfortunate patient in front of a school with children in recess, causing panicked pandemonium until teachers were able to herd the children inside (*San Francisco Chronicle,* September 4, 1868, 3). The reporter summed up his information rather more dramatically than the medical committee in saying that "such horrible outrages were committed, such terrible scenes transpired, such barbarity manifested that when the revolting details were brought to light, the indignation of the community was aroused as it has seldom been before" (*San Francisco Chronicle,* September 4, 1868, 3).

The community's purported indignation had little lasting effect, because reports during subsequent epidemics continued to depict abominable conditions and unprofessional care in the smallpox hospital. One especially wrenching scene was recounted by *The Call of San Francisco* during the final smallpox epidemic in 1888. A German immigrant's family was struck by smallpox during the Christmas season, the children first and subsequently, on Christmas Day, the mother. They were removed to the smallpox hospital, where the older child died by the end of the month. The mother and other child recovered, after which the mother recounted an incident that occurred while she was inside. Despite the fact that it was winter, only one stove heated the entire hospital; that stove was located in the nurses' bedroom. When the German woman huddled in front of this lone source of heat to keep her baby from freezing, a nurse entered the room and "attacked her with a two by four" (*Call,* January 11, 1888, 8). The same problem existed in the men's wards, as corroborated by a member of the board of health who visited the hospital — incidentally, the only time a board of health member visited the smallpox hospital during the last epidemic. He found fifteen men huddled in one small room with no heat and promptly ordered two stoves to be installed (*Call,* January 11, 1888, 5).

Damning as these reports were, it is likely that they served less to instill fear in people than to confirm fears already extant. Though the medical committee might have generalized the public's view of the smallpox hospital as one of gratitude that a containing space existed for smallpox, in reality public emotion was more complex. For one thing, smallpox was so virulent and spread with such alacrity that it is unlikely many would have thought in such myopic dualisms as "outsiders" versus "insiders." Given a day, a week, or a month, many would find themselves having crossed that real and symbolic boundary between the healthy and the doomed. Or even if they remained unscathed, many were forced to watch family members board the smallpox paddy wagon, to be carted away to misery and an uncertain chance of recovery. The fragmentation this act caused was severe and multilayered. On the emotional level, the potential comforts provided to the patient by the family and the home during the upheavals of an epidemic were nullified. And since removal to the pesthouse was considered all but a death sentence, it was far from certain that once family members were taken away, they would ever return. On the more practical level, removal to the pesthouse inevitably caused a disruption in economic livelihood, particularly since remaining family members were quarantined inside the home for several weeks (Municipal Reports 1872).

It is undoubtedly true that at one level, the smallpox hospital did provide a measure of comfort to a populace needing desperately to believe in the possibility of containing the disease within a delimited space. According to David Musto, quarantine laws were imposed often in response to public demand more than by the advice of physicians (Musto 1988, 72). But comfort was inevitably marred by ambivalence toward the hardships caused by the pesthouse and the suffering and death it symbolized. For these reasons, pesthouse incarceration was the most contested public health mandate during smallpox epidemics.

In one incident, for example, a businessman was approached by the health officer and informed that he had smallpox and would have to be taken to the smallpox hospital. The man's brother intervened and asked if the wagon (the special paddy wagon used to remove patients to the pesthouse) could wait until the end of the day, so that the brothers' shop customers would not become alarmed. The health officer agreed and sent the wagon that evening, only to find the smallpox victim had vacated the premises (*San Francisco Chronicle,* January 18, 1888, 8). A more confrontational incident occurred in Oakland only two days later, when health authorities tried to remove a woman to the pesthouse over the objections of her father. The father bargained with the health officers, saying he would agree to have yellow placards on his house and armed guards stationed to prevent anyone from exiting or entering. The officers refused and tried to remove the woman, only to find themselves faced with considerable "force . . . resist[ing] the taking away of the young lady." The officers finally gave up and left (*San Francisco Chronicle,* January 20, 1888, 5). On the other side of the bay, a health officer was dispatched to locate a reported smallpox case in a boarding house on Market Street. Upon arrival at the house, however, the inspector found that "the matter was kept so quiet by the inmates of the house that nothing could be learned of the whereabouts of the man" (*San Francisco Chronicle,* January 20, 1888, 5).

In their respective acts of defiance, the people in these stories engaged individualistically with the landscapes of contagion that confronted them. For some, this engagement consisted of willful refusal to acknowledge the real and symbolic transformation of city streets and buildings each epidemic brought. For others whose geographic imaginations encompassed both infectious and normative landscapes, there was a continual selectivity between the two, a dialectic driven by economic necessity and social need, on the one hand, and fear of infection, on the other. And finally, like the father protecting his daughter, there was a willingness to live within a zone of contagion rather than to allow the invasion of municipal authority into previously sacrosanct domestic spaces or to endure the impassable boundaries between family members created in the act of pesthouse incarceration.

Noteworthy as well is the fact that the health officer in this incident was forced to give up his effort to remove the daughter to the pesthouse. Fighting beleaguered health inspectors and their paddy wagons was the most violent manifestation of public ambivalence toward the pesthouse and toward the public health mandates that abrogated customary rules of privacy by breaking up the family and incarcerating the innocent. In San Francisco, these acts of open defiance appeared to remain largely individual, with single families defying public health authorities on their own or with the aid of a few friends. In other cities this was not the case. According to Judith Leavitt, in the Milwaukee smallpox epidemic of 1894–95, entire districts armed themselves and patrolled the streets in organized combat against health inspectors attempting to remove patients to the pesthouse (Leavitt 1985). Women, Leavitt notes, were the "front line guards" of these wards since the police and health officers were less willing to use their clubs against them. As observed by one newspaperman, "Mobs of Pomeranian and Polish women armed with baseball bats, potato mashers, clubs, bed slats, salt and pepper, and butcher knives, lay in wait all day for...the Isolation Hospital van" (*Milwaukee Sentinel*, August 30, 1894, cited in Leavitt 1985, 375). Similar uprisings occurred during the Montreal smallpox epidemic of 1885 (Hopkins 1983).

The second method of quarantine was also contested during epidemics, though actions against it were generally more surreptitious and less openly belligerent. When the smallpox hospital filled up, as was frequent during epidemics, or when the health inspector deemed it equally effective, smallpox victims were confined to their homes with no possibility of entry or exit for a period of two to three weeks. Yellow signs were plastered outside the house, a warning sign of contagion to anyone approaching the house. If less harsh than removal to the pesthouse, "yellow-flagging" nevertheless created economic and social burdens often outlasting the epidemic itself. Although a family was allowed to remain intact, it was forced to live with a degree of isolation and restriction unthinkable during normal times. The invisible boundary shutting them in and keeping others out was a constant reminder that they inhabited a liminal space, balanced precariously on the border between undesirability and nonexistence. Because their home was reviled and feared, it was assiduously avoided, eliminated as much as possible from local cognitive maps and physical pathways. In burning linens, draperies, and clothing, material testaments to the existence of those inside were obliterated.

Even if such a patient received aid from a doctor, every precaution was taken to keep spatial boundaries between physician and patient distinct, as exemplified by an excerpt from the quarantine rules of the Illinois Board of Health, adopted by San Francisco:

> Within a sick room, all draperies and rugs are to be removed...[and] sheets wet with disinfectant are to be kept over the doors....Before entering the sick room, a doctor or attendant should put on an outer garment closely buttoned up, and a handkerchief placed around the throat and neck which should be of linen or rubber. Exposure to the open air is the best disinfectant after leaving the sick room. (Printed in *Call,* January 20, 1882, 4)

Body boundaries potentially porous to viral intrusion were to be shored up through material reinforcement. The liminality of the smallpox patient's space was affirmed everywhere, from the shrouded room, the shrouded physician, the divestment of material belongings, and the stark contrast drawn between the sickroom and the healthy outside air.

Given the harshness even of the home quarantine, it was inevitable that some would find ways to circumvent it. In a report by the mayor during the 1868 epidemic, for instance, it was acknowledged that many times health inspectors could not find quarantined houses because as soon as members of the board of health flagged them, the yellow placards were torn down. It was resolved that the health officer, in order to mitigate this practice, would each week report to the president of the board of health the yellow flags placed for that time period (*Alta of San Francisco,* September 19, 1968, 1). Yet another reprieve for the smallpox victim came in a report a few days earlier that health inspectors were often lax in placing yellow flags on homes of reported cases (*San Francisco Chronicle,* September 16, 1868, 3).

More so than the smallpox hospital, the practice of quarantining small-pox victims in the home was contested by physicians as well as laity. Although many times protests were aimed at the supposed fallibility of the contagion theory, there were other motivations for their objections. One physician, for example, stated his theoretical disagreement with quarantining, asserting that smallpox was transmitted by miasmas and not person-to-person. Yet it becomes clear that his objections are based as much on emotional as epistemological arguments, when he derides the social isolation and obloquy imposed upon individuals under the onus of the flag:

> Were it simply useless, [the yellow flag] might be left to sport with the breeze; but as a symbol of disease, it becomes the means of shutting off the unfortunate family from society, depriving them of all human help, exciting fear in minds already too well disposed to be alarmed; it is, therefore, a danger in itself, ... a tyranny which necessity does not justify. (Aubert 1868, 1)

Flagging for Aubert was not a judicious use of public health authority in time of epidemic. On the contrary, it exemplified an ominous capacity to exert control over the use and signification of space in the name of public health, but with results both punitive and counterproductive. Yet the yellow flag had a long genealogy that spoke of the need to expropriate the culpable ill when dealing with terrifying epidemics. Before the eighteenth century, this was usually accomplished by the expulsion of the ill from the community. By the eighteenth and nineteenth centuries, however, municipal authorities had mastered the control and organization of space to the point of accomplishing exile within, or proximate to, city boundaries (Foucault 1965). Although incarceration in hospitals became the primary method of intraurban exile, quarantine served a similar purpose.

The objections of another physician spoke more to perceived structural impediments to flagging and the repercussions of deluded beliefs in its efficacy. Although he does not contest the plausibility of contagion in smallpox, he asserts that the practice of flagging was nevertheless "a perfect farce, . . . its novelty alone explaining why it was adopted by the Board of Health":

> If the yellow flag actually possessed the power of isolating the houses where it was exhibited, it might then be entitled to some considera-tion; but as, in a city, such houses are necessarily in close proximity to other houses, and in many instances on the great thoroughfares of trade, through which people must pass in spite of yellow flags, to transact business, the possibility of isolation under such circum-stances cannot for a moment be entertained. (*California Medical Gazette*, October 1868, 89)

For this anonymous author, the flag was not so much a symbol of disease as a "mysterious charm" lulling people into believing that its very presence could protect them from smallpox. For this reason was it indirectly "productive of very mischievous and fatal consequences" (*California Medical Gazette*, Oc-tober 1868, 89). To support his twofold argument against house quarantine, the author goes on to point out that despite (or because of) its implemen-tation, smallpox had increased in virulence, incidence, mortality rate, and geographic distribution within the city.

This physician's focus on the density of urban topographies illuminates the distinction between the symbolic meaning of quarantine, as depicted by Aubert, and its very real limitations within an urban setting. Though home confinement may have had a role in mitigating the spread of smallpox, this role was probably minimal — especially in poorer neighborhoods such as South of Market and North Beach, where every inch of space was taken up by cramped homes abutting each other, forcing people to use connecting cat-walks and communal laundry decks in order to gain street access. Avoidance of particular residences was difficult if not impossible, and the number of people living in each house made the spread of smallpox all the more likely. To borrow a term from the historian François Delaporte (1986), the localized "map of mortality" of these homes would have been exceedingly higher than in the more spacious homes of the upper and middle classes, with or without quarantine.

Even in lower-density neighborhoods, though, quarantined areas could not always be avoided. San Francisco's hilly terrain and limited throughways made alternate routes inconvenient, if not impossible. During the peak of epidemics, yellow placards multiplied and changed continually, creating a map of disease that was constantly changing shape and at times becoming al-most mazelike in its complex configurations of healthy and infectious zones. By the time a yellow placard was noticed, proximity might already have been reached, as is illustrated in the incident of a couple walking nonchalantly down a street until they had come upon a house with a yellow placard above the door. Upon seeing it, the two "of one accord . . . took to their heels, while they held their breath for fear of inhaling infectious atmosphere" (*San Francisco Chronicle*, December 30, 1888). Though the reporter's tone is rather glib in this account, the couple's terror was undoubtedly very real. Contagious boundaries were more encompassing and porous at a time when germs were perceived to waft through air and cling tenaciously to material objects. Not just the sick person within but the house and its immediate environs would have been perceived as potentially infectious.

Cartographies of Culpability

Feelings of fear and chaos for some were invariably facilitated by the contradictory actions of public health authorities and physicians. One reason for this was the theoretical squabble over how the disease spread and what responses were appropriate in mitigating it. Another reason was the social bias of some public health officers against the poor, as manifested in their more rigorous monitoring of lower-class over wealthy neighborhoods. One reporter following the activities of the public health office claimed that the abodes of poorer smallpox victims were usually marked by the flag, whereas "stately mansions and elegant brick buildings" were not (*San Francisco Chronicle*, September 16, 1868, 3). This even extended to the more expensive lodging houses of the city, whose unflagged "welcome" signs were still in place despite the residence of a smallpox patient (*San Francisco Chronicle*, September 16, 1868, 3). Although more subtle in the case of smallpox, once again the higher disease rates of the poor invariably brought upon them a disproportional degree of condemnation from a medical constabulary stymied in their efforts to control each successive epidemic.

The ineptitude of ward inspectors also meant that people were left ignorant of how to get assistance in cases of smallpox. It was generally known that all cases were to be reported and that public health headquarters were in the center of town. The result was that many people with active cases of smallpox simply showed up at the health office, having walked across town or used public transportation to get there. Ironically, in order to reach a physician's office within the public health headquarters, the infected person had to walk past the long lines of people waiting to be vaccinated against the disease (*San Francisco Chronicle*, September 16, 1868, 3). Not only did this facilitate infection; it also spawned greater chaos and fear. One newspaper article described the paranoia created by this practice during the 1876 epidemic:

> Large numbers of susceptible gentlemen for the past few months
> have been dodging fearfully around the streets in a vain effort to
> avoid their suspicious-looking fellow citizens who are afflicted with
> eruptive countenances, and... the much larger portion of the fe-
> male population of San Francisco have been confining themselves
> to home circles and timorously refusing to ride on the street cars lest
> they meet up with a smallpox case going to the Health Office. (*San
> Francisco Chronicle*, September 25, 1876, 1)

Paranoia also showed itself in assuming that anyone with a skin disturbance
of any kind should be shunned. One unfortunate young woman was evicted
from her lodging house and sent to the health office, only to be diagnosed
with a case of acne (*San Francisco Chronicle*, July 27, 1887, 5).

Evident in this account is the capacity of epidemics to strengthen the
demarcation of gendered spaces, claiming more firmly the domestic sphere
as feminine space and public streets as masculine. Less explicit is the effect this may have had on smallpox rates. Women as a rule did not work
in the nineteenth century unless they were widowed, single, or desperately
poor (Matthaei 1982). They were also not as visible on the streets, except for
those immediately surrounding the home; downtown streets were more the
purview of working men. But whereas the comparatively greater time women
spent in the home sometimes worked against them as regards tuberculosis, it
may have lowered their infection rates in the case of smallpox. The tubercle
bacillus stays alive for long periods outside the body, making protracted confinement to any space such as the home more conducive to infection. But
the smallpox virus does not live long outside the body, making person-to-
person contact essential for propagation of the disease. The relative isolation
of women in their "home circles," then, may explain why they appear to have
suffered proportionally lower smallpox rates than did men (Municipal Reports 1882, 1888). Out of 704 deaths in the 1868 epidemic, only 193 of them
were women (Municipal Reports 1868, 188); in the 1887–88 epidemic, 124
women were infected versus 444 men, over a threefold difference (Municipal
Reports 1888, 471) (see figure 3.1).

It must be emphasized, though, that this hypothesis is too simplistic to
be universally applied over the city. It is more likely to have held true for those
upper- and middle-class homes better insulated by space within and around
each residence than for the intensely crowded lower-class neighborhoods
where infection in one house was likely to spread to others. It is unfortunate that mortality and morbidity statistics do not allow for a more in-depth
analysis of spatial patterns in women's smallpox rates.[2] The absence of clear
information also makes it difficult to determine the extent to which different

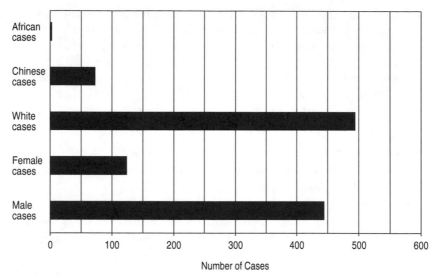

Figure 3.1. Smallpox deaths and smallpox cases by race and gender, 1888. Data from Municipal Reports 1888; created by Mark Patterson.

methods of treatment were applied to female smallpox victims. Reports of the Twenty-Sixth Street hospital (the smallpox hospital) show that far more men were admitted than women, as evidenced by the earlier comment that only one woman occupied the female ward of the hospital. During the 1868 epidemic, a total of 867 males were admitted into the smallpox hospital versus only 101 women (Municipal Reports 1868–69, 203). Either this indicates women in actuality suffered much lower rates of the disease, or it evidences a differential treatment of male and female patients. Men may have been sent to the hospital, in other words, while women were more apt to be treated at home.[3] For Chinese women, it can be more readily assumed that medical care was often not forthcoming. Chinese prostitutes in particular were usually not entitled by their employers to medical attention.

Compounding still further the uncontrolled feeling regarding the epidemics were the private physicians who, regardless of quality and degree of training, were relatively impotent to assuage suffering or stop the dissemination of smallpox. Like their public health counterparts, they debated epidemiologies and treatments. And as with almost any medical emergency, physicians were unable to care for all of those in need and were stretched too thin to be effective. Ethical questions arose as well, with some physicians refusing to treat smallpox cases for fear they would catch the disease themselves. And, finally, there were physicians who through ineptitude or inexperience simply misdiagnosed cases, even though smallpox had more distinctive symptoms than most diseases. Although error was more often on the side of overdiagnosing smallpox, sometimes the opposite occurred. These mistakes made life worse for those believing they had smallpox when they did not and in general added to, rather than diminished, uncertainties and fears concerning the disease. Needless to say, cases of smallpox left undiagnosed also further propagated the disease.

Many of these problems are exemplified in an account of a merchant on California Street during the 1876 epidemic. As the story was reported, the merchant left his shop after feeling somewhat ill for a few days and retired to his hotel, where he called for a physician.[4] After examination, the doctor pronounced the man's ailment to be a "bilious attack." Another physician was eventually called when the illness persisted, and the same diagnosis was rendered. Though the merchant in the meantime confined himself to his hotel room, relatives and friends came and went in ministering to his illness. When a third physician finally realized that the merchant had smallpox, "there was a general exodus from the room, and a remarkable amount of fresh air suddenly in demand, and those uninterested people who always linger around a sick bed...well nigh tore down the side of the hotel in getting out of the vicinity." Even the doctor diagnosing the case retreated in haste, explaining that he had promised his wife he would not treat cases of smallpox. Though a call subsequently went out to doctors and nurses throughout the city, all had too many patients already and could not call upon the sick merchant. Eventually, public health inspectors took him to the smallpox hospital (*San Francisco Chronicle*, September 25, 1876, 1).

The treatment received by this hapless man was almost certainly less than competent. It reflected, though, the exigencies of medical crises and the very human, if unethical, shortcomings of many physicians. Yet evident as well in this story is the fact that this man at least had family and friends to address his needs, and equally importantly he had the social standing and visibility to command care. For many, usually the poorest and most socially alienated, living through an epidemic was made even more hellish by an inability to access even those limited channels of care and treatment. For some, such as the Chinese community, those impediments to care spanned the social-political spectrum. It is no wonder that they hid their sick from punitive health inspectors and simply left their dead out in the streets for public health authorities to find (Municipal Reports 1876–77, 397; *Alta of San Francisco*, December 15, 1887, 3). But conditions were not much better for many other poor immigrants. One Italian family, for instance, was living in an alley between Broadway and Vallejo in impoverished circumstances. They spoke no

English and apparently had no family connections. When a reporter covering the epidemic discovered them, their three children had been suffering from smallpox for ten days with no medical attendance (*San Francisco Chronicle,* November 11, 1887, 6). For these people, lack of a common language, absence of social ties, extreme poverty, and ignorance of municipal public health programs combined to make the negotiated path through disease an even more terrifying, alienating, and isolated one.

Probably the cruelest irony of smallpox epidemics in San Francisco and elsewhere during this time was that an effective vaccine had existed since the eighteenth century. As with other cities in the United States,[5] San Francisco had its share of problems implementing vaccination, and the number of dead during each epidemic was partial testimony to the limited success the city achieved. One of the problems seems to have been on the part of the board of health itself. Although in its defense it eventually offered free vaccinations to the public during each epidemic, there is evidence that they were tardy in implementing the program. One censorious physician writing during the 1868 epidemic, for example, berated the board of health for waiting three months after the start of the epidemic to push vaccination. Had they only done so at the very beginning, he opined, the city "should long since have been relieved of the presence of this pestilence which is still killing so many of our citizens" (*California Medical Gazette,* October 1868, 90). Given Health Officer Meares's self-congratulation on saving hundreds of lives in the next epidemic by starting vaccination early, it seems the mistake was rectified (Municipal Reports 1876–77, 397).

Physicians and lay individuals posed their own obstacles. Smallpox vaccination continued to be questioned on both sides of the Atlantic despite evidence of its efficacy in lowering mortality rates (Hopkins 1983; Leavitt 1985).[6] For some, injecting smallpox virus directly into the body defied reason. For most, objection stemmed from fears that smallpox vaccination directly or indirectly led to other diseases. The most common beliefs were that vaccination could cause syphilis (Municipal Reports 1876–77) or mental degeneration or that it could increase mortality rates in other diseases (Shorb 1868, 59). One physician, exasperated with those who refused to take preventive measures and stymied by his own impotence to compel them, heaped opprobrium on unvaccinated smallpox victims: "For the living—those who have taken the smallpox and recovered—we cannot say we feel any particular amount of sympathy. That they are barely tolerated by their relatives and friends, and are repulsive to the public, that their faces are seamed, pitted and deformed, they have themselves alone to thank" (Shorb 1868, 60).

Although many of the fears concerning vaccination were born of ignorance or paranoia, they were also based to some degree in reality. Vaccination at this time was almost entirely unregulated. Some vaccine material was produced by various private companies, and some was even produced by physicians themselves. Either way, there was no institutional structure in place to supervise the production and regulate quality. As one physician put it, the more time that passed after the death of Jenner (the first person to produce smallpox vaccine), the more general the practice became and the more "the conditions of its success were to some extent lost sight of" (*California Medical Gazette*, March 1869, 158). Another physician expressed his fears of vaccination during the 1876 epidemic, explaining that supplies came in from various labs around the area and were immediately implemented without being first tested by the board of health. As a result, people lined up for the vaccine and later exposed themselves, thinking that they were immune when they were not (*San Francisco Chronicle*, August 13, 1876, 2). The physician had reason to worry. A company supplying large quantities of vaccine to the city was later found to be producing a placebo (Duffy 1990).

Such problems notwithstanding, thousands availed themselves of free vaccination during smallpox outbreaks. By the last major wave in 1887, the health office seemed quite practiced at vaccinating thousands of people in a very short period of time. Since vaccination was still not compulsory in California, they had been forced to develop a wide variety of outreach methods to encourage the practice. Physicians were hired in the beginning of the epidemic to go house-to-house persuading people to be vaccinated. Vaccination stations were set up in various parts of the city; advertisements were published in several languages in newspapers urging speedy vaccination; health inspectors were dispatched to public schools; and prison and almshouse inmates were vaccinated. Physicians were also sent to manufacturing plants to vaccinate laborers, and the health office maintained round-the-clock hours to accommodate as many people as possible (Municipal Reports 1887, 467–68). With each successive epidemic, so many people were vaccinated each day as to move one newspaper reporter to quip that the common greeting of "Hello, how are you?" had been replaced by "How's your scab?" (*San Francisco Chronicle*, July 29, 1868, 3). It is almost certain that despite its problems, vaccination played a significant role in decreasing mortality rates during each of San Francisco's epidemics.

Diminished Terrain

Although the epidemic of 1887 was not the last San Francisco would see of smallpox, the disease never gained ascendancy in the city again after that time. This gradually changed the way Chinatown was interpreted by the medical establishment as well as the public. Most notably, Chinatown lost over a period of time its synonymity with smallpox and other virulent diseases, though the plague epidemic of 1901 would reassert the tendency to ascribe epidemiological provenance of a feared disease to the Chinese community. This is not to say that Chinatown did not maintain its construct as a separate site within the city, inhabited by people still considered suspiciously foreign. The passage and renewal of the Chinese Exclusion Act are testaments to the continuing tensions between white and Chinese communities. Passed in 1882, the act prohibited any further immigration into the United States of Chinese laborers or their families and also prohibited the naturalization of Chinese residents (Saxton 1971). This law was renewed every ten years until its repeal in 1943 (Yung 1995). The number of Chinese living in San Francisco consequently dwindled, from a peak of approximately thirty thousand to between eighteen thousand and twenty-two thousand by 1890 (Municipal Reports 1890, 525; Saxton 1971).

The diminution of the Chinese population within San Francisco to some extent muted the fear with which Chinatown was regarded in the last few years of the nineteenth century. The ascendancy of bacteriology in medical theory also began making a gradual difference in discursive representations of Chinatown, although previous medical theories did not entirely lose their influence. Germ theory and environmental medicine continued to co-reside in reports of public health officers through the turn of the century. The authority of the physician also became more important to the maintenance of health, drawing attention away from the lifestyle of groups and their physical environments to the relationship of the individual to the physician. For the first time in 1891, a public health officer blamed Chinatown's high mortality rate on the fact that "they [the Chinese] are rarely ever attended by a physician" (Municipal Reports 1891, 525). Just the previous year, however, this same health officer was calling Chinatown a plague spot and congratulating himself for a thorough sanitary cleanup of the district (Municipal Reports 1890, 316). Clearer medical understanding did not entirely dissipate social and cultural interpretations of disease, in other words; it simply reworked them into the increasingly authoritative framework of medical and sanitary science.

One reason for the subsidence of smallpox in San Francisco was the general decline of the disease throughout the United States and much of Europe during the latter part of the nineteenth century. There were, in short, fewer sources of the disease in the form of migrants to San Francisco (Hopkins 1983). Combined immunities from vaccination (despite its problems) and previous exposure also diminished the pool of people vulnerable to the disease. As was seen in the mortality records for each epidemic in San Francisco, the number of cases, and of deaths, declined with each successive outbreak in the city. Though slow in coming, sanitation also improved during the last decade of the nineteenth century and the first decades of the twentieth.

One area where sanitation was forcibly improved for several years after the last epidemic was Chinatown. The epidemiological threat contained in its structures and the spaces between them remained a focus of public health authorities through the turn of the century, meaning that surveillance over and intervention into Chinatown's physical environment persisted as one perceived way to improve the health of the city as a whole. In 1890 the city's health officer reported that three times during that year house-to-house inspections were made of buildings and residences, rooting out supposed sanitary transgressions and rectifying them. Thousands of dollars were expended repairing buildings designated as problematic, or razing entirely those too old to refurbish and replacing them with brick structures. In less severe but more frequent instances, sanitary restructuring of interiors and surroundings was performed, not to mention a great deal of fumigating (Municipal Reports 1889–90, 316).

The rest of San Francisco benefited from a less vigorous but nonetheless energetic attention to sanitary reforms, spurred in part by the embarrassment of two smallpox epidemics in five years. In his report of 1890, Health Officer James Keeney claimed to have installed more new sewers in the city than ever witnessed previously. He also turned his focus on the more noxious industries of the city, such as the tanneries and dairies (Municipal Reports 1890). Several tanneries were purportedly condemned, and an ordinance was passed directing all dairies to be removed outside the city limits. Although some were consequently allowed back in, the dairy industry remained more highly regulated from this time on.[7] Food markets were also more intensively monitored, resulting in "consternation among the vendors" of those foods condemned for being substandard when in previous years they had probably passed inspection (Municipal Reports 1890). The only problems with which the health officer expressed continued frustration were the disposal of dead animals and garbage. Before the reforms of the early twentieth century brought these tasks under government purview, private companies were contracted to perform them; all too often, they did a less than commendable job (Municipal Reports 1890–91).

Partially because of these last problems, and the continued inadequacy of sewers, San Francisco still experienced a relatively high death rate from such infectious diseases as diphtheria and typhoid, even during years of low smallpox incidence. During 1890–91, for instance, there were 314 deaths from diphtheria and 137 from typhoid, and only 4 from smallpox. In 1901–2, there were 204 deaths from diphtheria and well over 1,000 cases (Municipal Reports 1891, 1902). Though these diseases never received the attention that smallpox did, the relative quiescence of smallpox reminded city health officials that even less dramatic but highly fatal maladies also needed attention. One answer to this came by the turn of the century in the form of an antitoxin for diphtheria; although it was not a preventative, it drastically cut down on mortality and received little if any resistance from the public. Better epidemiological tracing was also put into place. In his 1902 report the chief sanitary inspector, William Hassler, stated that inspectors had gone door-to-door in certain school districts with higher incidences of diphtheria and had found in one district alone thirty cases of the disease. After carefully tracing the contacts and family members of these thirty cases and excluding them from schools, new cases diminished (Municipal Reports 1902, 563). After the early 1900s, diphtheria ceased to be a serious health threat to San Francisco's children. For typhoid, the answer lay in the more gradual but persistent improvements in the city's water supply and sewer system. Although satisfactory performance levels were not reached for several more decades, each improvement brought proportionate decreases in typhoid cases until this disease, too, posed little threat to the city.

By the early years of the twentieth century, a more intriguing factor eroded the real and metaphoric powers once wielded by smallpox. In 1896, a strain of the disease was reported in Florida that was much milder and far less fatal than previous cases. The variety was termed *Variola minor* and was soon making its way across the country. By 1898 it had reached the midwestern states, by 1899 the northeastern, western, and northern states, and by 1900 it had reached California. It is not clear from the medical and public health records whether physicians in San Francisco realized the existence of this new variety of smallpox. Instead, they simply observed with mystification, and not a little satisfaction, the precipitous decline in mortality from the disease by 1901, attributing it to improved hospital facilities and medical care. The city physician in 1902, for example, claimed that though 206 cases of smallpox had been reported to him for that year, the extreme mildness of the disease probably resulted in many other cases being misdiagnosed as chickenpox (Municipal Reports 1902, 508). Of the 206 reported cases, only one resulted in death.

Though the more severe strain of smallpox occasionally reasserted itself in other cities during the next two decades (Hopkins 1983), it appears to have spared San Francisco almost entirely. The danger of the milder variety was in allowing it to spread virtually unhindered since it incited little fear or suffering. One particularly vivid example of this was a physician's discovery, during the chaotic aftermath of the 1906 earthquake, of a smallpox victim "in the advanced stages of desquamation" peddling doughnuts to inhabitants of the various tent camps set up over the city. Before the victim was apprehended, he had spread smallpox to at least fifty other people (Municipal Reports 1907, 518).

Despite such laxity in treating *Variola minor,* even this strain eventually diminished in incidence during the second and third decades of the twentieth century in San Francisco, as elsewhere in the United States. Cases continued to crop up from time to time, but their gradual decline into negligible numbers was evidenced by the abandoned plan for a new smallpox hospital. Though a tract of land was bought by the city in the early years of the century, the building itself never materialized because it became increasingly clear that not enough cases existed to warrant a separate facility. In addition, new "pavilion" designs had been implemented in some general hospitals by the early years of the century. By providing wings on the main building, and wards within each wing, those suffering from contagious diseases could be effectively isolated from other hospital patients within the same building, a feature not possible within the more communal designs of older hospitals. It was decided by the second decade of the century that these ward facilities would be adequate for handling any remaining smallpox cases (Municipal Reports 1916). The dreaded "pesthouse" finally became defunct.

During the final years of San Francisco's confrontation with smallpox, Chinatown was generally not targeted as the source of the disease. Rather, with the new focus and language of scientific sanitation, particular parts of Chinatown and habits of its denizens were deemed likely to propagate the disease. The only mention of the Chinese made by Hassler in his 1902 sanitation report, for example, was to assert "the importance of prohibiting the sleeping in the ironing room or storing of clothes in any portion of laundry used for such purpose" (Municipal Reports 1902, 565). The complaint of deleterious relations between bodies and their environments was an old one, reconstituted to fit better-understood epidemiologies and medical microtopographies. The mapping of infection changed with space now disarticulated, subdivided like the new hospital into its constituent parts for more effective pinpointing of dangerous zones and behaviors. Previously a dank basement, an especially narrow street, or an ill-ventilated laundry was proof of a larger malignancy, whereas by the turn of the century these were more frequently evaluated for their singular potential to harbor disease. Monitoring microspaces became the way to control the larger space. Only individual structures and highly specific behaviors now constituted a "morbid environment" (Delaporte 1986, 86).

Conclusion

Responses to smallpox beyond its ascription to Chinatown illuminate the personal fears incited by the disease and the spatial and social boundaries negotiated to deal with them. Smallpox forced the reallocation of personal and cognitive spaces within the city as houses were flagged with yellow symbols of contagious disease, vans moved through the streets carrying smallpox victims to the hospital, or vaccination stations were set up in various points throughout the city. Confronted with the chaotic boundaries created by these signs of infectious disease, individuals were forced to redraw life paths in ways that made sense to them. This meant negotiating the conflictual forces of personal fear, economic exigencies, and public health mandates by seeking the interstices among these. Some did this by simply defying boundaries of contagion, maintaining daily urban paths in an effort to retain a sense of normalcy despite the punitive spatial limitations created by quarantine laws. Others left intact those boundaries they deemed inviolable, while those considered more flexible were reshaped, suspended, or discarded. The boundaries of family, for example, were often considered sacrosanct even if that meant risking viral transmission to other family members. Business was another common priority, to the frustration of public health officials concerned with contagion to the exclusion of economic welfare. The resulting maps of meaning among individuals illuminated private values and contingencies holding primacy over notions of public good.

Smallpox and other infectious diseases would continue to generate trepidation among public health authorities through the turn of the century, even though 1887 was the last year a major epidemic took hold of the city. Minor smallpox outbreaks occurred through the first years of the twentieth century, but strict monitoring of urban spaces was maintained as a public health preventative to epidemic. So, too, were quarantine and vaccination. The 1902 health report conceded that San Francisco, "being a seaport town," had "given" during the preceding year "a great variety of contagious diseases consisting of diphtheria, tuberculosis, scarlatina, measles, smallpox, typhoid fever, beri-beri and bubonic plague" (Municipal Reports 1902, 495). None of these, with the exception of plague, became epidemic within the city, the health officer crediting the quarantine of incoming vessels to the port, the vaccination of over four thousand individuals against smallpox, and the increase of sanitary inspections over the preceding year from 5,881 to 15,278 (Municipal Reports 1902, 495).

Evident in this officer's report is a distinct lack of rhetoric against the Chinese for bringing these contagious diseases to San Francisco. This can be explained in part by the fact that they were not epidemic in the city. As Waldby notes, it is epidemics that "tend to be thought of as effects of poor social order, which must be brought under control through a social re-ordering" (Waldby 1996, 40). Absent the conditions of epidemic, Chinatown was carefully watched but not discursively represented as a malignancy in a threatened urban body. The greater understanding of etiology and epidemiology ensuant to the ascendancy of germ theory attenuated tendencies toward wholesale blame of a place and its residents. The plague epidemic of 1900, however, showed the limitations of new medical insights in moving away from politically informed interpretation of disease and its spatial provenance.

4

STRUCTURES OF SUSCEPTIBILITY AND THE
ARCHITECTURE OF DISEASE

The Plague Epidemics of 1900 and 1907

Bubonic plague, perhaps above all other diseases, possesses the richest genealogy of fear in the Western psyche. Endemic to certain regions of Asia, the disease surmounted topographical barriers and ravaged much of Europe from the fourteenth to the eighteenth centuries,[1] changing social and economic landscapes as a third of urban populations were decimated, agriculture was brought to a standstill, and economic production stagnated (McNeill 1976; Cipolla 1979; Calvi 1989). Extensive breakdowns subsequently occurred in spatial relations among individuals within cities, among cities themselves, and between the city and the countryside as a result of plague's destruction and of municipal attempts to mitigate it. It was perhaps the first disease to generate attention on the part of city authorities to the control of space as a means of controlling disease, yet subsequent public health policies did little to alleviate plague's capacity for social, moral, and religious devastation.

Unlike most other epidemic diseases, though, the fear of plague did not stem so much from its symptoms, which are painful but not particularly mutilating. Initial signs of the disease consist of fever, chills, and headache. The bacteria locate in the lymph nodes, and as they multiply they cause large swellings in the primary lymph sites of the groin, neck, and armpits — hence the name bubonic plague, from the Greek word for groin (Kraut 1994). Neither is plague highly contagious, since it is passed not from person to person but from infected fleas that generally turn to humans only when their preferred blood source, the rat, itself is decimated from the same bacterium, *Yersinia pestis.*

Rather, the fear incited by plague throughout history has stemmed from its astounding death toll, a mortality rate that has ranged from 60 to 90 percent of all cases regardless of whether epidemics occurred in the fourteenth century or the nineteenth (Kraut 1994). For pneumonic plague, where the bacteria enter the lungs rather than the lymph nodes, fatality rates were almost 100 percent. In contrast, even diseases such as smallpox or cholera had comparatively low fatality rates, the smallpox fatalities in San Francisco hitting a peak of less than 40 percent in the first epidemic. Even with fuller understanding of plague's epidemiology in the early twentieth century, fatality rates were not significantly mitigated until the advent of antibiotics at midcentury.

The history of plague is thus an account of economic disruption, population decimation, and social disorder unprecedented in the history of Western civilization. Consequently, its history is also an insight into the best and the worst responses to the multifarious upheavals of devastating disease. Some of the earliest public health laws in Europe were implemented in response to plague, including quarantines on incoming vessels and isolation of infected individuals within households or designated pesthouses (Cipolla 1979). The poor (Carmichael 1986) and Jews (McNeill 1976) were scapegoated at various places and times of epidemic, but any individual perceived as responsible for bringing plague into urban areas was not immune to the more violent outcomes of collective fear (Calvi 1989). Public health laws also compounded the dread of epidemic, often seeming more punitive than preventive in the severity of the restraints they imposed. As Giulia Calvi documents so eloquently (1989), the mandates limiting social relations, restricting movement within city boundaries, and preventing interurban and urban-rural commerce generated hardships from which it took years to recover. Consequently, plague epidemics were the sites of some of the first major contestations between individual and state concerning the extent of public health jurisdiction in time of crisis.

For San Francisco, smallpox was the first disease to generate such contestations. The two plague epidemics that struck the city in 1900 and 1907, however, caused an extension of public health control over bodies, behavior, and urban space to an unprecedented degree. This, in turn, intensified the contestation of medical authority beyond the relatively passive resistance encountered during smallpox epidemics.

Plague in San Francisco

The second epidemic in San Francisco was different for a number of reasons. First, the role of the flea and the rat in plague's epidemiology was fully understood. Second, the demographics of disease victims were almost mirror-opposite the first epidemic: virtually all cases and fatalities involved whites.

Third, the context in which the disease arose and thrived was the earthquake and fire of April 1906, after which much of the city burned or lay in rubble. Social turmoil, in other words, had already been generated by the quake; a plague epidemic merely exacerbated the chaos even as it altered its focus. Because the epidemiology of plague was better known in 1907, and because the victims were white, the public health campaign and the discourses informing it were of a different nature. Scientific method was invoked as the fundamental principle in the fight against the disease, and this translated into an unprecedented medical control over space as the macro- and microgeographies of the city were combed for infected rodents, and the social and economic practices of individuals were tightly monitored for their bacillus-breeding potential.

But the 1901 and the 1907 epidemics served another function in San Francisco. To varying degrees, they both changed the physical landscape of the city more than any other disease before it, and perhaps after it. One of the outcomes of the first epidemic was a sanitary makeover of Chinatown that it had not received even during smallpox epidemics. For a period of almost four years, inspectors and sanitary workers fumigated, sponged, gassed, and washed down the structures of the Chinese district. This had been done before, to a lesser extent. But this time, structural purging was not left to the powers of carbolic acid. By the end of the sanitary cleanup of Chinatown in 1904, over a hundred structures had actually been razed; streets had been cleared; and the balconies, wooden platforms, and decks built in between buildings had been removed. The look of Chinatown was more streamlined, moderately less dense, and scrubbed.

The second epidemic brought even more drastic changes to the rest of San Francisco. At the same time that buildings were being rebuilt after the earthquake, others were being torn down because they were made of wood, a material thought particularly suitable for harboring rats. The extensive pattern of backyard platforms, laundry decks, and sheds in poorer neighborhoods disappeared as these were systematically torn up or down. Stables too were demolished; chicken coops disappeared; wooden sidewalks became a thing of the past; and in general the face of San Francisco changed during the course of an antiplague campaign that was largely based on building a disease out of existence.

1900: Science and the Language of Susceptibility

Despite its episodic sweeps of Asia, Europe, and Africa, bubonic plague had never reached North America before the turn of the twentieth century. That changed on March 6, 1900, when Chick Gin, a Chinese resident of San

Francisco's Chinatown, was discovered dead in the basement of the Globe Hotel (Lipson 1972).[2] All Chinese who died unattended were required by San Francisco health authorities to have an autopsy performed (Report of Special Health Commission 1901), and accordingly Chick Gin received one. Suspicious factors led the attending physician, F. P. Wilson, to call in San Francisco's chief health officer, A. P. O'Brien, who in turn called in the city bacteriologist, Wilfred Kellogg. Kellogg suspected plague because of the appearance of the body and took samples from lymph glands back to the U.S. Marine Hospital Service laboratory on Angel Island, a facility run by Joseph Kinyoun. Eventually, a diagnosis of plague resulted (Kraut 1994; McClain 1988). This signaled the slow beginning of an epidemic that would last for four years, ending finally in 1904 after 121 cases and 112 deaths, almost all of them Chinese (Kraut 1994, 96).

By the time of the plague's first appearance in San Francisco, a diagnosis could be made of it not only by reading the signs of its presence on the body but more accurately by finding the presence of plague bacillus in tissue samples read under the microscope and by injecting samples of body tissue into laboratory rabbits and guinea pigs.[3] Confirmation came if these animals subsequently developed plague. The rising authority of bacteriology and the confidence generated by knowing the specific bacterium that caused plague inspired confidence in many public health officials that the disease could be easily controlled and even conquered in a short period of time. As confidently claimed in 1897 by Walter Wyman, surgeon general of the U.S. Marine Hospital Service,[4] plague "furnishes a striking illustration of the scientific advance of modern medicine. It was not until 1894 that positive knowledge of its true nature became known. Now its cause, method of propagation and the means to prevent its spread are matters of scientific certainty" (quoted in McClain 1988, 458).[5] In a relatively short period of time, science made remarkable strides in the arena of pathogen discovery,[6] and the knowledge that finally elucidated the mechanisms of disease did indeed bring with it a promise of power to subdue and to vanquish. Or so it seemed.

Wyman's confidence in the power of medical understanding to subdue plague was actually somewhat premature. In fact, plague's propagation was not entirely understood, as the bacillus was thought to be transmitted through the air into the lungs, or into the stomach. An individual was thought able to contract plague through the ingestion of contaminated food, through respiration of infected dust, or through contact with infected soil or with open abrasions on infected individuals. The rat was known to have some connection with plague, but its role in harboring plague-infested fleas that in turn bit humans was not known by 1900. According to Wyman and others in the medical field, though, there was one other factor in the epidemiology of plague, one that recalled the sanitary discourses of the previous century. Plague "was favored in its propagation by the presence of filth or other unsanitary conditions," thus evidencing that environmental theories of disease had still found a place within bacteriological discourse.

It was thus not only highly symbolic but trenchant that Chick Gin died where he did, in a basement room of a dingy hotel on Dupont Street in the heart of the Chinese district. Once again the discursive interpretation of an urban district as diseased, dirty, and depraved was confirmed in the discovery of a deadly and highly feared disease in its midst. A spatialized pathology was easily fit to the context of a new disease: if Chinatown produced smallpox, then it could just as easily produce plague out of the depths of its basement filth. Even if rhetoric had become more subdued in the specific nature of its spatial and behavioral targets over the last years of the nineteenth century, the fundamental idea that Chinatown still possessed the right combination, degree, and quality of characteristics to produce disease had never entirely faded. The advent of a new epidemic thus generated a renewed discourse on the sanitary deficiencies of the Chinese district and its limitless capacity to produce disease. Even with the knowledge that plague was caused by a bacterium, subsequent actions by health authorities testified to the continued medical construction of disease as produced by place.

Accordingly, the first reaction to the discovery of Chick Gin and the possibility of plague was the implementation of a cordon sanitaire around the entire district of Chinatown. This was done even before word of an official diagnosis from Kinyoun, who was waiting for the results of laboratory tests. As recommended by O'Brien, the board of health ordered police guards to surround Chinatown and to begin searching for more plague victims (Lipson 1972). All whites were removed from the district before it was cordoned off; thereafter only whites could leave Chinatown, but no one could enter it. Overnight, Chinatown had been effectively blockaded from the rest of the city.

This first quarantine did not last long, both because official diagnosis of plague was delayed and because reaction was negative from within and without Chinatown. San Francisco newspapers claimed, for example, that the plague scare was fabricated since no confirmation had come from Kinyoun's laboratory (Lipson 1972), while others claimed it was a ploy on the part of the board of health to garner a higher operating budget from the board of supervisors (Kraut 1994). Official confirmation of plague did come on March 11, but until this time health officers were vulnerable to these attacks. Within Chinatown, bitter opposition to the quarantine was widespread, and the Chinese consul general quickly issued a statement by March 7, including the remark that "it is wrong to close an extensive section like Chinatown simply upon the suspicion that a man might have died of the plague" (*San Francisco Chronicle*, March 8, 1900, cited in McClain 1988, 456). Bowing to pressure from many points, the board of health rescinded the cordon only sixty hours after it was imposed (Lipson 1972).

This was only the first of several controversial moves on the part of public health constabulary, however. The next action, coming shortly after the lifting of quarantine, was suggested by Walter Wyman. During his involvement in the plague controversy, Joseph Kinyoun reported events in San Francisco to his supervisor, Wyman, who in turn occasionally sent word back suggesting measures to take as the epidemic unfolded. His first such suggestions to Kinyoun on March 8 were to thoroughly disinfect Chinatown and to inoculate all Chinese with the Haffkine prophylactic vaccine (Kraut 1994). A vaccine might have seemed a humanitarian measure for a district perceived to be vulnerable to further cases of plague, but the Haffkine vaccine in 1900 was still experimental. It had been used on volunteers at a Bombay prison during the plague epidemic in India three years earlier, and after initially hopeful results had been distributed for use by thousands throughout India. Nevertheless studies had never been conducted on the vaccine's efficacy, and results as seen in the India example were mixed. Not only were inoculated individuals still sometimes vulnerable to the disease, but the side effects in themselves could be disastrous. Several deaths were reported after individuals in a Punjabi village were inoculated, and in less severe cases individuals could be incapacitated for days with painful symptoms. As Alan M. Kraut states (1994, 89), the Chinese were "nominated as the next guinea pigs by regulatory fiat."

The Chinese consul and the Chinese Six Companies[7] protested to the Chinese minister in Washington that forced inoculation might lead to violence, and lawyers for the Six Companies made last-minute attempts to convince the board of health to modify its policy of inoculation (Kraut 1994, 91–92). Despite these efforts, on May 19 a force of health inspectors descended upon Chinatown equipped with syringes and the vaccine. Whatever their expectations might have been, they found very few Chinese willing to undergo vaccination. According to Kinyoun, agreement had been reached between himself and spokesmen for the Chinese to the effect that cooperation would be forthcoming from Chinatown during the inoculation campaign. Instead, health inspectors found groups of angry men standing on street corners, merchants closing up shop in protest, and a general atmosphere of belligerence toward the health authorities (Kraut 1994).[8] It did not get any better over the next several days, and warnings posted by the board of health claiming harsher measures would ensue if the Chinese did not submit to inoculation only increased hostility.

Exacerbating the ill feelings was an auxiliary measure suggested by Wyman and promptly acted upon by Kinyoun forbidding travel by Chinese or Japanese outside of San Francisco without a certificate from the board of health stating that they had received the Haffkine vaccine. Since many Asians living in San Francisco traveled regularly to outlying cities and farms for business or family purposes, this limitation on movement threatened to create numerous hardships. The inclusion of Japanese in the ordinance also gave evidence to the way in which plague was being interpreted in its epidemiology.

Surgeon General Wyman's statements on scientific progress in elucidating plague and plague transmission are again insightful for the way in which susceptibility to plague was constructed. With the virtually universal embrace of the germ theory and concepts of bacteriology, the previous triumvirate of disease, dirt, and depravity was replaced at least in theory by a discourse that used epidemiological concepts to explain patterns of susceptibility. Even though dirt still held position in this language, susceptibility was figured more prominently by diet, heredity, or ethnic background. Previous concepts popular in environmental explanations of disease, then, were recouched into scientific language focusing on the body's internally prescribed vulnerability to germ access. In the case of plague, susceptibility was dictated by Asian origin and by a vegetarian, and more specifically a rice-based, diet. Plague was indeed termed a "rice-eaters' disease" by Wyman and others.

This in part stemmed from a general observation of various plague commissions. During the Asian plague pandemic of the latter years of the nineteenth century, American and European committees of physicians were sent to various loci of the epidemic in order to gain further knowledge of a disease whose etiology had just been discovered but whose epidemiology was still largely unknown (Kraut 1994). Their partial conclusion from observing the disease in India and Southeast Asia was that it seemed to affect those who did not eat meat. Susceptibility derived from rice-eating was in part, then, embedded in concepts of immune system vulnerability and the idea that meat strengthened the body's immunity to disease. Yet in the U.S. context, "rice-eaters' disease" became racially charged, an effective tool that again turned foreign designation into epidemiological explanation. It implied that no one but Asians could be vulnerable to the ravages of plague and indeed that all Asians were vulnerable. In this explanation comes the reason why whites in Chinatown were allowed to leave before the first blockade was established and why Japanese were targeted in the ordinance mandating confinement to San Francisco even though no Japanese victims of plague were to be reported for another year. All Asians had become potential carriers, and conversely it was unthinkable that whites could be vulnerable to the plague bacillus: diet became something of a proxy for reading susceptibility through physiognomic inscription.

How Wyman and other medical authorities actually explained this racialized framing of plague, and how they reconciled it with their knowledge of germ theory, is left to interpretation. For one thing, knowledge of how immunity worked was elementary given that it would take more powerful instruments later in time to begin unraveling the mechanisms of the human immune system. In the meantime, however, public health workers needed to explain why some individuals seemed to be more highly susceptible to particular diseases than others and why susceptibility seemed to show a pattern of family or regional groups.[9] Such explanations arose through a focus on particular behaviors and family backgrounds, and these explanations were geared to the patterns observed in each disease. Since Chick Gin was first discovered in March 1900, six plague victims had been found in the ensuing search of Chinatown. All of the victims were Chinese. The only other time plague hit U.S. soil was the epidemic of 1899 in Honolulu, which also affected almost exclusively the Chinese community. To some extent, then, Wyman and the San Francisco public health authorities had some basis for focusing their attention on Chinatown and the Chinese given the evidence they had before them. However, many white physicians had died in their own investigations of plague in Asia (Lipson 1972), rendering fallible an interpretation of plague epidemiology that left whites outside the mapping of vulnerability.

The Chinese community was well aware of the fallibility of public health authorities in their latest actions attempting to force inoculation and limit movement outside San Francisco. On May 24 a case went before the circuit court on behalf of a Chinese merchant, Wong Wai, against Kinyoun. The case mostly focused upon the vaccine program, with the complaint that the vaccine was experimental, was highly toxic, had dangerous side effects, and was thus inappropriate for use in San Francisco. The lawyers went so far as to argue that plague had not been proven to exist in Chinatown, and since the vaccine was only good as a preventive, its use in a plague-free area was uncalled for. Kinyoun and the other health officials furthermore had not proven that Asians were especially susceptible to plague, making their actions that much more discriminatory and arbitrary.

The lawyers for the Chinese complainant also raised the issue of travel, claiming that the ordinance forbidding exit from San Francisco by Asians without a certificate of inoculation was discriminatory and precluded the right of Wong Wai and other Chinese to pursue a "lawful business" (Kraut 1994, 91). It was further claimed that the ordinance made no sense from a public health perspective, since movement within San Francisco by all Asians was permitted. If the Chinese were considered such a health threat, allowing their free access to all points within the city highlighted the arbitrary nature of the mandate against traveling outside the city. Obviously this raised the question of what motivations influenced Kinyoun and the board of health. On the one hand, precluding movement outside San Francisco was designed to prevent the spread of plague to the rest of the state and to regions outside California. This was of particular importance given that the issue of plague had caused considerable political fallout within the state government. It had also caused geopolitical ripples outside the state, with quarantines of California products and passengers implemented by Texas (Freuch 1901), New Orleans, Colorado, Mexico, Ecuador, and Sydney (Haas 1959).[10]

On the other hand, the argument against the ordinance brought out the contradictions of a public health policy based more on racial bias than on epidemiological deduction. Bodies both live and dead were being monitored with some degree of rigidity within Chinatown. All Chinese dead were inspected by a medical officer who looked for signs of plague and reported cases accordingly. Interestingly, the vast majority of cases inspected died of tuberculosis, not plague (Blue to Wyman, May 15, 1903). Although no examinations of other Chinese were ordered, their immediate physical environments were being invasively monitored and altered. Plague was assumed to lurk, as had smallpox, in every dark crevice and filthy corner of the district. Yet the mapping of a disease onto racially inscribed bodies and habitats had its converse in the mapping of immunity onto white San Francisco, including immunity from those same diseased bodies that issued forth from Chinatown. Not examining the sick, allowing free movement within and without Chinatown, and not quarantining contacts of plague victims thus did not accord with the epidemiological understanding of plague as a disease transmitted from person to person, but followed the logic of a "rice-eaters' disease."

The judge hearing the Wong Wai case, William Morrow, agreed with the arguments of the lawyers for the Chinese. On May 28, Morrow handed down a verdict that vindicated the claims of the Chinese, agreeing that Kinyoun and the board of health had acted in ways that did not accord with the health situation as it had been stated. He agreed, for example, that allowing movement within San Francisco but forbidding movement outside of it was illogical and arbitrary. And the actions of the travel and inoculation campaigns, according to Morrow, showed a degree of racial discrimination that found no rationale in public health rhetoric. Finally, the Wong Wai case contested the power of the federal and state governments to police the behavior of individuals or groups in the name of public health. At this time it was generally agreed that states had power to create regulations to protect the public health and that local boards of health and municipal legislatures had broad powers to determine the nature and extent of those regulations. But in the case of Wong Wai, San Francisco's charter nowhere gave the board of health the authority to legislate without a majority popular vote.

Kinyoun and the board of health were thus forced to back down on their inoculation and travel limitation plans, but it was not long before the next controversial move was made. Almost immediately after Morrow handed down his decision, the state board of health met with railroad officers, local and outside health officers, and merchants. After lengthy discussion, a health officer from Texas, W. F. Blunt, claimed that the most logical idea from a public health perspective was to limit the movements of the Chinese to the Chinese district, thus precluding the intermingling of Chinese with white residents of the city. To lend weight to his suggestion, he added that only then would Texas agree to lift its embargo of goods and passengers from San Francisco. The state board of health voted to pass the suggestion on to the San Francisco health board, which in turn approved the measure. Kinyoun added his sanction to it, stating that Chinatown "would always be a focus of plague infection" (see McClain 1988, 485). After getting the approval of the board of supervisors, a quarantine went into effect on May 31, 1900.

As to why this seemingly race-based legislation did not contradict the decision made by Morrow, one state board of health member specified that the inoculation campaign targeted a particular race, whereas the quarantine targeted an urban district. Accordingly, the quarantine was approved not for Chinatown per se but for the blocks bounded by Kearny, Broadway, Stockton, and California Streets. When it was realized that there were whites living in some pockets of these boundaries, the lines were redrawn to exclude them from the quarantine. All buildings inhabited by whites were designated as lying just outside quarantine boundaries.

A *San Francisco Examiner* reporter toured Chinatown soon after and concluded that it looked like a besieged city. Stores were closed; business had halted; and people gathered on the streets voicing their anger over the newest public health action. Though the Six Companies did not immediately threaten legal action, the Chinese consul did inquire of the board of health why it made no accommodation to ensure the continued viability of the district and its residents by providing food or compensation for the loss of jobs and businesses. The hardships occurring as a result of quarantine conditions, including the loss of jobs for many Chinese who worked outside Chinatown as well as the loss of income to merchants within Chinatown, added to the air of a beleaguered city. Eventually, food shortages occurred within the district, and food prices consequently rose (Kraut 1994). Nevertheless, the board of health made no motion to compensate the quarantined district.

On the contrary, further measures were being discussed by the board of health and some of the city's newspapers. In a meeting of the board of health, it was agreed that inspection and fumigation of all Chinese laundries, no matter where they were located in the city, were necessary in case any Chinese who escaped from Chinatown were hiding in them. The board also agreed to ask the mayor's help in getting the federal government to assist in the designation of a site outside of San Francisco for detaining suspected Chinese plague cases (Risse 1992). The latter resolution was the idea of Kinyoun, who had himself asked about a few different sites and had concluded that Angel Island would make the best one for transporting Chinese having or suspected of having plague. Since Kinyoun claimed that thousands of Chinese would need to be accommodated on the island, Charles McClain suspects that Kinyoun's real plan was to transport all Chinese to the island while Chinatown itself was burned to the ground and rebuilt (McClain 1988, 492).

The latter idea had gained currency in the city among both scientific and lay constituencies as the plague scare continued. The *Call of San Francisco,* along with the *San Francisco Chronicle,* had at first continued to deny the existence of plague in the city. The *Call* went so far as to invite a New York physician, George Schrady, out to San Francisco to investigate purported plague cases and to confirm that in fact plague did not exist. After first substantiating the newspaper's position, Schrady was invited to attend the autopsy of a Chinese body, where evidence of the plague bacillus was seen under a microscope. Schrady, and consequently the *Call,* were forced to retract their previous positions and to admit the existence of plague. Schrady's method of avoiding a total loss of face was to reassure San Francisco residents that the few cases of plague evident among the Chinese did not mean that the average white resident was at risk, so long as homes were kept clean. The *Call* also concluded that, even if a few cases of plague among the Chinese did not make an epidemic, the city's best bet in avoiding the threat was to raze Chinatown.[11]

Using rhetoric very similar to that used during smallpox epidemics, the newspaper opined, in its about-face, that "in no city in the civilized world is there a slum more foul or more menacing than that which now threatens us with the Asiatic plague. Chinatown occupies the very heart of San Francisco

[and] so long as it stands so long will there be a menace...of every form of disease, plague, and pestilence which Asiatic filth and vice generate" (*Call,* May 31, 1900, 6). Once more the discourse of location and the association of vice and disease were invoked to rationalize the obliteration of Chinatown. The Chinese were in the very center of the city, strategically located to infect the rest of San Francisco with their diseases. It was interesting that the *Call* could so easily resurrect this discourse even though Schrady and the public health constabulary had, through their respective rhetoric and actions, indicated that whites in San Francisco were relatively immune to the threats of an Asiatic disease. Epidemiology clearly had little place in the newspaper's racial politics, which instead relied upon a more visceral invocation of the horrors of plague.

Razing Chinatown went beyond newspaper advocation this time, however. By June 1900, the board of health was making plans to vacate fifteen hundred Chinese to Mission Rock, having received permission from the California Dry Dock Company to use its docking facilities on the island. Discussions were still underway to get permission from the federal government to vacate a much larger number of Chinese to Angel Island. In addition, an even stricter quarantine was to take effect for Chinatown, with street cars not allowed to pass through the district and with an actual fence and barbed wire to be put in place around the quarantined area. The number of armed guards patrolling the quarantined district was also doubled.

The added threat of deportation spurred the Chinese Six Companies to action, and by early June they had taken the case to federal court. The basic complaint was similar to the former case, that is, that the actions of the board of health were based on race and not on the interests of public health. More specifically, the lawyers for the Chinese Six Companies pointed out the inconsistencies in the board's actions. First, the quarantined district's perimeters clearly saw-toothed around those buildings occupied by whites, even if they lay within the boundaries assigned for isolation. This showed that the quarantine was a targeting not of an urban district but of the Chinese. Second, the quarantine covered entire blocks of buildings in which not a single case of plague had been found, bringing into question the public health purpose of quarantine if healthy people were being isolated. Third, the board failed to isolate those houses in which plague had occurred, with the result that uninfected people within Chinatown were not being protected. In barring exit to those Chinese who had not been exposed, the board of health was further endangering residents of the district. The board also had made no compensations in the form of food or money for the hardships it caused the Chinese during the quarantine. Finally, the lawyers raised the issue of deportation, which the board was planning without adequate rationale and which the Chinese were to endure for an unspecified period of time.

The case was again under the jurisdiction of Judge Morrow, and again Morrow sided with the Chinese complainants. On June 15 he ordered the quarantine of Chinatown to be lifted, reasoning that it was indeed an act based more on discrimination than on maintaining the public's health. He did allow the board of health to maintain quarantine of those houses in which plague victims or their contacts resided, recognizing that the isolation of those known to be infected from those who were not was the true purpose of quarantine, not the cordoning of an entire district composed overwhelmingly of uninfected individuals. Within hours, the board of health had complied with the judge's orders, instructing the police officers to call in their men, to again allow entry and exit of people and transportation, and to dismantle the wooden wall and barbed wire encircling Chinatown. This was the last time that the board of health attempted anything so controversial in its efforts to curb plague in Chinatown, even though calls for the district's removal from San Francisco continued through the next few years.[12]

The (Non)Science of Sanitation

Recalling Wyman's epidemiology of plague evidences the ease with which the previous century's association of filth and disease imbricated with the newer world of germs. In the case of plague, the bacillus was assumed to lurk most commonly in soils and dirt, making an emphasis on sanitation still relevant despite the advent of microscopes and other laboratory equipment in the battle against epidemic diseases. Accordingly, almost from the time Chick Gin was discovered in the hotel basement a campaign of vigorous sanitary cleansing and monitoring began in Chinatown and continued on and off for the next four years. Only then, in 1904, was Chinatown declared safe from the threat of plague and safe from the possibility of infecting the rest of the city. Of course even the sanitary measures adopted by the board of health regarding Chinatown cannot be examined outside the context of the Sinophobia that was so heightened during the previous decades and still extant in 1900 (Risse 1992). As McClain states it (1988, 454), Chinatown had already been "invested by decades of public health iconography with the character of a discrete and undifferentiated hub of disease." The discovery of even one case of plague was enough, then, to warrant sanitary measures aimed at the whole district.

The first step in this process was the house-to-house inspection by medical investigators during the initial, short-lived quarantine. This inspection was both to check the sanitary condition of Chinatown and to uproot any more cases of plague that might exist. No more cases were found at that time

(Risse 1992). With the discovery of four more cases on May 15, however, sanitary monitoring was stepped up (Haas 1959). Inspection and disinfection commenced of buildings where infected persons resided, as did the generalized sanitary cleaning of Chinatown. This process continued through the proceeding inoculation campaigns, second quarantine, and deportation plans. Unlike their response to previous actions, however, the Chinese Six Companies and Chinese consul agreed to provide full cooperation with these measures (Risse 1992).

At first, it seems that sanitation followed similar lines to the sanitary purging of Chinatown during the latter smallpox epidemics. By 1901, however, the process became both more systematic and intensified. Following the denial of plague's existence by several factions including newspapers, Mayor James Phelan, city merchants, and Governor Henry Gage, a federal health team of leading bacteriologists was commissioned by the secretary of the treasury and sanctioned by President McKinley. This commission was to go to San Francisco, investigate the situation in Chinatown, and find out once and for all whether or not plague existed in the city (Municipal Health Reports 1901, 491). Consisting of Simon Flexnor of the University of Pennsylvania, F. G. Novy of the University of Michigan, and L. F. Barker of the University of Chicago, the team arrived in San Francisco and had established their own laboratory by January 1901. They proceeded to examine thirteen dead Chinese, and by March 2 they sent word to Gage that they had confirmed six reported cases of plague, examined a seventh, and had seen three additional cases that had not been reported to the local board of health (Freuch 1901, 6).

In the words of John Williamson, the president of the city board of health, the team's investigation "was so conclusive in its nature as to result in measures being taken to cleanse Chinatown" (Municipal Reports 1901, 491). This was something of an understatement. The newest "cleansing" of Chinatown was coordinated "in accordance with an agreement between the Department and the authorities of the State of California and City of San Francisco" and was carried out "by a corps of physicians and employees of the State and city, under the advice and direction of a surgeon and a corps of assistants of the Marine Hospital Service" (Municipal Reports 1901, 491). Physicians inspected Chinese individuals; cases of plague were sought out; attempts were made to trace contacts of those infected; and a corps of workers emptied buildings of their belongings, burned them, then proceeded to fumigate, hose down, and chemically purge their interiors. By the time this particular sanitation episode was considered complete on June 21, 1901, 1,180 houses or a total of 14,117 rooms had been disinfected (Municipal Reports 1901, 491).

The hiatus between sanitary interventions did not last long, however. The number of plague cases found between March 1900 and the beginning of July 1901 totaled thirty-four. But between July and November 15, sixteen more cases were found (Municipal Reports 1901, 491). The somewhat intensified spread of the disease prompted another round of sanitary cleansing. Again, the cleanup was an effort that employed the latest scientific techniques for disinfecting and the latest techniques in precise coordination of personnel and physical environment. Donald Currie, one of the supervising physicians of the antiplague campaign, kept a journal from 1901 to 1905. In his July 23, 1901, entry, he stated that "inspecting of Chinatown moved to disinfecting, distribution of lime; streets are to be sprinkled three times a week with HgCl2 solution after sweepings. An additional person is to come in to spray unclean rooms and floors and unsanitary closets with a 2.5 percent solution of carbolic acid. Another person is requested to remove accumulated garbage and filth from back yards and courts" (Currie, July 23, 1901). Everyone had a specified job; each part of Chinatown was designated for its particular sanitary intervention; and the methodical makeover of a diseased district proceeded.

These sanitary proceedings continued off and on for the next two years. Despite the efforts, however, cases of plague continued to occur. By March 1903, it was decided by Rupert Blue, the assistant surgeon of the U.S. Marine Hospital Service in San Francisco, and other health authorities that sanitizing was not sufficient; in order to head off further plague cases, parts of Chinatown needed to be demolished (Blue to Wyman, June 15, 1903). At this point, Blue, Kinyoun, and others were focusing some attention upon the rat. Although the exact role of the rat in transmitting plague to humans was not understood, it was becoming clearer that its role was nonetheless significant. Sanitary cleaning measures did not necessarily target the rat or the rat's habitat; demolishing specific portions of Chinatown that were thought to harbor rats would therefore be more effective. Currie's March 23, 1903, plague journal entry describes the visit of several physicians for the purposes of discussing "radical measures for the eradication of some of the unsanitary nuisances in Chinatown. It was agreed that all 'excrescences' or structures placed in back areas, courts and spaces between buildings, preventing the ingress of air and sunlight, should be at once knocked down and dragged out" (Currie, March 23, 1903).

The work began on March 30, with a gang of men "supervised by a competent person" descending upon Chinatown and with axes "and other suitable bludgeons" knocking out the balconies enclosing closets and kitchens in the rear areas of buildings in Chinatown (Currie, March 30, 1903). On April 5 the condemnation of another twenty-six structures was approved by the board of health, this time frame structures located in backyards of Chinatown buildings (Currie, April 5, 1903). They subsequently were destroyed. The height of surveillance in sanitation was attained by May 15 of the same year, when Currie describes in his journal a "new inspection system" whereby an inspector was assigned at least one name of a Chinese resident in a building. The health official consequently was to familiarize himself with the sanitary quality of the building occupied by that resident, keeping an eye on any sanitary transgressions or even perhaps more subtle degenerations of sanitary status. Currie designated the system a sort of census of the Chinese district (Currie, May 15, 1903). It is clear that the purpose of this personalized system was to more closely monitor the spatial relations of individuals and their physical environment in Chinatown and to more quickly be able to condemn those structures not maintaining adequate sanitary standards.

Between March and October, 1903, 160 buildings in Chinatown were destroyed and 70 houses vacated (*San Francisco Chronicle,* October 17, 1903). Similar proceedings continued well into 1904, before Rupert Blue finally declared Chinatown free of plague (Haas 1959). Although not as draconian a measure as quarantine, the sanitary onslaught on Chinatown, and particularly the last stage of demolition, nevertheless warrants a raised eyebrow for the ways in which it was carried out. First, there is the question of whether Chinatown deserved the scrubbing it got given the small number of plague cases reported over the four-year period. In defense of the health authorities, one explanation of this might lie in the behavior of plague as observed in epidemics in Sydney and Calcutta. In those cases, plague also began tentatively, with only a few cases reported for two to three years before any significant outbreak finally occurred (Haas 1959). Yet the health authorities showed no compassion or sense of responsibility where hardships among the Chinese were concerned. The chemical agents used to disinfect Chinatown were themselves highly noxious if not toxic. As Currie himself stated, the chlorine gas escaping from the chlorinated lime compound used on the inside of houses "often sends the inhabitants of a house out to find fresh air" (Currie, March 1, 1903). Most structures would have been uninhabitable for a period of time after such treatment. The long-term health consequences of repeated use of chlorinated lime, carbolic acid, bichloride of mercury, and other noxious substances on the structures of Chinatown can only be guessed.

The demolition of structures was also a curious blend of older sanitation discourse and a new motivation for sanitary restructuring. Within the commentary by Blue and by Currie on the destruction of balconies and other added building structures there is a repeated mention of letting sunlight and air into the alleyways and byways of Chinatown. This is curious only in that sunlight and air were part of the sanitary discourse of the latter nineteenth and early twentieth centuries having to do with better health in general and with combating tuberculosis in particular. They have little to do with killing rats. In the next epidemic, the sanitary restructuring of the rest of San Francisco was very similar to that of Chinatown, but the language describing it was more accurate in targeting the demolition of structures because they were thought to harbor rats or to make optimal nesting sites for them. In this case the actions of the public health constabulary were similar, while the discourse behind them suggested divergent viewpoints about the urban districts being restructured. In the case of Chinatown, rhetoric still focused upon a political anatomy of body and landscape that was pathologized beyond plague.

The politics of plague and its attendant discourses cannot be complete without some mention of its broader context. In the case of San Francisco's first plague epidemic, the racialization of disease was mediated by a simultaneous attempt to deny its existence in any form or within any space in the city. This denial came from multiple parties, primarily city merchants, the governor of California, and eventually the California State Board of Health. Subsequent friction between state officials and city administrators is beyond the scope of this analysis, but the reasons for the denial are easy enough to locate in the forbidding psychological authority of the disease. For the commercial and administrative factions, the existence of plague in San Francisco signaled in effect the quarantining of the whole state of California from the rest of the country and the world. Commerce would end; trade would come to a halt; goods would no longer come into the state; and local products would find no out-of-state markets. It signified the death of California's economy. The danger of pretending that plague did not exist is easy enough to see now, and it was equally easy for public health officers to see at the time. Public health ultimately won out, but the point here is that for some, even plague's spatial concentration in a marginalized community did not preclude a much wider area of economic influence. Contestation of medical authority was greater here than in the case of smallpox, yet those who fought the racial framing of plague in 1900 did so in support not of the Chinese but of their own economic interests.[13]

Control, Contestation, and the Culture of Medical Knowledge

The actions taken by the federal and local health authorities against the Chinese constituted something akin to what Matt Hannah calls the "imperfect panopticon" (Hannah 1997), a system functioning much the same as Foucault's conceptualization of a panoptic environment, a "hierarchical structure of command unifying...three 'moments' of control: observation, judgment, and enforcement of behavior" (Hannah 1997, 347).[14] Yet the imperfect panopticon needs no institutional walls to reorder behavior, and in the case of plague in Chinatown, it did not stop at disciplining individuals but focused as well upon reordering physical surroundings. Paraphrasing David Armstrong again, this new gaze identified disease not just in the physical body but in the social body and its material terrain (Armstrong 1983, 8). It also identified the control of disease increasingly as an agenda of spatial control. A team of inspectors, city workers, and physicians thus constituted the "authoritative subjects" (Armstrong 1983, 8) who presided over the disciplining of an entire urban sector that once again, less than twenty years after the last smallpox epidemic, was designated as a center of epidemic disease. The more plague lingered, the greater the need to maintain a tight surveillance over spatial relations within Chinatown. Never before had these relations been monitored with such precision in the name of public health. In a missive from Assistant Surgeon Rupert Blue to Surgeon General Wyman in June 1903, Blue reports that a directory of permanent residents of Chinatown was being drawn up so that "a useful check can be had on the movements of the Chinese from place to place in the city" (Blue to Wyman, June 15, 1903).

On the one hand, this system served the purpose of tracing contacts of infected individuals, a task that made epidemiological sense but frustrated health officials for months. On the other hand, underneath its scientific mantle the rigid surveillance of Chinese individuals and their habitations exemplified the vestigial need to depathologize an urban district by normalizing its landscape and its residents. In other words, despite the new language of scientific elucidation, the need to normalize a deviant sector of society was still an imperative of public health. In this case, the conception of deviance focused less upon Chinese bodies than upon their physical surroundings. The rhetoric behind public health actions had largely shifted since the smallpox episodes to one of bacterial elimination, but the agenda was still heavily informed by miasmatic and moralistic theories of disease. The discourse of plague in 1900 was still very much one of normativity versus pathology, not one of bacterial transmission.

This focus was one of the parallels between the first plague epidemic and the smallpox epidemics of the previous century. Another was in the way that individuals reacted to public health policy. The Chinese did not just use the judicial system to contest the actions of local and federal health authorities during the four-year plague episode in Chinatown. As in smallpox epidemics, they also engaged in other tactical maneuvers that evidenced a profound distrust of public health authority. For example, the Chinese often hid their sick and dying in order to avoid the intrusive eyes and scalpels of white physicians, to the sustained frustration of the latter. The correspondence of Assistant Surgeon Rupert Blue with Surgeon General Wyman and the plague journal of Donald Currie are both peppered with commentary concerning the tendency of the Chinese to hide the bodies of their dead and to secret their sick to places where health inspectors were not likely to find them. In a May 9, 1901, journal entry, Currie recounts finding a sick Chinese child the previous day and reporting it to Blue, only to find the child gone the next day and its father refusing to tell where the child was hidden (Currie, May 9, 1901). In a letter to Wyman, Blue bemoans that "it is almost impossible to catch the Chinese contacts. They seem to know a suspicious case, and depart, like the fleas, before the body cools off" (Blue to Wyman, October 18, 1901).[15]

Part of the reason for the elusive behavior was the fear of quarantine and its attendant hardships. As in smallpox epidemics, many Chinese preferred the risk of infecting more members of their families by hiding their sick to the deprivations of enforced isolation. It became obvious enough during Chinatown's quarantine that public health officers had no intention of compensating the needs of those restricted to the district; neither was there reason to believe that compensation for home quarantine would be forthcoming. Symbolically, flagging Chinese homes forefronted a status already liminal because of ethnicity but made even more so by inscriptions of plague. It is no wonder that a family paid one hundred dollars to remove their plague-infected son from San Francisco to Oakland in order to avoid a quarantine and disinfection of their home (Blue to Wyman, September 24, 1901).

Other parallels to smallpox epidemics are obvious as well, including the focus on a racialized landscape in the production of disease, the subsequent calls for Chinatown's excision from the city, and calls for its sanitary purging. There were dissimilarities as well, though, the most significant perhaps being the absence of a district-wide quarantine in Chinatown during any of the smallpox epidemics. The even greater fear generated by plague probably played a role in driving this more drastic measure. The better understanding of germs and germ transmission during the plague epidemic probably contributed. The more contentious theories regarding smallpox as either a contagious disease or one derived from faulty sanitation might have acted as a curb on quarantining the entire district, even though Chinatown was seen as producing the disease. Whatever the theories used to explain each disease, however, the first plague outbreak must be seen in its larger historical context as an epidemic that struck a district already heavily imbued, to recount McClain's words, with an iconography of disease and of irreversible depravity. Rather than cut through the discursive depths of this iconography, medical knowledge displayed its own embeddedness within a widespread racial politics.

In this way the 1900 plague epidemic in San Francisco warrants comparison, in another historical direction, to the recent epidemiological interpretation of AIDS. The parallels have their obvious limitations, but on two particular counts they are instructive. The first involves again the social embeddedness of epidemiological interpretation, proving an inherent inability of medical science to act outside a political economy of the corporal (Foucault 1977).[16] In both plague and AIDS, a cultural politics of race and sex influenced an epidemiological framing of disease focusing attention upon the infective possibilities of social category rather than upon those urban political ecologies that would better support the logic of pathogenic transmission. What Cindy Patton says about AIDS holds true for both diseases, that "the central trope of normal, white, middle-class, adult health" became the normative model against which AIDS and plague were defined, and against which the deviant body was pathologized (Patton 1995, 341).

In both cases, too, epidemiological interpretations persisted despite evidence contradicting their validity. The earliest evidence of AIDS, for example, occurred in Los Angeles among five openly gay men in 1981. These men had come down with *Pneumocystis carinii* pneumonia (PCP), a condition that usually occurs only in those with defective or suppressed immune systems; there was no reason to believe that any of these young and otherwise healthy men should be vulnerable to PCP. By the next month a report had been published in the Center for Disease Control's *Morbidity and Mortality Weekly Report* (June 1981, 2) describing the condition of the five men. As an accompanying editorial noted, "the fact that these patients were all homosexuals suggests an association between some aspect of a homosexual lifestyle or disease acquired through sexual contact and *Pneumocystis* pneumonia in this population" (cited in Oppenheimer 1992, 53). As Oppenheimer comments, the hypothesis that homosexual status predisposed individuals toward immune deficiency was based on all of five cases from one community (Oppenheimer 1992, 53). Unspoken but implied is the probability that if similar cases of PCP had been discovered initially in young and otherwise healthy heterosexuals, initial epidemiological conclusions would not have focused upon sexual practice but upon other possible explanations.

Regarding this point Patton (1995, 340) makes the interesting comment that it was the depathologization of gays in the late 1970s and 1980s that even allowed the appearance of medical anomalies among gay men to be designated as a disease. She argues that had these cases occurred a decade previously, the still dominant pathologization of homosexual status would have offered sufficient explanation for why these men were dying. But though the later search for an etiologic agent for this syndrome supports Patton's contention, she overlooks these earliest, and sustained, epidemiological pro-nouncements concerning the intrinsic capacity of homosexual sex acts to cause disease. Poirier (1991) offers a contradictory contention that the des-ignation, and naming, of AIDS offered further ammunition to the idea of homosexuality as a disease. His analysis finds greater reflection in the actions following these first cases.

Yet cases did occur among heterosexuals early in the immune-deficiency scenario, the first only three months after the initial five cases. By June 1982, the *Morbidity and Mortality Weekly Report* stated that heterosexuals comprised a full 22 percent of those diagnosed with PCP or Kaposi's sar-coma, the other illness marking immune deficiency among the young and otherwise healthy (Oppenheimer 1992). Almost a third of these heterosex-ual cases were women (Oppenheimer 1992). Despite this significant pattern, the centuries-old association of disease and deviance continued to take prece-dence as epidemiologists focused undivided attention on finding connections between immune suppression and male homosexual sex. When the pathol-ogization of particular sex acts was not always supported by evidence from case studies, attention was turned to the other primary form of behavioral deviance among gay males, the use of recreational drugs such as amyl ni-trite. Despite conflicting evidence obtained in studies, associations between drug use, homosexual status, and immune suppression continued to find representation in the medical literature (Oppenheimer 1992).

With the added clarity of hindsight, it seems apparent that limiting epi-demiological focus to a still marginalized population served to place palatable limits (for those outside gay communities) on a disease terrifying both for its symptoms and for its lack of medical prevention or cure. For many commen-tators on the AIDS epidemic, the epidemiological history of the syndrome cannot be understood outside homosexuality's concomitant criminalization and pathologization.[17] As Poirier notes, the fear was/is one not just of phys-ical but of moral contagion from the gay community (Poirier 1991, 139). A new disease thus intensifies constructs of homosexual pathology, presenting an authoritative tool to reinforce socially constructed boundaries between the normal and the deviant. As in the case of plague, however, HIV/AIDS has also provided a means of contesting these boundaries. Groups such as ACT-UP have forced awareness of the many travesties perpetrated around the AIDS issue because of its perceived locus in the homosexual community. The sluggishness of federal reaction to the problem of HIV/AIDS, the lack of sufficient funding for medical research, the focus upon medical prevention over public health education, and the prudish nature of national outreach campaigns have all been protested over the course of the past fifteen years

(Watney 1986; Gilman 1995; Shilts 1987). Such movements have served less to break down the barriers erected between the normal and the marginalized and more to illuminate the questionable ideological foundations of those barriers.

The designation of plague as an Asian disease was made on even flimsier evidence. Previously mentioned was the historical precedence for presuming vegetarianism as a predisposing factor for the disease. Basing on one case the conclusion that plague would affect only the Chinese and Japanese communities in San Francisco was nonetheless not only unprecedented but scientifically fallible since white cases of plague had already occurred. Perhaps these previous cases were easy to ignore because they occurred in geographically distant places. Harder to discount were the white cases that occurred within San Francisco, but unlike early heterosexual cases of AIDS these abrogations were accommodated within the dominant epidemiological framework by tracing connections between infected whites and the Chinese community.

In one letter from Blue to Wyman dated September 23, 1901, Blue recounts the case of Alexander White, a seaman who came down with plague while on a ship transporting hay from northern California to San Francisco. In a subsequent letter dated September 25, Blue clearly indicates that he has been trying to find the missing factors connecting White to the Chinese community. Failing to place him anywhere near San Francisco's Chinatown, he concludes that White also visited the California Powder Works at Pinole, "where large numbers of Orientals are employed" (Blue to Wyman, September 23 and 25, 1901). Interestingly, Blue does not specify whether any plague outbreaks had occurred among the Pinole Chinese; the mere fact of their ethnic status was sufficient to implicate plague's presence. On October 4 of the same year, another missive from Blue to Wyman confirmed the death of another white patient, this time a woman. Again Blue bemoans that the source of infection was not easy to trace, but clearly this case provided more abundant possibilities for him. First, the woman's father and son were teamsters, their work frequently taking them in and out of Chinatown. The father in particular had just hauled goods for a Chinese merchant. And then, too, the family lived in the Hotel Europa, located just one block north of Chinatown (Blue to Wyman, October 4, 1901). The source of infection must surely be located in either of these possibilities.

Indeed Blue states outright what few, if any, epidemiologists in the AIDS epidemic would explicitly articulate: the actual *desire* to keep a disease limited to an undesirable community. In the September 25 letter to Wyman, Blue states his preference for finding a Chinese origin to the White plague case, a desire that explains why he looked so hard for Chinese links to the white cases of plague and consciously ignored other possible sources of infection (Blue to Wyman, September 25, 1901). Blue's explanation for this desire derived from the greater difficulties of containing a more dispersed epidemic. In so stating the case, however, Blue revealed the underlying preference to keep dominant the simultaneous inscriptions of disease and social deviance on the bodies of plague victims (Patton 1995, 340). Plague, after all, had become part of the lexicon defining the Chinese as a separate community and social category. As with smallpox in the nineteenth century, plague at the turn of the new century was an integral component to keeping clearly demarcated the boundaries of a foreign entity within the urban body. Epidemic dispersion to white communities thus would allow at least the possibility of a dissolution of these boundaries and the integration of Chinatown into the normative social body.

A second parallel between the plague of 1900 and early AIDS epidemiology lies in their degree of spatialization, each disease localized in and therefore transforming areas associated with the respective target populations. In the case of AIDS, a pathologization of sex acts and recreational activities inevitably led to a public health focus on those nonprivate spaces in which such activities were likely to take place. Gay bars, discos, dance halls, and bathhouses subsequently were reproduced from relatively marginalized loci of celebratory deviance to highly stigmatized nodes of deadly disease. Previously the mainstream heterosexual public either had paid little attention to these places or had raised various degrees of concern over the scandalous excesses said to go on inside these urban spaces of gay sexual liberation. The emphasis was a moral one centered on the type and degree of sexual activities, but also on the fact that these had broken out of the private bedrooms of America into more accessible public spaces. The early AIDS epidemiological focus on these spaces provided medical authority the opportunity to reconstruct them not just as moral nuisances but as points of contagion threatening to disseminate a still-mysterious but deadly affliction to more "mainstream" locations. Excision of such threats from the urban landscape seemed the only option. The later inclusion of intravenous drug use as a signifier of risk meant a parallel production of inner-city neighborhoods as not only marginalized but contagious locations. In this case, the newer layer of meaning rationalized policies of neglect or a variant of sanitary overhaul — gentrification.

The sanitization of Chinatown, the closing of gay bathhouses, and the neglect of inner cities all exemplify Alan Pred's contention that struggles over power are inevitably struggles over space (Pred 1984). The power relations here were largely shaped by medical knowledge couched as scientifically objective, yet embodying social ideologies of normativity that informed subsequent public health actions. The need to confront and reform the spatial representations of *non*normativity exemplifies Lefebvre's question, "What is an ideology without a space to which it refers, a space which it describes, whose vocabulary and links it makes use of, and whose code it embodies?" (Lefebvre 1991, 44). Medicine's authority, in other words, was and is grounded in its ability to pathologize spaces. In so doing, it invests in them particular meanings that create the need for control by public health or epidemiological agencies. But pathologization also rationalizes the normative *re*production of these spaces. Medical authority thus not only makes use of the vocabulary of particular spaces but appropriates and reissues it in a different code that signifies a "healthy" (i.e., safe) return to the mainstream. As the above three examples attest, however, the pathologization of space is not necessarily a predictor of how it can be reproduced, since the processes of normalization are multiple and varied. The next epidemic of plague in San Francisco illustrated the medical success of this process, at the same time that it forced a complete respatialization of plague's pathology.

1907: The Architecture of Redemption

On Wednesday, April 18, 1906, San Francisco was hit in the early morning hours with an earthquake that left much of the city in rubble. The damage left hundreds of people homeless, a good deal of the city's infrastructure paralyzed, damaged, or defunct, and services strained. Recovery began almost immediately but was slow, the process of cleaning up coinciding with the need to build tent cities for the homeless, to resurrect needed services including hospitals, and to address fractured infrastructures such as transportation. Not surprisingly, the sustained urban ruins signified to health officials a nightmare of public health hazards that did not take long to materialize. Two problems causing the greatest trepidation were the broken sewer lines and water pipes, meaning that much of San Francisco had neither potable water for everyday use nor a functioning septic system.

But as with many posthazard situations, it was not infrastructural problems alone but the broader scenario of devastation that created the right conditions for public health disaster. Descriptions of the city made by the city health officer in 1907 give some indication of the state San Francisco was in and the degree to which the lives of its residents were reconfigured and placed in jeopardy of disease. "The squares, public parks and vacant lots were packed with the stricken multitude, and without sanitary conveniences of any kind. . . . Sick and well were confusedly packed together; water supply cut off; sewers broken and no protection from the elements, which were unusually severe for this time of the year" (Municipal Reports 1907, 515). In addition to the victims of the earthquake, hundreds of workers poured in to the city from surrounding areas to help in the rebuilding process. These, too, were housed in makeshift tent cities (Todd 1909). All available public plots of land previously intended for the health and recreation of the city ironically were turned into overcrowded, poorly sanitized, and unhealthy refugee camps. In addition to being crammed into every available public space, the homeless were also quartered in streets, stables, and those basements left intact. Temporary latrines were set up next to tent camps, but these were found by teams of inspectors to be unscreened, uncovered, and close enough to the camps to present health hazards. The onslaught of flies engendered by the latrines was exacerbated by the overflow and the consequent deposit of excreta on surrounding areas (Municipal Reports 1907, 519). Makeshift kitchens were often found to be located close to these latrines, sharing the same army of flies and, given the lack of sanitation, helping to propagate infection through the food they produced.

The disease most likely to flourish in these conditions was typhoid fever, and accordingly the number of cases soared in the months following the earthquake. In April 1906 there were 7 cases of typhoid under observation; by June of 1907, 1,279 cases had been reported, with 228 deaths (Municipal Reports 1907, 518, 524, 590). Diarrheic diseases also rose to 108 deaths from a 1902 figure of 63 (Municipal Reports 1907, 590; 1902, 745). Typhoid cases were treated aggressively, a "rigid inspection" system initiated to locate each case, keep it under control, and trace contacts (Municipal Reports 1907). Latrines were disinfected and emptied more often; kitchens were inspected; flies were targeted; and arrests were made for unscreened food stores and butcher shops. Finally, a ward for typhoid cases was opened in the City and County Hospital (Municipal Reports 1907). Cases gradually diminished due to these efforts, and over time as people began moving back into rebuilt homes and potable water again became available, typhoid reverted to negligible numbers.

As it turned out, typhoid and diarrheic diseases were not the worst problems with which public health officers would have to contend. On May 27, 1907, over a year after the earthquake, a sailor died from plague in the U.S. Marine Service Hospital. By the end of September, there were 38 positive cases, 21 suspicious cases, and 22 deaths from the disease (Blue to Glennan, September 22, 1907). The second epidemic to hit San Francisco was more dispersed, infected more people, and took greater efforts to control than the previous epidemic, even though it proved less costly in terms of lives. By the time it was over in October 1908, 160 cases had been reported, and 78 were dead (Todd 1909). The good news in those numbers was a reduction in mortality rate from over 95 percent in 1900 to just under 50 percent, a difference attributed to earlier detection and treatment (Todd 1909, 9).

In terms of the localized symbolic and literal mapping of plague, the most significant difference between the two epidemics was that in the second, almost all of the victims were white. Although the initial focus seemed to hover in the North Beach Italian district, it soon became apparent that virtually every district in San Francisco was affected except for three: Sunset, Richmond, and Chinatown (Todd 1909, 9). On the one hand, it is difficult to explain why the first two were not impacted, except that they were located at some distance from the center of the city, where the initial focus of disease occurred. They were also newer and therefore less densely populated than those districts closer to downtown. Finally, they were farther from the main centers of earthquake destruction around North Beach, South of Market, and downtown. On the other hand, it became apparent that Chinatown was not affected because of the thorough nature of its sanitary makeover during the previous epidemic. It was scoured and streamlined, and even though it also took a beating during the earthquake, many of its foundations and secondary structures had been built over with cement in the sanitizing campaign of 1900–1904. The state of the city, and the configuration of the epidemic, had in essence become mirror-opposites of 1900: Chinatown was the "normalized" district, the one to be emulated as the rest of San Francisco tried to climb out of its sanitary morass and curtail the epidemics confronting it. Typhoid was expected, but plague brought with it an entirely different cognitive map for many residents of the city.

As Frank Todd philosophically stated it in his firsthand account of the 1907 epidemic, "One of the peculiar characteristics of plague epidemics ... is the readiness with which a community will believe some other community has it, and the distrust it has for any evidence of its own infection" (Todd 1909, 34). Plague in the lexicon of the general populace was still an Asian disease, an affliction that did not impact white society and to which white districts of San Francisco should have been immune. Evidence to the contrary was incontrovertible, yet much of San Francisco did not want to admit that the discursive epidemiological rendering of the disease and its attendant physical and symbolic mapping might have to be reconfigured. As further articulated by Todd, "plague no longer [was] a typically Oriental disease, nor wholly a filth disease, nor the peculiar affliction of vegetarians. Yet it was curious how hard these ideas were to dispel, even in the face of the evidence furnished by white men's funerals" (Todd 1909, 38). Convincing came during a large gathering of businessmen and other citizens called to a meeting on the floor of the Merchant's Exchange in January 1908 to hear about the state of the epidemic.

A map of cases was shown to the audience, and "to the mortification of many present, the only sanitary part of San Francisco except a couple of outlying districts, appeared to be Chinatown" (Todd 1909, 54).

A shift in the spatial focus of public health response to plague came as well with the elucidation of its epidemiology in 1905. Based on the studies of the Indian Plague Commission, the role of the flea in transmitting plague to rats, and subsequently to humans, was finally understood (Todd 1909). By 1907, the commission had published its findings, and the role of humans in the dissemination of plague receded to make room for the role of the flea and the rat (Risse 1992, 269). Elaborating on Todd's claim, the language of susceptibility focusing on behavioral mechanisms such as diet or racial status no longer could sustain credibility in the face of epidemiological evidence tracing plague from fleas that were brought into contact with humans through infected rats. The language of susceptibility subsequently shifted to focus on possibilities of exposure to infected rats. In so doing, public health attention began to focus on those built structures, building materials, and architectural styles that offered greater possibility of harboring the bacillus.

Since the earthquake, the number of rats had indeed been growing exponentially, the destroyed areas of the city serving effectively as a breeding ground for rodents. In a letter from Rupert Blue to Wyman in September 1907, Blue describes the rat situation with a keen eye to San Francisco's microgeographies: "The ruins and piles of building material, and the broken and choked sewers form excellent nesting places, while the warehouses and uncollected garbage furnish an unlimited food supply. In addition, the houses for the most part are unprotected against the ingress of rats and other vermin" (Blue to Wyman, September 22, 1907). The burnt-out areas suffered the highest encroachment of rats, but Blue was quick to specify that the situation was in fact widespread, few areas of the city being immune to the rodent or its fleas. Worst hit of all were the refugee camps and tent cities with their sanitation problems and overcrowding (Blue to Wyman, September 22, 1907). As Guenter Risse states it, rats became the most visible reminders of the recent earthquake and the state of physical and sanitary ruin still characterizing the city (Risse 1992, 269).

An epidemiological breakthrough helped mitigate plague's psychological impact, yet the second wave of epidemic in six years caused some panicked movement within San Francisco. Within the first few months, a small exodus of urban residents occurred, particularly among the Italians, whose district seemed at first to be the locus of the disease (Blue to Glennan, September 27, 1907). But the greatest area of concern, as with the first epidemic, came on a larger scale. The prospect of an embargo on San Francisco goods, either by the rest of the state, by the United States, or by foreign countries, was a threat that needed immediate attention from public health authorities and city and state administrators. The improved worldwide surveillance of the disease this time precluded any possibility of denying its existence in San Francisco, and in fact no attempts were made to do so. Greater honesty, however, made more urgent the economic imperatives of eradication given San Francisco's struggle to regain its status as a major city of commerce and finance after the devastations of the earthquake (Risse 1992).

The recall to San Francisco of Rupert Blue signaled the first serious move in the direction of eradication. Not only was Blue already familiar with the disease in San Francisco, but his arrival also meant the addition of much-needed funding from the U.S. Public Health Service and the U.S. Marine Hospital Service.[18] One of Blue's early communications to his superiors in Washington indicated the daunting task he felt lay ahead of him this time around (Blue to Glennan, September 27, 1907). The fears expressed during the last epidemic, that the disease would spread to multiple sites of infestation, had in fact occurred beyond expectations, as articulated in Blue's statement that "the bacilli are to be found all over the city" (Blue to Glennan, September 27, 1907). Any thoughts toward containing the spatial purview of the bacillus were thus pointless, leaving the campaign the task of limiting cases and addressing the numerous spaces already harboring rat populations. To a disconsolate Blue, it would "take many months to eradicate the infection; possibly years" (Blue to Glennan, September 27, 1907).

In the few years since his work on the 1900 plague epidemic, though, Blue had kept up with the latest epidemiological and bacteriological studies of plague, and his new plans reflected the increasing representation of science in the application of antiplague tactics. Unlike the mixed discourse behind the 1903 Chinatown sanitation campaign, the citywide rat extermination plan of 1907 would be carried out with "the accuracy born of scientific knowledge" (cited in Risse 1992, 273). Science, in this case, meant the translation of epidemiological knowledge into the reproduction of space, as the primary means of obliterating the plague bacillus came through reconfiguring the built landscape. It also meant an increased authorization for medical control over space. Whereas previous public health purview extended over sanitary practices, antiplague efforts now rationalized its surveillance over the structural foundations of domestic and economic practice. The previous epidemic engendered this increased surveillance, but only for a delimited district; the second campaign extended medical control over an entire city. As such, the campaign was sweeping in reach, targeting every district, area, building, and microspace known or thought to be capable of housing rats. It was also uncompromising in the degree to which it transformed these areas, either through obliterating them entirely or through rebuilding them with different building materials and, when applicable, different architectural styles. Elaborating upon Foucault's contention that disciplining the body was the response to the outbreak of epidemic diseases (Foucault 1977, 138), in the case of the second plague epidemic it was above all the disciplining of space that took precedence, with the disciplining of bodies a necessary corollary. The result was a reconstitution of the city's domestic and economic landscapes.

Increased control over urban space was evident in the first step of the antiplague process, involving a division of San Francisco into thirteen sanitary districts (Blue to Glennan, September 27, 1907). Monitoring of each of these was facilitated by the assignment of an office, a surgeon, and a corps of inspectors who traced cases of the disease and their contacts. A team of laborers was also assigned to each district to begin the process of trapping and exterminating rats, but this task was also spread to the public at large. Responding to the pervasive reach of the epidemic and its rodent transmitters, Blue's tactic this time was to elicit the public's aid in widening the net of public health authority. As figure 4.1 illustrates, billboards encouraged all citizens to do their part in fighting the epidemic by building domestic defenses against the rat. The dispersion of responsibility increased surveillance of residential areas, but in case the menacing picture of a rodent did not spur enough people into action, a pecuniary reward was offered for every rat brought in to municipal laboratories for inspection (Risse 1992, 274).

In the meantime, quarantining the infected in their homes was made difficult by the breakdown in infrastructure and the fact that many victims were homeless. The City and County Hospital, long a source of shame to the city, was finally condemned after the earthquake, and a makeshift contagion pavilion for plague victims was erected. This structure was located on the grounds of the old hospital and consisted of several small buildings built on stilts. Raising buildings off the ground was an architectural adaptation that prevented rats from nesting by exposing the ground underneath and allowing cats and other rat-eating animals access (Blue to Wyman, September 22, 1907). The plague hospital was in turn surrounded by a fence of galvanized iron eight-feet high, preventing the ingress of rats but also sending the clear signal that the hospital was a site of contagion to be avoided by anyone other than medical personnel and patients (Blue to Wyman, September 22, 1907). The homes of plague victims, when there were any, were invaded by the district inspectors who rid the houses of fleas, sanitized them, and when necessary tore down those structures such as cellars and backyard decks offering the best opportunity for rat-breeding (Risse 1992).

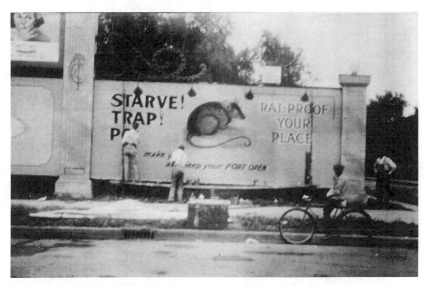

Figure 4.1. "Rat-Proof Your Place." Courtesy of the National Archives.

Blue's tactics of scientific surveillance and community participation seemed to be working when viewed through the declining numbers of plague cases. Sixty confirmed cases occurred during September, followed by thirty-one in October, forty-one in November, and only eleven in December (Risse 1992, 276). The decline caused Blue concern, however, because he was afraid that improved statistics would lead to lethargy among residents of the city — a dangerous prospect with the coming of summer and its favorable conditions for flea infestation. Accordingly, Blue intensified his outreach to the public, initiating educational meetings to inform the public of the disease and its epidemiology and pressing the city government to pass initiatives that would make mandatory the previously voluntary cleanup of residences. By March 2, 1908, an ordinance was passed "providing sanitary regulations . . . to prevent the propagation and spread of the bubonic plague" (Ordinance 1908).

The new regulations were thorough in their specifications for recon-struction. All walls of basements and buildings, storerooms, warehouses, residences, and other buildings; chicken yards, pens, coops and houses; and barns and stables were to be rebuilt to make them impervious to rats. This meant that wood would have to be replaced with concrete or other rat-proof building material, and floors replaced by concrete or gravel. Walls of stables had to be made of concrete at least three inches thick, and the manure had to be placed in galvanized iron, tin, or zinc boxes. Chicken coops and pig sties

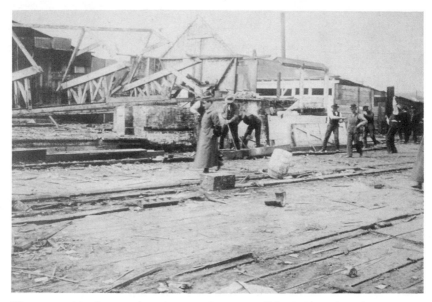

Figure 4.2. Tearing up the wharves. Courtesy of the National Archives.

had to have concrete floors and wire enclosures, and even wooden laundry decks — abundant particularly in working-class areas of the city — had to be destroyed and replaced with concrete. Building foundations were required to be constructed of concrete or brick and to extend one foot above the surface, and even markets were to be repaved in cement. Every residence and business was required to keep rat traps, and the dumping of garbage anywhere except in regulation garbage cans with tight-fitting lids was prohibited. Finally, the 1908 ordinance gave inspectors the authority to enter any building or private residence between the hours of nine and five to monitor its sanitary state and to present fines or make arrests in the event of transgressions (Ordinance 1908; Todd 1909).

Accordingly, during 1908 the majority of the city's numerous wooden structures were razed. The waterfront and industrial areas changed appearance as warehouses were torn down and replaced with reinforced concrete, and the wharves were repaved in cement (figure 4.2). Commercial zones changed as wooden sidewalks were torn up and replaced by concrete slab (figure 4.3); markets were cemented; and stall owners rebuilt their portable businesses to fit specifications. Working-class residential neighborhoods in particular were reconfigured as commonplace wooden laundry decks were torn down and replaced by cement or gravel, foundations were rebuilt, and

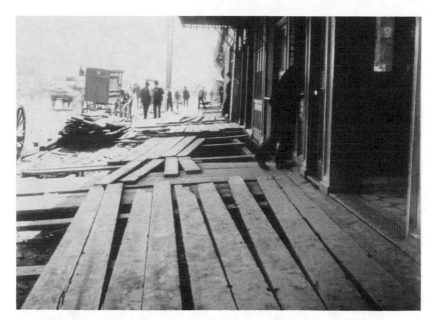

Figure 4.3. Replacing city sidewalks. Courtesy of the National Archives.

stables were torn down or adapted (figure 4.4). Blue's ardent wish was being realized: "The disease [was being] built out of existence. This is the hope of San Francisco and in time that city will be one block of concrete throughout" (Todd 1909, 218). Few individuals other than public health officials would look upon this prospect with such obvious satisfaction, but the result of San Francisco's transformation into a modern landscape of cement preeminence was indeed a lower population of rats.

For many the transformation meant loss of economic means when the cost of restructuring proved prohibitive. The most visible example of this was the virtual extinguishing of San Francisco's domestic chicken industry. Prior to the 1907 plague epidemic, a significant proportion of the city's supply of chickens came from backyard growers supplementing their incomes. The necessity of building new coops with inches-thick concrete floors and high-grade wire mesh was a larger capital outlay than most of these small producers could afford. The city's chicken supply consequently shifted to Petaluma (Todd 1909). Similar closures occurred with other small retailers, whose unconverted stands of merchandise and food items were boycotted by consumers newly aware of the hazards of wooden structures (Todd 1909).

The new sanitary method of spatial dissection was especially evident on the domestic front, where previously private facets of household structure and

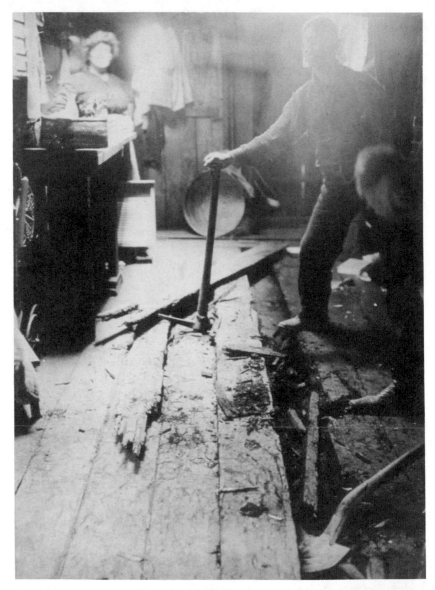

Figure 4.4. Tearing out the laundry deck. Courtesy of the National Archives.

domestic practice were scrutinized. For this, Blue found the "conscientious housewife" (Todd 1909) a more effective agent than medical inspectors, and he accordingly pressed these housewives into action in their neighborhoods. According to Risse, women volunteers served as perhaps the most energetic surveillance force during the last year of the plague campaign (Risse 1992, 280; Todd 1909). They monitored their neighbors to make sure that garbage was placed in regulation cans, laundry decks were rebuilt to specification, rat traps were properly laid, and domestic premises were kept sanitized. They called mothers' meetings to preach the word of sanitation. But they also extended their policing purview to educational and commercial fronts where they "woke up" schools and got them cleaned, inspected hotel kitchens, candy stores, factories, and restaurants, and monitored the state of street cars and lodging houses (Todd 1909, 110). They even pressed to have trash cans placed in parks and on city beaches (Todd 1909, 112). The reach of this organized force was pervasive and enduring, their efforts according to Todd resulting in a change in the garbage disposal practices of an entire city (Todd 1909, 112).

On their part, the Society of Elks encouraged their male members to cooperate with the team of federal and city health inspectors and to do their part "in suppressing the scoffer, the man who laughs in his ignorance, and who in that ignorance wants to trifle with a situation like this" (cited in Todd 1909, 254). A mass meeting was also called by the merchants of San Francisco in January 1908 to better educate themselves about the epidemic and its prevention tactics and to offer material support for the campaign (Todd 1909).

The spirit of self-surveillance and dispersed policing was indeed strong in the last year of the campaign, and by all accounts it seems to have paid off by ending the campaign earlier than might have been the case had the medical inspectors been left to manage the task by themselves. By October 23, 1908, Blue reported the last plague-infested rat in the San Francisco laboratory, and the campaign to fight the epidemic was effectively ended soon after (Risse 1992). San Francisco could not be characterized as one entire block of cement, and indeed much still remained to be done in the way of rebuilding after the earthquake. But Blue's hope of building an epidemic out of existence was realized, proving that at least in the case of this epizootic the most effective public health measures centered on space and its regulated reproduction.

Conclusion

Though many of the public health actions taken during the first plague epidemic were similar to those enforced during smallpox epidemics, there were differences that bear investigation. A primary one was epistemological. Unlike smallpox, there was relatively good understanding of plague's etiology even in 1900, with an extensive embrace of the germ theory by the turn of the century and the discovery of the plague-causing bacterium in 1894 (Kraut 1994). Yet the capacity of scientific understanding to be influenced by cultural practice became evident with the way in which the first plague epidemic in San Francisco was racialized — a throwback to the smallpox epidemics even though this time public health authorities had the tools of better etiologic understanding and bacteriological investigation to aid them. What changed to some extent was the language of racialized discourse, still accommodating the older association of depravity and disease while introducing a more medicalized language of susceptibility centered on diet and racial background.

A second difference was the reaction of the Chinese to the consequences of a racialized interpretation of disease. More than once, Chinese authorities challenged in federal court the actions taken against Chinatown by both municipal and federal public health authorities. Each time, they won. These contestations did nothing to change the ways in which Chinese diet and hygiene were taken as epidemiological explanation of disease and used ultimately to signify a pathologized collective Chinese body and district. Yet they did successfully mitigate the material consequences of this medical framing, thwarting the more severe practices and spatial monitoring by municipal authorities and managing to create for the Chinese a semblance of equal treatment in the face of inequitable scientific interpretation.

The contestation of public health authorities' interpretations of plague illuminates as well the multiplicity of discourses constituting the experience of disease. This was true for smallpox, but in the case of the first plague epidemic a contravention of dominant medical discourse came from another authoritative source, the legal system. The Chinese won their cases in court because the judge in each instance undermined medical authority in pointing out the racist political agenda of public health action. The setback was a minor one, however. Medical discourse remained dominant because physicians were considered the most authoritative source of disease interpretation, and as a consequence the racialized interpretation continued to receive widespread public support outside the Chinese community. The 1900 plague epidemic is thus instrumental in showing the difficulty nondominant discourses have in gaining support, even when they have authoritative institutional provenance. It also shows the difficulties of undermining medical discourses when they so obviously resonate with the ideological needs of a particular place in time (see Gilman 1988). The parallels to AIDS are apparent, which is to say that the many constituencies opposing dominant epidemiological interpretations of AIDS have succeeded in illuminating the political location of these interpretations, but not in eliminating their social influence. Medical discourses are many times enduring precisely because they have the capacity to work hegemonically, eliding political agenda with scientific understanding and promoting a politics of the normal in the name of public health.

The second plague epidemic emerged from a different social and scientific context than the first, meaning that different questions were raised concerning its impact and different responses were generated against its assaults. In the few intervening years since the first plague campaign, bacteriology had gained preeminence among medical practitioners, public health officials, and even the public. The full elucidation of plague's epidemiology made clearer the measures needed to prevent further cases of the disease and to quash the hold of the bacillus within the city. It informed the need to focus attention more on infected rodents and their territorial domains than on infected individuals in preventive efforts. It consequently shifted the discourses of susceptibility away from the personalized invectives of racial origin to the depersonalized arena of spatial relations.

Yet the degree to which medical knowledge alone eliminated social discrimination from plague's interpretive context needs questioning. The history of epidemics has rarely shown the capacity of medical authority alone to purge discrimination from social responses to disease even when epidemiological understanding is extensive. In the case of the second plague epidemic, equal weight must be given to the fact that most of the city except Chinatown was overrun with rats, and only 3 out of 160 victims of the disease were Chinese. The spatial focus of the second epidemic, in other words, necessitated a change in its discursive framing.

The racial delineation between infected and immune largely dissolved within San Francisco, but this in part simply shifted the boundaries of culpability. Finishing Blue's statement on preventive measures, his desire was to cement the city so that "the gateway to the Orient [would be] closed against plague" (cited in Todd 1909, 218). Even if whites were now susceptible to the disease, its origins remained predominantly Asian. The modus operandi of public health action was to make the city not just healthy for its residents but safe against further bacteriological attack from a still-threatening if more distant Oriental "Other." To some extent Blue's statement was justified economically and epidemiologically because plague at the time was perceived to be endemic to India (Todd 1909, 218). The degree to which San Francisco engaged in trade with Asian countries could make the city constantly vulnerable to infected ships from Asian ports and subsequently economically vulnerable to trade embargoes from other countries. Yet Blue's rhetoric did not extend to other geographic regions, including Australia and parts of Europe, which were impacted by plague on a periodic basis and with which San Francisco interacted commercially. In essence Blue was engaging in a common practice of placing geographic boundaries on a disease still threatening despite its subjection to medical control (Gilman 1988). There was still the threat that plague would return, even if the source was now exogenous rather than internal.

The plague bacillus in fact remained relatively close by, spreading across San Francisco Bay and settling into the rodent population of much of California and the Southwest. It remains there still, but the cement barriers of San Francisco's cityscape, begun in 1908 and continued thereafter, have continued to hold off further incursions of the bacillus. The second round of plague was the last major episode of epidemic disease with which San Francisco would contend until the appearance of AIDS eighty years later. This left public health officials to focus their attention on a more long-standing and costly health problem, tuberculosis.

5

REFORMING BODIES

Poverty, Discipline, and the Sanatorium Experience

But this deprivation, into which millions are born and hundreds of thousands are dragged by impoverishment, does indeed disgrace. Filth and misery grow up around them like walls, the work of invisible hands.
— Walter Benjamin, *Reflections*

The turn of the century brought with it shifts in medical and social agendas, each of which was integrally related to the other. On the medical front, tuberculosis took center stage nationwide. The subsidence of infectious epidemics such as smallpox, plague, and cholera meant that public health officials could focus their attention on the less dramatic but more insidious problem of tuberculosis. Robert Koch's discovery of the tubercle bacillus in 1882 and the subsequent acceptance of tuberculosis as a contagious disease contributed as well to dissolving the previous century's complacency concerning this disease. By the early twentieth century, the pervasive hold of tuberculosis over urban populations[1] was increasingly recognized, particularly with the help of better statistics and better diagnostic capabilities.[2] The mortality rate for tuberculosis nationwide in 1900 was 201.2 per 100,000 population, accounting for 10 to 15 percent of all deaths. Among those fifteen to forty-four years old, tuberculosis still accounted for one-third of all deaths.[3] It was finally being decried as the most important public health topic of the times, and the antituberculosis campaign consequently was born. By 1904 the National Tuberculosis Association was formed, and many states followed suit with the establishment of state and local tuberculosis associations.

But the antituberculosis campaign cannot be analyzed outside of its larger social context. During the last years of the nineteenth century and the early years of the twentieth, the attention of municipal administrations, welfare agencies, private philanthropic organizations, and the new breed of professional sociologists was increasingly fixed upon one thing, the city. Across the country, cities registered huge increases in population in the early decades of the new century (Boyer 1978, 189). Not only did the increase of industrial manufacturing attract migrants to cities from surrounding rural areas, but migration from Europe picked up pace after a brief lull in the 1890s. From 1900 to 1917, 17 million immigrants entered the United States (Boyer 1978).

But it was not just the degree of growth but the nature of it that worried officials and social commentators. First, a higher proportion of those migrating into the country went to cities and stayed in them, making this latest wave of immigration a particularly urban phenomenon. Always the largest magnet for European newcomers, New York City added 2.2 million people in the first two decades of the twentieth century (Boyer 1978), but every other major urban center of the country gained significant new constituencies as well. Second, a significant proportion of those migrating in the early twentieth century were impoverished workers from poor regions of southern and eastern Europe. These individuals crossed the Atlantic in search of better fortune, but more often found grinding poverty in their new urban habitats. The swelling of cities thus translated into the sizable increase of an urban underclass and an urban landscape disproportionately filled with tenements, lodging houses, shanties, and other structures of poverty. This shift in the social and physical landscapes of cities in turn brought about a new interpretation of their meaning within the context of American society.

One of the dominant discourses at this time concerned the crisis of order in American cities, a crisis unleashed by the proliferation of poverty and its attendant blights of urban degradation — crime, welfare dependency, and disease (Boyer 1978; Ward 1989; E. Wilson 1991). Cities were becoming metaphors for a particularly ominous brand of chaos as fears focused upon rising numbers of unemployed, increased awareness of infectious disease among slum-dwellers, and the sense that the growing ranks of the "have-nots" could eventually rise up in organized confrontation with the "haves." It was in part a problem of boundaries. Poor neighborhoods were no longer contained and relatively diminutive portions of city maps. Slums were now often themselves imaged as infectious diseases, threatening to take over middle- and upper-class domains as they advanced inexorably across urban topographies. Streets were spaces where class boundaries dissolved, the massive numbers of poor mingling promiscuously with the moneyed, threatening to degrade better-groomed bodies and minds in their proximity and sheer numbers (E. Wilson 1991). American society was for the first time a predominantly urban society, but according to many the quality of urban life was heading precipitously downward.

The discourse was both class- and ethnicity-based, the perception of urban problems centered on lower classes that in many cities were increasingly represented by southern Italians, Poles, Russians, and Jews (Boyer 1978). According to turn-of-the-century rhetoric, these groups were living degraded lives in tenements and lodging houses largely unfit for human habitation. New York represented in many respects the epitome of immigrant poverty. The photographer Jacob Riis, for example, brought to a disparate audience at the turn of the century an awareness of New York's poorest sectors with his moving photographs of tenements, back-alley squatter shacks, and their largely immigrant inhabitants (Riis 1971 [1901]). Others captured similar scenes in cities like Chicago, Philadelphia, and Boston (Klein and Kantor 1976). The simultaneous expansion of heavy industry and urban populations created these images and realities of unhealthy cityscapes, typified by smoke-belching factories giving way to squalid lower-class neighborhoods.

A carryover from nineteenth-century discourse, the physical environment of the slum was still considered to have a deleterious impact on the physical and moral health of those individuals living in them. Tenements bred vice, dirt, and immorality as much as they bred disease. The environment of poverty would thus always reproduce itself by continually molding new individuals to lives of depravity. The corollary of this discourse was that at the turn of the century poverty was still connected to moral defects within the individual (Ward 1989). Reform of character through the inculcation of middle-class values thus joined reform of the physical environment in policies toward poor neighborhoods (Ward 1989).

With the rise of the Progressive Movement in the early decades of the twentieth century, a different discourse emerged to join, but not to supersede, the discourse on environment and character. The poor were still considered relatively irresponsible, but Progressive reformers were beginning nevertheless to look at external reasons for why the poor were poor — reasons having to do not with the influence of their domestic environments or their immorality but with structural factors (Ward 1989; Boyer 1978).[4] These included industrial exploitation, substandard housing, and government corruption, but disease increasingly came to the forefront as a leading cause of poverty and vice versa.

As one author stated in his analysis of poverty, "We found that disease produces poverty and now we find that poverty produces disease; that poverty comes from degeneration and incapacity, and now that degeneration and incapacity come from poverty. Yet it is not without benefit that we trace the whole dismal round of this vicious circle, for it well illustrates the interaction of social forces" (cited in Ward 1989, 98).

Perhaps more than any other disease, tuberculosis came to symbolize the early twentieth-century city. It was both cause and outcome of urban decay, a sentinel of what was wrong with programs of municipal reform, and a symbol of the consequences of profound poverty. Tuberculosis became linked with slums and the underclass most specifically, as better statistics illuminated the vast discrepancies in tuberculosis rates between lower-class and upper-class urban neighborhoods (Rosner 1995). In New York City at the end of the nineteenth century, a wealthier Upper West Side district had a tuberculosis mortality rate of 49 per 100,000, versus a rate of 776 per 100,000 for an impoverished tenement section in lower Manhattan (Rothman 1994, 184). In a larger sense, though, tuberculosis became associated with the increasingly unhealthy nature of cities in general. As industrialization deepened, crowding escalated, and two major depressions hit within four decades, images of urban insalubrity intensified throughout the United States. Poor quarters came to represent not departures from, but exacerbated versions of, the city as a whole. The insidious spread of tuberculosis became a metaphor for the physical decline of the American city in the minds of some early-twentieth-century social and medical thinkers. As one historian remarks, to have tuberculosis was to "dramatize in your own body the traumas of the nation" and the decay of the nation's cities (Caldwell 1988, 65).

To stop the spread of tuberculosis, then, meant nothing short of a restructuring of urban social and physical landscapes. If cities were the active incubators of the disease, they would also have to be the antidote. Progressive ideologies coming to the forefront at the turn of the century helped shape the subsequent framing of the antituberculosis campaign. The Progressive agenda, among other things, was based on the "conviction that the moral destiny of the city would be most decisively influenced through . . . a fundamental restructuring of the urban environment" (Boyer 1978, 190). Some Progressives approached this by attempting to reform the structural bases of poverty such as poor housing and substandard sanitation. They also agitated for shorter workdays and the implementation of workmen's compensation and other laws providing laborers a minimum standard of living (Ward 1989). Other Progressives continued the older focus on what Boyer calls "positive environmentalism" (Boyer 1978), the idea that providing particular kinds of uplifting environments such as parks and playgrounds would raise the discipline of the underclass to middle-class standards and entice them to live as cultivated, socially responsible citizens (Boyer 1978, 190).

The antituberculosis campaign in limited ways exemplified Progressive agendas through its two main prongs, the sanatorium movement and domestic restructuring. In the first case, it focused upon inculcating middle-class values in tuberculous individuals through the control of their physical environment and their behavior; in the second case, the objective was to reconstitute the domestic environment. In part the inability of researchers to find a vaccine for the disease necessitated the focus on environmental restructuring, despite general public health trends toward bacteriology (Rosner 1995). As the evidence became clearer that deleterious environmental conditions facilitated the spread of tuberculosis, so too did it become clear that ameliorating those conditions was a necessary antecedent to improved tuberculosis morbidity and mortality rates. Many reformers sought to target the most blighted sectors of an ever more degraded urban landscape, wanting to see a threatening urban wilderness replaced with a healthier, "well-regulated city within a city" (quoted in Rothman 1994, 186). Or as Boyer states it, the "task was to replace the demoralizing detritus of years of urban growth with a consciously planned urban environment" (Boyer 1978, 180). As will be seen in this and the next chapter, however, how to accomplish this change could be flexibly interpreted.

The endurance of morality and the newer discourse of social order in the discussion of poverty might predict in turn a continuation of nineteenth-century rhetoric condemning the poor for their disease. To a certain extent, it is true that blame was not excised from the connection between disease and poverty by the turn of the century. As Naomi Rogers discusses in her account of polio in the first two decades of the twentieth century, "The germ theory and the new scientific medicine did not magically dissipate the influence of cultural prejudice in defining the relationship among disease, environment, and individual behavior" (Rogers 1992, 6). This was particularly true for those diseases such as tuberculosis and polio that remained without a cure despite the increasing authority of bacteriological medicine. In lieu of such cures, and informed by dominant discourses of poverty, public health personnel still tended to fall back upon characterizations of the poor as morally and intellectually weak and to some degree responsible for facilitating the onset of disease by their questionable hygiene (Rogers 1992; Ward 1989).[5] This discourse in turn informed the antituberculosis campaigns in San Francisco and the rest of the United States for several decades.

Individual blame was only a partial explanation of tuberculosis, but it nevertheless generated a corollary emphasis on social control and order in Progressive-Era medical discourse. Although certainly not new (see Rosenberg 1992a), the focus on environmental and social regulation as an antidote to disease was dominant during the first three or four decades of the century. Not until the advent of HIV would society again be faced with the contradiction of a scientific explanation for the most feared disease of the time without the corresponding medical clue to a cure. The connection with behavior and environment in the epidemiology of tuberculosis provided guidelines for treatment recommendations. To control the disease meant to reform the individual as well as to restructure the environment (Caldwell 1988; Rothman 1994). The result was an unprecedented degree of authority by physicians over the tuberculous patient from the turn of the century until the discovery of antibiotics in the 1940s (Rothman 1994, 180).

The Campaign in San Francisco

In San Francisco, the discourse of urban degradation was not as strong as it was in older cities such as New York. For one thing, San Francisco was not as heavily impacted as eastern and midwestern cities by the latest wave of immigration from Europe. Rather than arriving in the millions, immigrants arrived by the thousands: the population increase between 1900 and 1920, for example, was approximately 168,000,[6] a mere fraction of New York's gain of 2.2 million persons in the same time period (Boyer 1978, 189). Immigrants who arrived in San Francisco also frequently did so with a little more money in their pockets, many of them having stayed in eastern cities until they saved enough to move west (Walker 1995). The 1882 law precluding immigration of Chinese to the United States also meant not only that few Chinese were added to San Francisco's population but that the resident population slowly dwindled during the twentieth century (Issel and Cherny 1986; U.S. Census 1910). The history of housing in San Francisco was also somewhat different than some eastern cities in that large tenement houses for the poor, although present in the city's landscape, did not predominate. Rather, lodging houses and tenements in the downtown, Western Addition, and wharf areas were mixed with large areas of single-family dwellings in the South of Market district. The fervor of tenement reform that swept New York in particular during the last decade of the nineteenth century (Ward 1989; Klein and Kantor 1976) thus came to San Francisco in a much attenuated form, and only in the early years of the twentieth century.

Different cartographies of poverty did not, however, prevent San Francisco from being highly concerned with its still-significant underclass and with the tuberculosis it harbored. Poverty was an issue at the turn of the

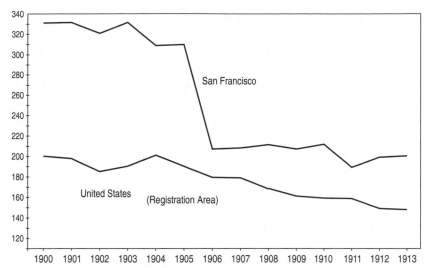

Figure 5.1. Tuberculosis cases per 100,000 population, 1900–1913. Data from San Francisco Tuberculosis Association 1915; created by Mark Patterson.

century in San Francisco, and as in the rest of the country it was an issue integrally related to the problem of tuberculosis. As figure 5.1 attests, San Francisco's tuberculosis rates prior to 1906 were in fact significantly higher than the national average. While rates for the United States averaged over 200 deaths per 100,000 in 1900, San Francisco weighed in with 330 (San Francisco Tuberculosis Association 1915). Even worse, San Francisco's tuberculosis mortality rate was higher than New York's in the first decade of the century, with New York averaging 248 deaths per 100,000 for the combined years 1901–5 versus 319 for San Francisco (Hiscock 1930, 42). These were shameful statistics for public health authorities whose recent predecessors had lauded the greater salutary quality of San Francisco compared to eastern and midwestern cities.

The antituberculosis campaign in San Francisco consequently was as serious an affair as in the larger and more densely populated cities to the east. Lodging houses and tenements were known to be sites of transmission, but so were other lower-class neighborhoods such as South of Market. San Francisco's antituberculosis campaign thus took the same two-pronged approach as did those in much of the rest of the country, focusing on the provision of sanatorium beds for incipient cases and on restructuring domestic environments and providing more adequate hospital facilities for those who were not sent to sanatoriums.

Despite the rhetoric on environmental reform, however, the outcomes of the antituberculosis campaign in terms of real changes in the structural causes and outcomes of poverty were limited. Like the nineteenth-century French social hygienists mentioned by Barnes (1995), it might be said of those reformers of the Progressive Era who concentrated their attention on tuberculosis that their newfound statistical capabilities were used more to illuminate conditions among the underclasses than to change those conditions in any profound way. It was certainly desired that tuberculosis be contained, and in fact it was necessary if a productive workforce were to continue sustaining the growth of industry. At the same time, medical reformers, Progressive or otherwise, wanted to achieve this task without significantly changing the status quo in class relations. Environmental control in the context of the tuberculosis campaign meant primarily the *improvement* of existing structures within their own limits and a change in how individuals chose to configure those structures. It did not mean the obliteration of substandard housing and its replacement with more salubrious habitats and the means with which to maintain them.

In other words, obliterating structural causes of poverty and its material accouterments was nowhere in the antituberculosis discourses of the first decades of the twentieth century in San Francisco or in most other cities, and this distinction is important to make. The nature of tuberculosis prevention programs thus raises questions concerning motivation and desired outcome. In his analysis of tuberculosis in interwar France, France Lert asks whether an extension of the medical body into the previously civic domain of working-class lives was not at stake in the tuberculosis prevention program. Alternately, did the huge extension of public health authority have as its ultimate aim a greater regulation of behavior among the poor and the functional reproduction of the status quo (Lert 1982, 2)? These might seem cynical questions aimed at attempts to diminish the world's most deadly infectious disease, but they do raise some important concerns.

First is the issue already discussed vis-à-vis epidemic episodes concerning the boundaries between public health authority and individual autonomy. To reiterate Rothman's comment, the degree of authority held by public health officials and sanatorium physicians over individual behavior was relatively unprecedented during the antituberculosis campaign in the United States and Europe. In light of resurgent tuberculosis today and the debates over appropriate treatment, it is not irrelevant to ask whether this authority was necessary given the task at hand or whether less-intrusive approaches would be equally effective. The second issue again addresses the intersection of social values and medical knowledge, recognizing that public health policies not only are not always separate from the social agendas of dominant cultural groups but in fact often play key roles in operationalizing them. Referring back to Lert's inquiry, the public health campaign medicalized the social practices and lifestyles of the poor in conjunction with tuberculosis, providing a rationale for extensive medical interventions into working-class behavior that benefited upper-class desires for a more orderly, and thus less fearful, stratum of urban poor. The question then is whether the public health campaign had as its primary motivation the medical agenda of diminishing tuberculosis or the social agenda of controlling an unruly underclass while maintaining the status quo of class relations.

These questions will be explored in this chapter and the next in the context of the sanatorium regimen and urban prevention approaches, respectively. The rest of this chapter examines briefly the establishment of the sanatorium system in the United States before concentrating on those sanatoriums local to San Francisco residents. Focus is placed in particular on one sanatorium built near San Francisco in 1911, the Arequipa Sanatorium for Working Women. The experience of women in sanatoriums has been addressed recently by historians such as Sheila Rothman (1994), but insufficient attention has been paid to ways in which a specifically female tuberculous body was produced and subsequently acted upon in a sanatorium setting. The differing social and economic functions of women must have necessitated within the sanatorium a different type of discipline and ascription of normalcy from that employed with men. As such, working within the Foucauldian framework used below, analysis will focus upon how a specifically female docile body made a difference in the institutional treatment of tuberculosis.

The City Away from a City

To some extent, the twentieth-century sanatorium, like its nineteenth-century precursor, was still an institution whose location outside a city was integral to its function as a retreat for the tuberculous by-products of urban life. Yet by the early twentieth century, sanatoriums in the United States had changed significantly. The sanatoriums of the latter part of the nineteenth century had been retreats for the upper classes, places to come for rest and relaxation, reprieves from the city. The sanatoriums of the early decades of the twentieth century were the ideal embodiments of medical control in the name of tuberculosis prevention. Their isolation afforded a degree of supervision over the tuberculous patient not possible in an urban setting, and their relative spatial compactness enabled environmental conditions — from cleanliness to architectural design — to be carefully overseen and regulated.

The increasing authority of physicians and of medical science, coupled with a profound fear of the disease, largely explains why patients allowed a degree of control by their physicians rarely replicated before or after the first half of the century.

The idea for a closed sanatorium, one with a supervised regimen where patients were not free to come and go as they pleased, originated with the German physician Peter Dettweiler in the 1870s. His ideas were introduced to American physicians by Paul Kretzschmer a decade later. In the Dettweiler model, doctors were adjured to establish complete supervision over the tuberculous patient if he or she was to be cured. The sanatorium regimen should be based upon outdoor rest, supplemented by a nutritious and bountiful diet, mild exercise, and regular physical examinations by the supervising physician (Rothman 1994, 196). These ideas were not readily embraced, nor did they go uncontested by some American physicians (Rothman 1994, 197).[7] It took until the turn of the century for the "closed" sanatorium to take off, by which time the idea resonated with the recognized need for environmental and behavioral control in mitigating the spread of tuberculosis. Once the idea was widely accepted, sanatoriums proliferated for the next three decades, from approximately 34 in 1900 to 536 in 1925, with an estimated 673,338 beds (Rothman 1994, 198). Though form and regimen came to have at least equal importance to location, sanatoriums still tended to be built in the mountains of the Northeast and the arid regions of the West.

From the early years of the sanatorium's ascendancy, close attention was paid to its architectural form, an essential factor in incorporating the proper treatment regimen and the necessary degree of supervision over the patient. In accordance with these new socio-spatial prerogatives, the single behemoth building style of early German sanatoriums was rejected as not fulfilling either objective of treatment and regulation. A more open-aired and panoptic style was needed and was found in two architectural variations that came to characterize most sanatoriums in the United States. One was the cottage style, first utilized by Edward L. Trudeau[8] at his famous Saranac Lake sanatorium in the Adirondacks of New York. In this variation, small cottages for patients were arranged within close proximity to a main administrative building where dining facilities, infirmary, medical offices, and examination rooms were housed. The cottages' main feature was a large porch, usually facing an attractive view, where patients spent a preponderance of their time lying in "rest" chairs regardless of weather conditions. The second style (sometimes called the lean-to style) was a compact modification of the first, with one-story wings attached to either side of a main building, and porches lining each wing. Extensions could be added to accommodate an increase in patient numbers, but the ob-

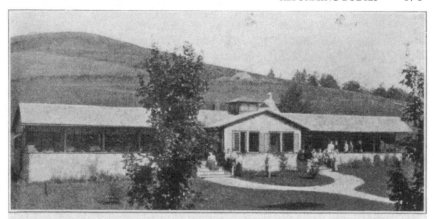

Lean-To Type—Capacity 16 Patients

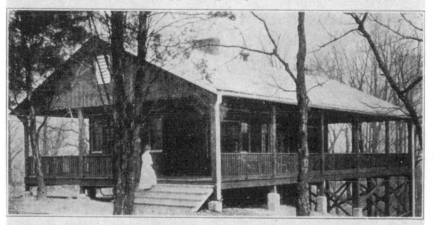

Courtesy, "Hospital Construction"
Cottage Type—Capacity 12 Patients
QUARTERS FOR EARLY CASES OF TUBERCULOSIS
San Francisco Needs at Least Two Hundred Beds for Incipient Cases,
Preferably in the Country.

Figure 5.2. Cottage-style and lean-to sanatoriums. Courtesy of The Bancroft Library, University of California, Berkeley.

jective again was to ensure the relative proximity of all patients to the main administrative building. Figure 5.2 illustrates these two styles of sanatorium.

These two simple architectural forms encompassed to near perfection the tenets of the antituberculosis campaign. In both models, the design of cottage or wing was purposefully minimalistic for two reasons: patients were to spend most of their time outdoors,[9] and the unobtruded cellular design meant increased capacity for supervision even when patients were inside their rooms. The diminution of niches, corners, and crannies also meant fewer places where dust could harbor tubercle bacilli. The proximity to administrative and medical facilities meant that the enfeebled tuberculous patient did not have far to go for medical examinations, meals, and regular weigh-ins. The close arrangement of the structurally more diminutive cottages or wings around the imposing administrative building also symbolized the power and authority vested in the physician over the sanatorium patient (Caldwell 1988, 88–89). Segregation of the sexes, a regulation of most sanatoriums, was implemented through the arrangement of single-sex cottages or wings and enforced through the same panoptic design facilitating observation at all times.

The grounds of the sanatorium were designed with similar objectives in mind. Benches where patients could quietly sit were placed strategically, including along the paths created for those patients able to exercise. Walkways between buildings were maintained, and the areas immediately surrounding cottages and buildings were kept manicured and were easily negotiated. The effect was a combination of bucolic rusticity with well-regulated and maintained order. The former represented the vestige of geographic influence in the tuberculosis campaign, the attempt to simulate the "tapestry of rural informality" (Caldwell 1988, 91) and to galvanize the city-weakened tubercular, psychologically if not physically, along the path to robust health through the hearty abundance of nature. The latter reinforced the Progressive notion that well-regulated behavior and a well-regulated environment were the most important elements in combating tuberculosis (Caldwell 1988; Rothman 1994). Everything about the sanatorium, in effect, was designed not only to regulate patients while they resided within the institution but to instill by constant example and teaching a desire for cleanliness, order, and outdoor recreation even after returning to the city.

In design as in ideological predication the sanatorium epitomized, as perhaps no other medical institution in recent history other than the insane asylum,[10] Foucauldian concepts of discipline and control through the organization of space (Foucault 1977, 1975). In *Discipline and Punish* (1977), Foucault discusses these concepts as evolving in Europe in the eighteenth and nineteenth centuries. Yet in the case of tuberculosis in the United States, it was the early-twentieth-century public health physician who recognized that the key to stemming the disease lay in "the ordering of every detail of individual and collective life." The way to accomplish this was through "distributing individuals in space" in such a way as to map and thus to regulate them at all times. The sanatorium achieved this objective in the precise method outlined by Foucault: it constituted a space "closed in upon itself, . . . the place

of disciplinary monotony"; and within this it incorporated a careful partitioning of individuals into given spaces, in order to "eliminate the effects
of imprecise distributions, the uncontrolled disappearance of individuals,
their diffuse circulation." Finally, there was further imposition of authority
through the codification of other spaces into sites of supervision and examination (Foucault 1977, 198, 141–44).[11] Through his meticulous control of space,
the sanatorium physician could in turn impose upon his individual charges
the peculiar combination of discipline and compliance deemed imperative
to combat tuberculosis and the social disorder out of which it formed. This
imposition of discipline and control constituted something of a paradox of
the sanatorium modus operandi. The sanatorium regime was geared toward
producing vigorous bodies from weak ones, bodies that could again become
productive components of an industrial society (in Foucault's terms, they
would repossess "bio-power"). Yet, paradoxically, vigorous bodies could only
be produced through the coterminous production of docile bodies.

The creation of docile bodies was made easier given that twentieth-
century sanatoriums catered largely to the poor. If the sanatorium setting
enabled a "meticulousness of the regulations...[and] the supervision of the
smallest fragment of life and of the body" (Foucault 1977, 138), the poor patient was thought to provide its most successful object, an individual already
made docile through persistent conditioning to his or her social status. The
predominance of poor tuberculars in sanatoriums by the early part of the
century was a consequence of recognizing that stemming tuberculosis meant
aggressive targeting of those with the highest rates of the disease. But the
poor were also sent to sanatoriums with higher frequency because they were
thought to lack not only the resources but the discipline to seek a cure on their
own (Rothman 1994, 206). Either way, the early-twentieth-century sanatorium was often a class-coded institution, not just in targeting the poor but
in gearing the physical design and regimen of the facility to the presumably
different temperament of the poor tubercular.

First, the physical design and setting of a sanatorium for the poor could
be especially minimalistic, since the poor were unaccustomed to lavish or
even comfortable surroundings. Thomas Carrington, author of a respected
early-twentieth-century book on sanatorium planning, advised that sanatoriums for the poor be inexpensive and humble in design, stating that "this class
of institution returns patients to their homes without making them unduly
discontented with the environment and life to which they belong" (quoted in
Caldwell 1988, 93). Second, sanatoriums catering to the poor also frequently
implemented work programs into the treatment regimen for all of those patients ambulatory and able to perform light industry. The rationale behind

such a program was twofold: along with the humble surroundings, a regimen of light labor kept the poor tubercular accustomed to the type of work routine to which he or she must eventually return, while staving off the proclivities toward idleness presumed characteristic of most urban poor. Third, a work regimen was usually geared either toward an industry that could earn the sanatorium sorely needed funds, such as craft production, or toward agricultural production that could save the sanatorium money by supplementing food supplies (Bates 1992; Caldwell 1988). For the private upper-class sanatoriums, such rationales did not exist; accordingly, in most of these the strict regimen of rest and inactivity was enforced.

Even within sanatoriums for the poor, distinctions were made among the worthy versus the unworthy, the cases with potential versus those that were hopeless. In most states, there were institutions privately funded by employers, philanthropists, or social reformers targeting incipient cases of working-class tuberculars who could not pay for sanatorium treatment on their own. The most famous example of this class of institution was Saranac Lake; another was the White Haven sanatorium run by Lawrence Flick outside Philadelphia (Bates 1992). Because they were private, these sanatoriums could screen their patients, rejecting either those who did not display an adequate degree of pliancy or those who had progressed too far in their disease to benefit from sanatorium care. As Flick and Trudeau often bemoaned, the more advanced cases cost these perennially fund-strapped facilities too much money by their lengthier stays and additional medical needs (Trudeau 1916; Bates 1992). The completely impoverished, along with the advanced and dying cases, usually ended up in city and county sanatoriums or in the tuberculous wards of city hospitals (Rothman 1994). These in effect replaced the nineteenth-century almshouse in providing an institutional setting for the preparation for death.

San Francisco's Sanatoriums

By the closing years of the nineteenth century, San Francisco public health authorities were also recognizing the benefits of sanatorium care. Not only did it remove tuberculous individuals from insalutary surroundings, but through isolation it prevented them from infecting other individuals. At an annual state sanitary meeting in 1896, one participant proposed the view that tuberculosis cases be isolated in medical institutions such as hospitals, a practice generally not adhered to prior to that time (California Department of Public Health 1934). By 1906, the secretary of the state board of health, N. K. Foster, clearly aware of the established connection between tuberculosis and the environmental conditions of poverty, recommended the accessibility of sanatoriums for all who needed them (California Department of Public Health 1934, 17).

Part of Foster's motivation for such an appeal was the number of tuberculars who continued to come to California seeking a recovery from their disease. By the turn of the century, most of these migrants were heading for southern California rather than for San Francisco, a fact reflected in the higher tuberculosis mortality rates of southern California cities: in 1907 Los Angeles had a mortality rate of 324.8 per 100,000 compared to San Francisco's substantially lower rate of 209.3 (San Francisco Tuberculosis Association Annual Reports 1912).[12] Statistics of length of residence at the time of death show that, for the state as a whole, almost one-third had lived in California for fewer than nine years, 8.2 percent for less than a year. For San Francisco, these figures were 9 percent and 2.1 percent, respectively (California State Board of Health Reports 1910, 106).

More importantly in Foster's mind, many tuberculous migrants came at the last stages of their disease, with no or little funding to support themselves or to obtain treatment (California Department of Public Health 1910). Realization of the severity of the disease, the potential for public alarm, and the problem of caring for so many indigent tuberculous is reflected in his regret that so many came to California when they "could get air and sunshine and good food at home" (California Department of Public Health 1910, 19). At least for this physician, the lack of facilities and funds to care for the number of tuberculous in California had turned the state's image as a health resort into a nightmare. He was clearly not alone in thinking this, for in the 1920s the state board of health issued a flyer aimed at those "traveling for health." In an about-face from the nineteenth-century stance on California's salubrious climate, the flyer claims that a change of climate is not as important as rest, food, and fresh air in mending tuberculosis. Above all, it warns tuberculous individuals not to consider coming to California unless they had adequate means to support themselves during their stay, because the state was lacking in any public institutions for the treatment of their disease (California State Board of Health Reports 1930).

Foster proved more farsighted than most in calling for state-supported sanatorium facilities. Such appeals would be repeated by other physicians who were concerned with the lack of care for the indigent tubercular, who considered tuberculosis the responsibility of the state, or who found shame in California's poor record of indigent care when other states had already funded state sanatoriums.[13] These appeals were to little avail. A bill was introduced into the state legislature in 1904 asking for an appropriation of $150,000 for a state sanatorium, but the bill failed to pass (California State Board of Health

Reports 1916, 26). In 1915, a measure was again introduced to the legislature asking for a state-funded sanatorium, and again it was voted down. This time, the legislature passed instead a measure to subsidize counties maintaining tuberculosis hospitals, agreeing to pay three dollars per individual per week for those indigent patients otherwise being funded by cities and counties for institutionalized care of their tuberculosis. Efforts to provide sanatorium treatment to the urban poor in California therefore remained a private endeavor initiated by physicians who saw a need to remove underclass patients from their home environments and from the city.

From Factory to (Panoptic) Finishing School

In San Francisco this initiative was led by a physician named Philip Brown, who ran the San Francisco Polyclinic, which provided health services to the city's poor. With the development of better diagnostic capabilities for tuberculosis, Brown realized the extent of the disease among patients coming to his clinic and the inadequacy of treatment options available to them. A representative of his time, Brown recognized the seemingly insurmountable obstacles facing poor working-class tuberculars. They lived, as Brown described it, in unhygienic environments that precipitated the onset of tuberculosis; they delayed seeking care for their disease partially because they knew how atrocious was the care at the city hospital; and out of necessity they continued working despite their illness. Those who were sent to the City and County Hospital invariably left before they were healed and returned to the same squalid lodging home or crowded frame house that facilitated their disease in the first place (Brown 1911b). To make the situation worse, according to Brown, the city's poorer neighborhoods were even more conducive to the spread of tuberculosis after the earthquake and fire of 1906 because of further increases in crowding and dust (Brown, n.d.[b]).[14]

More unusual at this early date, for San Francisco and elsewhere, was Brown's focus on poor women and the different epidemiological mechanisms of infection that applied to them. Chief among these was the greater amount of time spent indoors in unhealthy environments, both at home and in the workplace. Employment opportunities for women had expanded to a limited degree by the turn of the century, but the choices still largely were restricted to clerical, nursing, teaching, factory, and domestic jobs (Rothman 1978; Broussard 1993). Especially in the years prior to workplace regulations, the vast majority of urban working women still labored indoors for protracted hours under less-than-optimum conditions. For some, like the San Francisco women in a turn-of-the-century sewing factory (figure 5.3), conditions were appalling. The caption under the photograph states, "the naked light bulbs

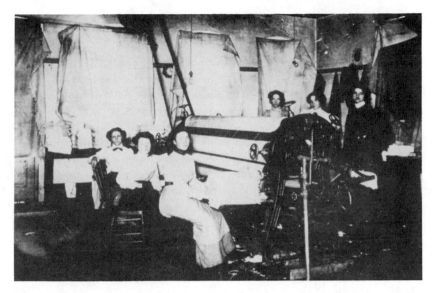

Figure 5.3. Female factory workers, turn of the century. Courtesy of The Bancroft Library, University of California, Berkeley.

and the muslin sheeted windows created a sweatshop reality for these women" (Olmstead et al. 1979, n.p.). Stated another way, the organization of space in these workplaces could not have been more conducive to the spread of tuberculosis. Ventilation was minimal; dirt was abundant; and female workers were crammed into the smallest possible space of production. Many men suffered similar working conditions, but in Brown's opinion

> the opportunities that are open to women are distinctly against them, not only being conducive to the acquiring of tuberculosis, but offering a minimum of opportunity for recovery under the present conditions. As dressmakers, stenographers, clerks, factory workers, etc. they are often where the most unsanitary conditions in business life are found. The outdoor occupations, which are plentiful for men in California, are hardly open to them at all. (*San Francisco Chronicle,* April 6, 1911)

Furthermore, women were required to spend more time inside the home fulfilling their domestic duties, whether or not they were also employed outside the home; men had no corresponding obligations.[15] The consequence, according to Brown, was a mortality rate from tuberculosis among working women twice that of men (Brown 1911b).[16]

Brown's solution to this situation was to set up a sanatorium for working

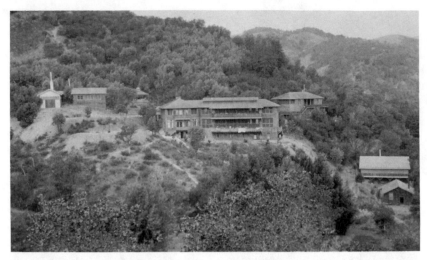

Figure 5.4. Arequipa Sanatorium. Courtesy of The Bancroft Library, University of California, Berkeley.

women in Marin County, an area close to the city yet still rural in character. The idea for the initial institution was to acquire a modest frame home with a large veranda that could house a small number of women and accommodate them outdoors. Farming and raising chickens would be pursued to offset costs and "continue the economic viability" of the patients (Brown n.d.[a]). The funding for this sanatorium would come in part from the women themselves, but mainly from their employers, with the rationale that a healthy employee would be a more productive one in the long run.[17] Care would be provided by nurses who themselves had tuberculosis but who could care for other patients two to three hours a day in return for lodging in a separate facility at the sanatorium. Finally, the sanatorium itself would be located adjacent to Hill Farm, a municipally funded outdoor home for sickly children. Since tuberculous parents were still thought to produce children themselves more vulnerable to the disease, the proximity of the two facilities was considered propitious (Brown 1911b).

In September 1911, the Arequipa Sanatorium for Working Women opened its doors to a select few of San Francisco's tuberculous working women of modest means. The institution as realized was somewhat larger than originally envisioned, with an initial capacity of forty patients and a large two-story structure to house them. The design of Arequipa's buildings, as well as their specific location and placement, exemplified the Foucauldian assertion of institutional control through mapping the individual in space.

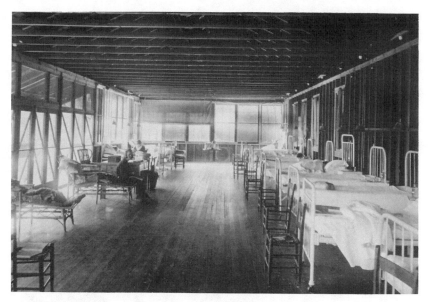

Figure 5.5. Sleeping ward, Arequipa Sanatorium. Courtesy of The Bancroft Library, University of California, Berkeley.

The first objective of this disciplinary cartography, the space "closed in upon itself [to affect] disciplinary monotony" (Foucault 1977, 141), was achieved through locating the sanatorium in an isolated and relatively uninhabited area. As seen in figure 5.4, the rugged hillside location effectively prevented any extensive forays from the institution, and its distance from town or city assured the relative isolation of its patients from society, and conversely of society from its patients. Disciplinary monotony came in part, then, from turning the institution into the only social and experiential context of the sanatorium patient.

In addition to the sanatorium's isolation, the architectural structure of the buildings ensured a relatively unfettered observation of patients at all times, preventing the "uncontrolled disappearance of individuals" in the institutional context and allowing sanatorium staff to see whether and when patients were following the prescribed treatment regimen. As figures 5.5 to 5.8 show, Arequipa achieved an operationalized panopticism through incorporating huge windows into its outer walls, especially in sleeping areas, constructing few internal walls to obstruct vision or movement, and keeping patients contained in one main building that served administrative, medical, and residential purposes. Of course Arequipa was also designed to accom-

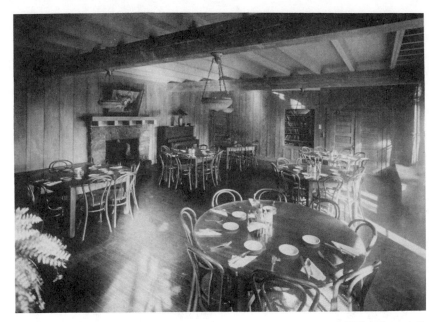

Figure 5.6. Dining ward, Arequipa Sanatorium. Courtesy of The Bancroft Library, University of California, Berkeley.

modate the environmentally based theories for treating tuberculosis that included exposing the body as much as possible to fresh air and sunlight. Yet the disciplinary regimen that coordinated with the internal layout suggests motivating factors beyond fresh air and sunshine to explain the panoptic institutional design of Arequipa.

Indeed, the "imprecise distribution of individuals" was circumvented at Arequipa, as at many sanatoriums, by a rigid schedule that coordinated every movement of the patients through time and space from the moment they arose in the morning until they went to bed at night. Every patient was required to adhere to the schedule or risk being discharged. The day started for everyone with a "rising bell" that rang precisely at 7:30. Meals were participated in by everyone and occurred at the same time everyday, breakfast at 8:15, dinner at 12:15, and supper at 5:15. The small number of patients at Arequipa, together with communal dining tables, enabled the monitoring of every patient at every meal, except for those who were confined to bed rest. Rest hours were mandatory for every patient and occurred twice a day from 11:00 to 11:45 in the morning and 1:00 to 2:45 in the afternoon. Lights-out was promptly at 9:00 (Regulations, n.d.).

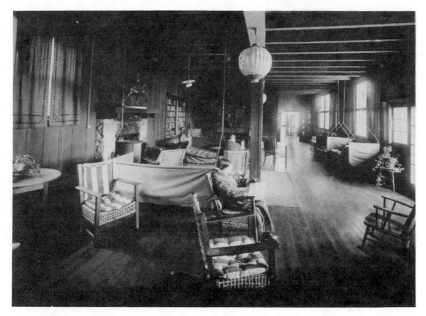

Figure 5.7. Recreation area, Arequipa Sanatorium. Courtesy of The Bancroft Library, University of California, Berkeley.

The Three *R*s: *R*est, Self-*r*egulation, and the Work *R*egime

But Arequipa did not just instill order through the design of its buildings or the coordination of its time clock. Several other means were also used to en-sure the successful inscription of productive values onto patients, namely, admissions policies, institutional regulations, and the patients themselves. Looking at admissions policies first, simply being working-class and having tuberculosis were not enough to assure a woman's admittance into Arequipa. She also needed to display the seeds of feminine docility and malleability before she got there. According to Philip Brown, these qualities, particularly among the working class, were not always easy to find. "This class," he stated, "is discouraging any way one looks at it. They are irresponsible as a rule and unattached and drift from place to place scattering disease as they go. If sent to the county hospital they leave as soon as they feel a little better and rarely return until forced to by a bad return of their symptoms" (Brown 1911b, 7). Granted, this discursive fictioning of the poor and their very real impedi-ments to health and health care was applied equally to men and women. Yet Brown further specified the type of woman he would allow in to his new sanatorium.

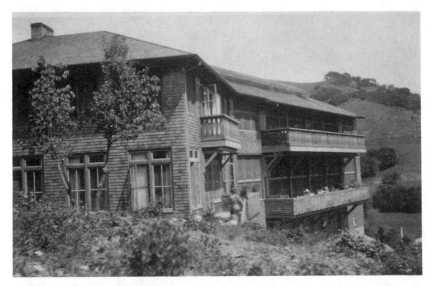

Figure 5.8. Outdoor decks, Arequipa Sanatorium. Courtesy of The Bancroft Library, University of California, Berkeley.

First, the women could not be indigent; besides financially draining the sanatorium, this class was considered beyond reform and better handled at the City and County Hospital.[18] Second, women had to be relatively young and, until about 1940, white. A 1930 report from the sanatorium's city office mentioned among its applicants a Negro woman who "could [thus] not be accepted," while another woman past sixty years old "was advised to consider some other sanatorium" (Arequipa Sanatorium [physician and staff correspondence] 1930, n.p.). Third, in addition to the applicants' possessing the baseline attributes of proper class, race, and age, Brown specified that among them "only the intelligent, teachable type is selected, and only those allowed to remain who prove amenable to discipline and willing to cooperate. This policy results in a student body of fine character which becomes in time a group of loyal alumnae and a very real force in public health education" (Brown 1911b, 17).

Once the carefully screened and presumably malleable patient arrived at Arequipa, however, she had to be fictioned in a somewhat different way. If the sanatorium were to function as a site for the embodiment and subsequent social deployment of middle-class values, the sanatorium patient had to be seen as lacking those values to begin with. Hence in a report from 1914, a resident secretary claims that "almost every patient coming to Arequipa presents, in addition to her lung trouble, problems of a financial, temperamental, social or moral nature.... With the exception of two or three cases, morally incorrigible because of lack of proper early environment, almost every problem has been met through the efforts of the staff" (Arequipa Annual Reports 1914, 10). It might be presumed from this statement that despite having a job and the "correct" attributes of youth and Anglo heritage, these women nonetheless contracted their "lung trouble" at least in part through their class-coded moral failings.

The secretary's comment is in fact rife with meaning, summing up one early-twentieth-century interpretation of tuberculosis epidemiology. The first part of her statement evidences the persistent notion that degraded environments produced morally degraded bodies, as distinct from producing particular diseases. Yet in a second-stage process, tuberculosis evolves out of—in fact seems an inevitable outcome of—the moral shortcomings produced by these lower-class environments. Tuberculosis symbolizes more than anything here the social, moral, and economic failings of a particular class. Unlike the racially coded interpretations of smallpox and plague, in its lexicon of temperament, morality, environment, and disease the discourse represented in the secretary's comment pathologizes class and turns into etiologic explanation the fictional deviance of chronic poverty. Hence the necessity of attacking tuberculosis through the reproduction of class values.

The second of the three means of disciplinary control, institutional regulations, directly tackled these real and imaginary shortcomings. Besides the strictly kept timetable of meals, rest hours, and sleep, movement within the sanatorium and the degree of social interaction were similarly regulated, again mirroring Foucault's analysis of individuals being subject to an "ordering of every detail of [their] individual and collective lives." Patients, for example, were not allowed to go from one ward to another without permission, and in the interests of "speeding the cure," they were encouraged to speak in a modulated voice, to not whistle or sing, and to learn what was dubbed the "arequipa crawl," that is, a slow walk. Visiting periods were limited to two two-hour periods during the week and one three-hour period on Sundays; patients were not allowed to go into town or leave the grounds without permission; and complete inaction — including not reading or talking — was enforced during rest hours. In addition, no food was ever allowed in the wards or to be brought to bedridden patients without permission of the superintendent, and each mobile patient was responsible for keeping her bed made and her room tidy and clean (Regulations, n.d.). Though many of these regulations were necessary for treating tuberculosis, a significant proportion appear to be aimed at quashing those "problems of a moral nature" through complete acquiescence to the authority of the physician and to the sanatorium regimen. Those who did not acquiesce were asked to leave.

Typical of most working-class sanatoriums, Arequipa residents who were not confined to bed rest were also required to perform every day a few hours of an income-generating activity. Although partly driven by the need to supplement chronic shortages of funds for the sanatorium, this activity too had its class- and gender-based ideological undergirding. To quote Brown's own rationale for a work regimen at Arequipa:

> There is a certain moral advantage to be gotten out of requiring work of the patients, to which I believe more attention should be given. The objection raised to the sanatorium cure of tb cases is that the absolute rest upon which much stress is laid brings about habits of idleness which the patients never overcome. While the work done might not be of much value in supporting the institution, it will certainly be of inestimable value in maintaining the economic efficiency of the patients. (Brown 1911b, 7)

Admittedly ineffective as far as tuberculosis was concerned, the work regime's therapeutic value lay in "rearrang[ing] not only the complex of interests proper to *homo oeconomicus,* but also the imperatives of the moral subject" (Foucault 1977, 122–23).

Not any work regime would do, however. For women at Arequipa, work was carefully selected to fit middle-class notions of the type of work suitable for female pursuit. In Brown's own words, only those occupations that "appeal to the feminine instincts of personal adornment and homebuilding" (Brown, n.d.[a], 3) were undertaken, including pottery making, basket weaving, millinery and dressmaking, typing, and shorthand. The irony of these choices was that their distinctly feminine and middle-class quality as pursued individually within the sanatorium bore little relation to the industrial settings in which many Arequipa women would need to pursue them after their discharge. It is also worth noting that Brown framed his selection of pursuits in terms of a gendering process rather than in terms of their greater suitability for weakened tuberculous bodies.

The last of the three prongs of productive discipline involved the role that patients themselves played in instilling "right" attitudes and behavior. The Arequipa newsletter, entitled the *Hi-Life* and written by the patients themselves, evidences the degree to which older patients assigned themselves the task of teaching the newer patients the ways of sanatorium life and the benefits of acquiescing as quickly as possible to the work regime, the rigid choreography of movement, and the authority of the resident physician. As one patient wrote in the March 1932 *Hi-Life:*

Becoming a resident of Arequipa calls for an adjustment which is not altogether the task of the incoming patient alone. A responsibility is bestowed on the old-timer which, if it is conscientiously carried out, may be of great value to the new-comer. Surely no one understands better the difficulties confronting the beginner than we do and if we have profited at all by our experiences we should be of real help to the new patients. (*Hi-Life,* March 1932, n.p.)

Another patient, writing in the September 1931 *Hi-Life,* outlines the process more specifically. To the question of how the Arequipa "graduate" learned the tenets of a permanent cure, she responds:

By two methods. The first of which one is barely conscious in the daily routine which stresses rest and includes a specially arranged diet and ordinary precautions in one's habits. The second method, one really pedagogic, consists of informal talks by Dr. Owen [the resident physician] pertaining to the essentials of the rest cure as well as advice concerning one's life in the world. (*Hi-Life,* September 1931, n.p.)

The method this patient left out, of course, was the pedagogic function of the *Hi-Life* itself. Within its pages patients were constantly reminded of how to behave. They were advised, for example, to maintain cheerful attitudes, to keep appearances neat, clean, and decorous even when confined to bed rest, and to learn patience, tolerance, and consideration for fellow patients. The January 1932 edition printed the winners of the "Arequipa's Perfect Girl" contest. The perfect girl seems to have been a composite portrait featuring "a smile like Phyllis," "sweetness like Carmen," "a sense of humor like Barney," and so on. At least here was the implicit acknowledgment that the perfect girl was unrealistic as constituted by a single individual.

Poetry was clearly another means by which patients were urged to safely channel their concerns while continuing to nurture their cheerful attitudes. One poem, printed in the March 1932 *Hi-Life,* poignantly tells of the obvious loneliness and isolation of sanatorium life while dispelling any lasting effect through its optimistic endnote:

And so you think us lonely when the throng
Has ceased to come? We used to be—
The one road blocked by tourists, no company!
How stillness hurts you town folks cannot know.
The chores and housework none, time dragged along.
It's different now. Of course we're shut in still,

But we've a radio with which to fill
The ice-bound chinks of silences with song. (*Hi-Life,* March 1932, n.p.)

Despite the poem's turn toward optimism, the sentiments in it make very real the term "disciplinary monotony." By all accounts, life in the sanatorium for any class of individual could be excruciatingly lonely, isolated, and even boring.[19] The average stay for patients at Arequipa was six to ten months (Arequipa Sanatorium Annual Reports 1912, 1914), and the exact same routine was performed every day for that time period. The routine itself, too, was bereft of any but the most superficial means of entertainment and mental stimulation. The private sanatoriums had more money to ship in various forms of distractions for their residents,[20] but the working-class institutions in general did not possess as many means to do this. Many physicians also did not think the stimulation of too much entertainment physically beneficial. Ironically, it was this hazard perhaps more than any other that drove people away from finishing their residencies.[21]

Alta Sanatorium: A Middle-Class Sanctuary

Though the poor received more attention for their higher tuberculosis rates, they did not have a complete monopoly on the disease. Sanatoriums also catered to the middle and upper classes, and it proves instructive to look briefly at one of these in order to highlight further the particularities of the working-class sanatorium. The Alta Sanatorium for Early Tuberculosis, located in Placer City, sixty-eight miles east of Sacramento, was a facility for the middle- to upper-middle-class tubercular. It was a cottage-style sanatorium, with one central structure and five cottages for patients, in addition to support facilities. All structures were designed for "rendering practicable the outdoor life," with large windows, sleeping porches, and minimal indoor features. Women were housed on the second floor of the main building, while male patients occupied cottages in groups of five or ten. Two cottages were designated as "suites" and were located further up a hill. Although somewhat unusual for a sanatorium, it appears that these suites were for married couples or families, their location "affording more privacy, but preventing entire isolation" (Alta Sanatorium Reports 1909). No one, even at an upper-class sanatorium, was allowed exemption from the panoptic gaze of the resident physician and his or her staff.

The main difference between the Alta and Arequipa Sanatoriums, the primary factor marking Alta as a middle-class institution, was the absence of a work regimen for its patients. At Alta, emphasis was placed on complete rest and relaxation, broken only by the short walks allowed those patients showing improvement and absence of fever. Economically, the fees of the sanatorium (one hundred dollars per month for a private sleeping porch; eighty dollars for a private dressing room and shared porch; or seventy-five dollars for a shared porch and dressing room) obviated the need to generate extra income from patients. Socially, it was not considered necessary to instill a greater work ethic in the middle- and upper-middle-class patient. However, the same degree of submissiveness and pliancy was required at Alta, the same complete relegation of will to medical authority while within the gates of the sanatorium.

Education was also an important part of the middle-class sanatorium regimen, as for the working-class sanatorium. For those patients who returned home before they were completely cured, it was necessary to teach them how to avoid infecting other members of their family. For all patients, certain rules of sanitation and personal habits needed to be instilled to maintain healthy living and prevent recurrences of disease after leaving the sanatorium. While some of these rules of hygiene were not class-coded, others were part of the changed lexicon of contagious practices illuminated by bacteriology. Use of communal drinking cups, for example, a common domestic and public practice for all classes in the nineteenth and early twentieth centuries, had to be dissuaded (Bureau of Tuberculosis 1916). Proper eating habits were also emphasized, but for the middle and upper classes this meant instruction in the nature and preparation of fortifying foods such as milk, eggs, and meat. It also meant combating what the state Bureau of Tuberculosis described in 1927 as a teenage and female fad of "dieting in order to look like the poorest people in Europe to whom we contributed shiploads of food after the war" (Bureau of Tuberculosis 1927, 4). Nutritional instruction was similar at Arequipa, with the difference that the affordability of such foods was questionable for the working-class family.

Perhaps as a correlate to the long hours of enforced inactivity, the importance of landscape to the cure regimen also tended to be more emphasized at upper-class sanatoriums. The location of the Alta Sanatorium in the Sierra foothills, for example, was chosen for both medical and aesthetic reasons. The elevation of 3,600 feet was thought sufficient to stimulate the patient's appetite and cause an increase in the red and white blood cells; in addition, it was thought to increase the lung capacity by stimulating better breathing, thereby building up the "muscles of inspiration" (Alta Sanatorium Reports 1909). The patient was supposed to benefit not just from the salubrity of the location, however, but from its beauty and tranquillity. Since nervousness, fretting, and overwork were considered detrimental to improvement, the serenity of the wooded hills, it was hoped by physicians, would help keep patients calm and optimistic. As the century wore on and the pace of life quickened with the advent of faster forms of transportation and communication, the serenity of rural sanatoriums served as an example to the patient of the wisdom of slower living. After reprimanding patients for living the "ultramodern life" with its "highstrung existence" and "crowded speedways," a 1941 newsletter from the St. Helena Sanatorium in Napa claimed that "there is nothing like a great peace-drenched mountain with its deep sunbathed pensive valleys to calm [the patient] down. If one lingers in the hills enough, he will feel presently the cool touch of mother nature's fingers drawing the fever from his life" (*Saint Helena Sanatorium News,* August 1941, 1). Even for the moneyed tubercular, the absence of effective chemotherapy rendered Nature the most hopeful antidote to a relatively hopeless disease.

The Postgraduate Highlighted

Arequipa was relatively unusual in catering strictly to female patients, as evidenced by the increasing referrals it received from physicians in other parts of California and the United States (Arequipa Sanatorium Annual Reports 1917). It was typical, though, in its combination of medicine and social control, the authoritative manner in which its staff located ideologies of proper behavior and moral conduct within the boundaries of medical prophylaxis. The distance between the sanatorium and the city in a sense symbolized the agenda of the treatment regimen: it constantly reminded the patients of the distance between how they were perceived and how they needed to be before they could expect to return to the city without regressing back to a diseased state. Although a degraded environment was seen to have precipitated their disease, the poor — and particularly poor women — were seen as abetting that degradation through ignorance and poor domestic hygiene. In other words, there was still ample space in the interstices of bacteriology and environmental medicine for behavioral interpretations of disease, and this space was clearly mapped out in the underlying philosophy and treatment regimen of Arequipa.

The difference between Arequipa and other working-class sanatoriums was that in the former the inculcation of middle-class behaviors was highly gender-coded. A woman was discharged having learned skills of good hygiene, nutrition, and a proper work ethic, all of which she would need to keep herself healthy and to perform adequately her role as the health gatekeeper of her family. The irony here is that being female directly and indirectly caused tuberculosis through social constraints and institutional exploitation. Yet the key to *curing* tuberculosis, according to Brown, also lay in the cultivation of penultimate "femaleness." The cure lay in the redefinition and deployment of the cause, and in this Brown felt himself successful. Writing in 1938, he states: "In brief, here is an institution that has restored physical and social value to countless girls, an experiment that has proved its worth" (Brown 1938, n.p.). The alternative, of course, was to change the structural and social causes of women's higher tuberculosis rates, and neither Brown nor anyone else involved in the San Francisco antituberculosis campaign embraced such a proposition.

If a Foucauldian framework has left an obvious hole in not addressing the issue of resistance, it is because feminists of late have tended to over-emphasize and dilute the meaning of this term, a matter on which I agree with Susan Bordo (Bordo 1993). It is true, as she states, that to a certain extent "resistance is perpetual and hegemony precarious" and that we need to "acknowledge adequately the creative and resistant responses that continually challenge and disrupt" regimes of truth (Bordo 1993, 193). Through their letters, their poetry, their attitudes, and their actions women did in fact display to one degree or another a perpetual resistance to a regime that few of them denied was controlling. Women could, and did, leave Arequipa because they chose not to abide by its inflexible rules. They also left because they missed their families, hated the isolation, and chose to finish their cure in the comfort of their own homes and away from a stifling and rigid atmosphere. For those who stuck it out, the poetry they wrote and the humor that infuses many of their writings were not simply therapeutic but indeed creative disruptions of a regimented existence. It should also be noted that some women enjoyed their stay at Arequipa, and of course many appreciated the health it restored to them.[22]

It needs to be emphasized, however, that creative disruption was not the same thing as effective reconfiguration. These collective negotiations did not result in any serious disruption of the "regime of truth" that prevailed at Arequipa and at other sanatoriums. The combination of bacteriology, environment, and behavior in the interpretive epidemiology of tuberculosis persisted until the advent of antibiotics in 1946 and the subsequent closing of sanatoriums. A necessary corollary of this epidemiology was the absolute authority of the resident physician, and this also remained relatively unchallenged until effective chemotherapy obviated the need for so much control over behavior and attitudes.

For most patients at Arequipa, resistance was obviated by the way in which their choices were framed. Within the convincing precepts of medical doctrine, to acquiesce to the imperatives of discipline, forceful good cheer, and cleanliness meant to embrace the only chance of healing a highly fatal disease. To resist meant to risk life itself. As the patient Ruth Ashby's poem entitled "Life in a Lung Resort" (n.d.) illustrates, it is not hard to guess which choice most women made:

> Do not talk
> do not walk
> easy does it
> always sit
> do not stand
> nor raise a hand
> above your head
> stay in your bed
> to cut your bill
> you must be still
> then to a man
> eat all you can
> soar your weight
> slow your gait
> take your rest
> tis for the best....
> well I've tried
> to abide
> by the book
> and by hook
> to gain my health
> and keep my wealth
> I'll cut my pace
> and win this race.

Body Politics at the Industrial Crossroads

Quoting Bordo again (1993, 195), an emphasis on resistance also does not help us to "describe and diagnose the politics of the body" within a particular culture at a particular moment in time, and the gendered body politics of early twentieth-century tuberculosis deserves some further diagnosis. Women such as those at Arequipa were bodies-in-the-making (Haraway 1995) at the nexus of a range of material forces and ideologies. Women as gatekeepers of health, notions of social-urban disorder, and behavioral components of tuberculosis as opposed to structural facilitations of it generated a politics that produced the female body as especially culpable but also key to the prevention of tuberculosis. As discussed in chapter 1, women were seen as pivotal components of health maintenance, a vital if unprofessionalized public health constituency that translated medical doctrine into healthful domestic hygiene for their families. But as Brown and others made clear, for the working-class tubercular and in particular the poor tuberculous woman, poor domestic habits derived from ignorance in large part were held responsible for causing tuberculosis (Brown 1911b). In other words, what David Barnes claims for late-nineteenth-century France was true of early twentieth-century America and San Francisco in the context of sanatorium treatment: rather than the dangers of slum housing, medical focus turned to the dangers of slum residents' ignorance of hygiene (Barnes 1995, 17), thus fixing blame on the individual rather than on the individual's structural environment.

Delving further into this contradiction and its gendered configurations, a body politics of tuberculosis needs to take into account a politics of labor versus domesticity, an oppositional that placed lower-class women in a particularly contradictory position in late-nineteenth- and early-twentieth-century society. On the one hand, the participation of women in the labor force, even at the turn of the century, was not a particularly new phenomenon of industrialization in the United States. Their entry into manufacturing and other industrial jobs was considered by employers a key to increased profits through lower wages, thus affirming David Harvey's statement that women's "insertion into the circulation of variable capital...has to be seen as a powerful constitutive force in distinctively capitalist constructions of gender" (Harvey 1997, 10). Though ostensibly the maintenance of productive bodies was necessary to sustain industrial production, in reality such "capitalist constructions of gender" rendered their own pathologies in the form of exhaustion, undernutrition, and tuberculosis.[23]

On the other hand, the representation of women in the labor force in the early twentieth century "still posed (and continues to pose) a fundamental challenge to many traditional conceptions of the family and of gender roles" (Harvey 1997, 10). The upper classes largely saw women's place as remaining in the home regardless of economic imperatives. The "cult of domesticity" had risen and waned over the past century, but it rose again in the early twentieth century, having embraced the mantle of science in the pursuit of more efficient housekeeping.[24] A dispersion of the germ theory to the general populace subsequently informed tenets of housekeeping, emphasizing hygiene and cleanliness applied both to bodily practice and home maintenance. Medical discourses concerning tuberculosis further assisted this ideology by producing women as necessary components in the antituberculosis campaign. Scientific housekeeping was not just vital to the reproduction of healthy American families — it was necessary more specifically for tuberculosis-free families. Yet women could only properly serve the function of health gatekeepers from the confines of the home while pursuing their proper roles as wives and mothers.

Tuberculosis in this analysis was thus at the center of a paradox: the outcome of one process and the tool of another. Phillip Brown seems to have understood this, not so much as a contradiction but as an explanation, on the one hand, and a solution, on the other. Brown never went so far as to urge graduates of Arequipa not to go back into the labor force; he was too well aware of the economic imperatives facing these women and their families. His solution, rather, was to reconcile the paradox by fully embracing tuberculosis as a tool for reconstructing gender and class behaviors in an effort to open up more healthy employment opportunities for these women, thus stopping the cycle of industrial pathology. In the absence of industrial reconfiguration, the reclassing and regendering of tuberculous bodies thus could be construed as a necessary if authoritarian step in the prevention of tuberculosis. Reworking a comment by Donna Haraway (1995, 515), for working women (or men) tuberculosis was a measure of incommensurability with an economic system and a regime of truth designed to be commensurate with the majority. Everyone, in other words, had a place in the capitalist production process, a process that could run smoothly only if everyone did their part and that promised rewards to each who successfully maintained their role within the system. The sanatorium regimen was not a point of resistance outside domination, but instead was a way of reworking a particular kind of fitting within the boundaries of a dominant construct.[25]

Besides a keener focus on gender, San Francisco's body politics of tuberculosis differed from that of many other U.S. cities by not being particularly racialized. As Alan M. Kraut records, the Jewish immigrant was targeted in New York as being less clean and more diseased than other immigrants living in slum tenements. The statistics showing that Jews had the second lowest mortality rates of any immigrant group (next to Swedes) did not deter these perceptions (Kraut 1994, 146). In many large eastern and midwestern cities the association of poverty with immigrant groups in general, and the association of tuberculosis with poverty, resulted in constructions of the tubercular as southern or eastern European (Kraut 1994; Rothman 1994). Tuberculosis in these cities, then, was a disease not just of poverty but of ethnic poverty, and the tuberculous body in public health construction was often a racialized one.

In the medical discourses concerning tuberculosis in San Francisco, such racializations were largely absent. Poverty was fixed upon as a primary causative factor of tuberculosis and as a social construct of the tubercular, but the poor for the most part were assumed to be white. In fact, as will be discussed in chapter 6, public health authorities in San Francisco perhaps did not focus enough attention on the racial aspects of tuberculosis. Statistics gathered at various times by the city's tuberculosis association showed that African Americans and Chinese suffered considerably more from the disease than did whites (San Francisco Tuberculosis Association 1915, 1937), yet little was ever done about this problem in terms of intensified public health intervention, better hospital care, or material assistance. Indeed, as hospital and sanatorium rosters show, ethnic minorities had disproportionately low representation in those institutions that might have provided them a chance to beat their tuberculosis. This might provide one reason for their higher mortality rates. The tuberculous body was not racialized in social and medical discourses, but in grim irony the real tuberculous body in San Francisco was disproportionately racialized through economic discrimination and public health neglect.

Conclusion

The Question of Infringement

The question posed above of whether the sanatorium regime was a necessary infringement of medical authority on personal space can be answered only vis-à-vis the larger political and socioeconomic context in which the sanatorium was embedded. There is little doubt that the sanatorium for working-class patients in San Francisco and the United States was seen in part as an antidote to unprecedented urban growth and, more specifically, to an alarming aggrandizement of the urban poor in the last decade of the nineteenth century and the first decades of the twentieth. Certainly by 1900, tuberculosis was seen as a disease of poverty (Rothman 1994; Dubos and Dubos 1987), a real and symbolic manifestation of everything that was going wrong in America's cities in the eyes of the middle and upper classes. It was also symbolic of underclass pathologies and the environment in which they were produced and reproduced — an environment not only of deprivation but of ignorance and disorder. Tuberculosis was, in a way, the ultimate early-twentieth-century disorder in the medical but also the social contexts of that term. Within this discourse, the sanatorium was designed to provide the antidote for both epidemiological interpretations of the disease. It was as much a finishing school as a medical institution, providing the means to take the poor away from the wretched environments that were degrading them morally as well as physically. It incorporated rigid discipline to instill order out of disorder and to educate the pathologically ignorant. It was an institution that simultaneously catered to a disease of the poor and the dis-ease of the middle class.[26]

But to end conclusively with this critique is to show only part of the picture. As any analysis of the Progressive Era attests, there were multiple discourses attempting to make sense of the ills perceived as characterizing American cities and to diagnose the pathologies of the poor. Even in the sanatorium context the discourse of blame and patronization of the poor was not the only one informing physicians and the treatments they implemented. Tuberculosis, for one thing, was not just a symbol of poverty and urban disorder. Some physicians such as Phillip Brown recognized that tuberculosis was a disease of industrialization, emerging from the particular configurations of industry that became for men and women "a pestiferous source of corruption and slavery, [where] the worker exists for the process of production and not the process of production for the worker" (Marx 1976, 615, cited in Harvey 1997, 10). The sanatorium in its rural setting offered a reprieve from those deleterious conditions in which most working-class individuals labored and because of which their bodies had degenerated into diseased states. The disciplinary regime within this discourse was framed as a necessary tactic to ensure that an abundant amount of rest, sunlight, and fresh air was received by every patient and that a tendency toward overstimulation did not threaten the progress of healing. It was also necessary as an educational tool to make sure that when patients eventually returned to their everyday environments, they would be better able to protect themselves from further physical degeneration by paying attention to their diets, resting as much as possible, keeping windows open, and keeping their domestic premises clean.[27]

Yet even with an awareness of occupational causes of tuberculosis, sanatorium physicians and the public health constabulary in general did not attempt to confront the ways in which industry produced tuberculous bodies. Despite Brown's astuteness in pointing out the cause of working women's tuberculosis, there is no record showing that he campaigned for better working conditions or for better standards of housing for the working poor. Like other sanatorium physicians, he worked within the status quo remaking bodies to be more commensurate with a system of class relations and industrial output that changed somewhat through the efforts of other Progressive reformers but that remained largely undisturbed. In Brown's case more specifically, he changed female bodies into more refined forces of production less suited for industrial labor and better suited for occupations — such as seamstress, stenographer, or lab assistant — that were more conducive to health but also more middle-class in their domestic derivations. In other words, the sanatorium played an important role in early-twentieth-century American society in reinscribing gender and class onto lower-class bodies while retaining inequitable class relations. Referring back to Lert's questions concerning the motivations behind the antituberculosis campaign, the answer must be that the sanatorium regimen accommodated both social and medical agendas through its extensive interventions into the lives of its patients.

The Question of Success

How effective the sanatorium was, to what degree the fastidious organization of space and the regendering of bodies succeeded in improving tuberculosis, is difficult to determine. Indeed one irony of the entire antituberculosis movement is that by the time it was under way, tuberculosis rates were already declining in the United States and Europe (Shryock 1957; L. Wilson 1990). Rates continued to decline, but the role of the sanatorium in effecting this is virtually impossible to tease out from other simultaneous factors such as nutrition, housing, wage levels, and hospital care. Indeed there are continuing debates over the role of sanatoriums versus public health and social factors in the diminution of tuberculosis over the first half of the century.[28] For those arguing that sanatoriums played a significant role in this process, the benefits of isolation are emphasized (cf. Bryder 1991 and L. Wilson 1990). Sanatoriums did not always cure their patients, but isolating them for long periods of time during an infectious stage of their disease is thought to have at least helped prevent infection from spreading to members of the patients' families and others with whom they would normally come in contact. Acquiring definitive statistics to prove or disprove this assertion is virtually impossible, however. Even evaluating the rate of cure within sanatoriums was made difficult by the length of time over which the disease stretched (during and after sanatorium care), the subtlety of its symptoms, and the mobility of former patients.

Arequipa nonetheless attempted to determine its success rate, recording the condition of its current and former patients every few years. In 1914, out of fifty-nine patients discharged, twenty-three were listed as "apparently cured"; ten had arrested cases; eleven were improved; and fifteen were unchanged (Arequipa Sanatorium Annual Reports 1914, 7). Seventy-five percent of what were called third-stage cases, those with advanced disease, had died within one to two years of discharge (Arequipa Sanatorium Annual Reports 1914, 12). In 1917, the rate had improved to some extent, with 63 percent of third-stage cases found to have died after discharge, compared with only 7.3 percent of first-stage cases, and 22.5 percent of second-stage cases. However, of those first-stage cases found alive, only nine of forty-one were reported cured; the rest were still in the tenuous state of "arrested" or "improved" disease (Arequipa Sanatorium Annual Reports 1917, 6–9). The 1922 comprehensive study found, over the sanatorium's ten-year history, a total of 53.6 percent of seven hundred women alive and well. Fewer women were dying, the study claimed, because more of them were learning how to monitor their condition once they had gone back to urban life (Arequipa Sanatorium Annual Reports 1922, 6–7). Arequipa's record seems to compare favorably to other sanatoriums in various parts of the country. The U.S. Public Health Service kept statistics from nine sanatoriums that followed the progress of their discharged patients. Combining the data from all nine institutions, in 1922, 74 percent of 520 were dead at the end of 10 years; 85 percent were dead at the end of 15 years (Whitney 1922). Clearly even for those lucky enough to find a space in a sanatorium, their chances of effectively stopping the progress of their disease was slight.

The inherent problem of the sanatorium, of course, was that eventually the patients had to return to the deleterious urban conditions that had originally precipitated disease. The skills learned while in residence would help discharged tuberculars reconfigure their home conditions as advantageously as possible, but particularly for the poor patients, the battle was unevenly waged.

The most chronic problem plaguing sanatoriums was their inadequate capacity to treat all of those in need. Most sanatoriums, Arequipa included, accepted only or predominantly first-stage cases, that is, those patients who had the initial, mildest form of the disease. The reasons for this were twofold. First, chronic shortage of sanatorium beds meant that most institutional directors wanted to reserve openings for those who stood a better chance of benefiting from sanatorium treatment (Bates 1992; Rothman 1994). It was recognized early on that the efficacy of rural surroundings and the sanatorium regimen was severely reduced for more advanced cases (Trudeau 1916). For working-class sanatoriums especially, the length of residence for advanced patients and the need for more expensive medical intervention also made the treatment of these cases untenable. Those whose disease had progressed beyond the first stage were thus usually relegated either to the tuberculosis hospital or to almost certain death at home. Even those with first-stage disease could not always be accommodated, as the long waiting lists at Arequipa and other sanatoriums attest (Arequipa Sanatorium Annual Reports 1914–24; Bates 1992; Rothman 1994).

Although rarely stated, it is also unlikely that nonwhite ethnic minorities ever found the doors of most sanatoriums open to them. African Americans were technically permitted to use San Francisco's health facilities (Broussard 1993), but Arequipa, Alta, and St. Helena were private institutions, as were all sanatoriums outside San Francisco until the second decade of the twentieth century. Except for Arequipa, they were also far more expensive than the vast majority of African Americans living in San Francisco could afford. With annual incomes for African Americans in 1939 averaging four hundred to six hundred dollars (Broussard 1993, 35), a typical stay of about seven months at the Alta Sanatorium would cost more than a year's income. Not until a municipal sanatorium was finally built outside the city in the mid-1920s would this group have better access to sanatorium care. This was more than was available to the city's Chinese population, which continued to be excluded from most health care outside Chinatown until well into the century (Trauner 1978). All ethnic groups were excluded from Arequipa until only a decade or so before the institution closed its doors around 1950.

For all of San Francisco's poor and working class suffering from tuberculosis, institutional space continued to be acutely inadequate even after municipal sanatorium care was implemented. In 1935, the municipal tuberculosis hospital and sanatorium combined provided only 57 percent of the National Tuberculosis Association's recommended bed capacity for tuberculars (Works Progress Administration 1937). For the majority of San Francisco's actual and potential tuberculosis cases, solutions within the city would have to be sought as an alternative to the expense of sanatorium care.

6

REFORMING THE CITY

Domestic Restructuring and the Tuberculosis Hospital

If it was impossible to sequester the body of the tubercular in a sanatorium in every case, then alternatives within the city needed to be devised. Informing the campaign for lower urban tuberculosis rates were the same ontologies of poverty and epistemologies of health undergirding sanatorium care. If anything the 1906 earthquake exacerbated the perception of a city out of control, or conversely a city needing desperately to reshape itself into something at once more orderly and less plagued by the blight of disease. The two were clearly related in the minds of many Progressive reformers and public health officials. The directions taken by the campaign against tuberculosis, in San Francisco as elsewhere, reflected the belief that to diminish the numbers of tuberculars meant a systematic program of targeting the poor to screen out infectious cases, controlling these cases, reeducating them into middle-class notions of behavior and hygiene, and monitoring their progress in this endeavor. As stated in the third annual report of the San Francisco Association for the Study and Prevention of Tuberculosis, "The disease can be stamped out as soon as all consumptives are reached, controlled and specially instructed, and public measures against infection enforced" (Arequipa Sanatorium Annual Reports 1910, 6). Two assumptions are evident here: the poor were generally irresponsible and ignorant, and tuberculosis was a function of this.

In San Francisco, as in the rest of the United States, control and reeducation were undertaken via two primary means: reconfigurations of housing and domestic practices by visiting field nurses and the isolation of advanced cases in hospitals. The role of each of these in diminishing tuberculosis rates is difficult to assess, but it is likely that both were relatively ineffectual given their limited scope and the constraints under which they were carried out. Like their sanatorium counterparts, it was clear in the structure of the antituberculosis campaign and in the discursive rendering of the target population that public health authorities in the city had no intention of disturbing the status quo of class relations or the structural undergirdings of the underclass. Addressing a disease rooted unmistakably in poverty without truly addressing poverty would seem to be a difficult undertaking, but the effects of germ theory were to reconstruct the purview of public health as limited to individual behaviors divorced from their wider economic context. The rest of this chapter will expound upon this and the campaign as a whole, after a description of San Francisco's poverty and tuberculosis.

Urban Structures of Disease

Elaborating from the last chapter, San Francisco did not so easily fit the image of the gray, industrial city of the eastern United States. Much of the heavy industry such as steel, sugar, and machine production previously based in San Francisco relocated to the East Bay by the turn of the century (Walker 1996; Issel and Cherny 1986). In its place the economy was based primarily on finance, shipping, construction, canning, and crafts — occupations that were certainly not all white-collar, but that did not elicit the grim images of factory and sweatshop labor emerging from other urban areas at this time (Walker 1995). Phillip Brown was right to point out that these main occupations in San Francisco were overwhelmingly male, leaving many of the lower-paying domestic, service, and small-scale manufacturing jobs to women and ethnic minorities (Brown 1911b; Broussard 1993). Nevertheless, these less-optimal occupations did not dominate the economic landscape.

Images of San Francisco's poorest districts also did not conjure up the desolation and hopelessness of New York's tenements or Pittsburgh's factory-fringe shanties. As seen in the earlier photographs of South of Market, frame houses predominated San Francisco's lower-class neighborhoods at least until after the turn of the century, with the exception of Chinatown. Though run down and spaced close together, these frame houses appeared better able than huge tenement buildings to admit light and ventilation. As many public health workers were discovering, however, single-family dwellings could be just as efficient in the spread of tuberculosis when they were characterized by crowding (Rosner 1995; Ward 1989). In some poor districts of Philadelphia, for example, tuberculosis rates were as high as those for New

York's tenement zones, even though like San Francisco, frame houses characterized Philadelphia's poorest neighborhoods (Ward 1989). A 1936 study of tuberculosis in San Francisco found the number of tuberculosis cases in one household to be directly proportional to the size of the house and the number living in it rather than the type of dwelling (Works Progress Administration 1937). For San Francisco, crowding in South of Market had already become acute by the turn of the century, with eight, ten, or twelve people living in a house originally meant to accommodate four (Olmstead et al. 1979). High real estate prices, middle-class flight to new suburbs, and a large percentage of properties owned by landlords more interested in property income than upkeep caused deterioration in a significant proportion of San Francisco's housing by the early decades of the century (Broussard 1993).

The effect of the earthquake on tuberculosis rates is difficult to determine, although from statistics it is clear that rates dropped significantly between 1905 and 1906: from 308 per 100,000 to 209. One explanation for this decline was the open-air lifestyle forced upon thousands of San Franciscans with the destruction of housing stock; though residence in tent camps was temporary, the shift in accommodation may have effectively prevented transmission. The earthquake also wiped out numerous "breeding places" such as schools, theaters, and workplaces, even though these were subsequently rebuilt with architectural designs not radically different from before. One of the most significant factors behind the decline was the exodus of people moving either temporarily or permanently out of the city after the earthquake. Exact numbers are unknown, but, according to the report cited above, they were large enough to reduce the pool of people at risk (San Francisco Tuberculosis Association 1928, 20).

Housing improved for some after the 1906 earthquake, but it worsened for others. A special corporation was set up in the summer of 1906 to administer loans and grants to those needing to rebuild their homes destroyed during the earthquake and for those who had not owned homes before the earthquake to enable them to do so (Kahn 1979). At the end of the loan-granting period, however, it became clear from a survey of relief efforts that the corporation had assisted primarily those middle-class persons who had some means already at their disposal. For those of lower economic standing, the corporation ended up funding 5,610 "temporary" cottages and nineteen tenements with two-room apartments (Kahn 1979, 151). When surveyed a year after the earthquake, these cottages were found to be crowded together, lacking inside toilets or bathtubs, with the majority lacking water. Why more assistance was not proffered those of lower incomes was answered by the authors of the relief survey, and in their response is revealed the attitude of distrust in which the poor were held:

> Those who possessed vacant lots, or other property, or who could command means with which to build, gave tangible proof that the foundation of previous thrift and enterprise would serve as a guarantee of wise use of aid from the relief funds. The applicants who had owned no property, possessed no savings, and whose standard of living was low, could offer little, if any, guarantee of a wise use of funds.... Had a body of expert social workers been engaged... [to teach] each to be a good householder, a more liberal housing allowance could have been safely granted. (Cited in Kahn 1979, 153)

The absurdly flawed logic of this statement could only seem reasonable if viewed through an ideological lens construing the poor as childlike and privileging the abilities of the expert. A "culture of poverty" argument was added for good measure, however, when the authors concluded that the "poorest class of homeless refugees [was]... accustomed to comparatively low standards of living" (in Kahn 1979, 152). The relief organizers, like their counterparts in public health, were not interested in disturbing the class status quo.

In other areas, the destruction of housing stock resulted in hasty construction of larger multiunit buildings and increased segmentation of larger apartments. The Western Addition, an area north of Market extending from Larkin to Divisadero, was such an area. Residents from harder hit districts flooded to the Western Addition, and buildings quickly were converted into cramped apartments. Basements, storage rooms, and attics were even made into living quarters in an effort to meet the overwhelming demand for space. Industries also entered the area, often operating in close proximity to living spaces. The result was that "every condition that would make a modern city planner shudder was soon to be found in the Western Addition in exaggerated form: indiscriminate mixture of land uses, excessive density of population, substandard housing, traffic congestion" (Scott 1959, 111). Sections of the Mission suffered a similar fate as older homes left intact by the earthquake were refitted to accommodate more occupants. In the process, "faulty room arrangements and bad lighting and ventilation resulted" (Scott 1959, 111). By the 1930s, the Western Addition had become home to a large proportion of the city's small but growing African American population, most of whom were working-class. Russians and eastern Europeans also moved into this area in the early years of the century (Godfrey 1988).

The formerly middle-class enclaves of Bernal Heights and Potrero Hill became more working-class in character as poor Italian and other unskilled laborers moved to these areas to be closer to factories, railroads, and warehouses (Godfrey 1988). Many Italians and other immigrants after the turn of the century also moved to North Beach, dramatically increasing the degree of crowding in that area. In 1900, the North Beach district bounded by Montgomery and Kearny Streets and the Bay contained thirteen thousand people; by 1910, there were twenty-two thousand, half of whom were foreign-born (Cinel 1982). The middle and upper classes, in the meantime, continued the pattern of outward movement into newly created suburban fringes. In the first decades of the century, the Sunset and Richmond districts and the area west of Twin Peaks became the new middle-class zones of disengagement (Godfrey 1988), as did the Peninsula, Marin County, and the East Bay (Walker 1995).

Even South of Market's topography changed significantly by the 1920s and 1930s. After the 1906 earthquake and fire destroyed much of South of Market's mixture of cottages and lodging houses, rebuilding followed a pattern that better accommodated the district's changing demography. Though not a new phenomenon, the number of single, male migrant laborers residing in South of Market was growing (Wollenberg 1975). The district's hobo population also increased between 1880 and 1920 as men sought inexpensive lodgings while working intermittent jobs in industry and on the railroads or while simply waiting out the winter in the city until agricultural work opened up again in the spring (Averbach 1973). By 1914, a survey of the district found approximately forty-thousand single men living in South of Market during the winter (Groth 1994, 153).

Accordingly, a significant proportion of rebuilding after the earthquake took the form of larger, high-density flats or tenements and cheap residential hotels (Groth 1994; Godfrey 1988; Averbach 1973). A predominance of single men was of course not the only factor dictating a proliferation of high-density living accommodations in the area. Financing, and the acute shortage of housing after the earthquake, also shaped the erection of larger buildings. As Langley Porter, president of the San Francisco Housing Association, pointed out in 1911, "The people wanted shelter, the workmen needed wages, the contractors in many cases had to rebuild shattered financial standing, and lot owners were anxious for the same reason to get the greatest possible income from their property.... Merely that a building would not fall was all they asked. Thus tenements, not homes, were built" (cited in Scott 1959, 112).

These buildings, like their counterparts in other cities, were constructed with little regard to building codes or the tenets of public health and sanitation. They were designed to render the maximum number of individual cells within a given space with a minimum amount of upkeep. The cubicle and dormitory ward designs met these standards most efficiently. The former was characterized by a large rectangular building filled in with thin partitioning, usually not more than seven feet high, comprising rooms of five by seven or six by eight feet. Each room contained a single bed or cot and was topped by chicken wire to prevent men from accessing the rooms without paying (Groth 1994, 144). Dormitories had even fewer structures and were characterized by large empty rooms with perhaps canvas hammocks or wooden platforms for sleeping (Groth 1994, 144). Ventilation in these buildings was virtually nonexistent, standards of cleanliness poor, and the possibilities of tuberculosis transmission rife.

As part of a report on conditions in South of Market, a State Relief Administration worker in the 1930s described the inside of a typical cubicle hotel:

> Room #88 was an inside room, about the center of the house, size 6 by 8. Walls were 6 feet high with chicken wire overhead. The room contained a cot with a dirty straw pad, and three, very dirty comforters. The linen was clean. A small clothes closet contained five empty liquor bottles. . . . A lighted match, applied to cracks in the partitions, scattered bed bugs in all directions. (Cited in Olmstead et al. 1979, 259)

The disease and fire dangers posed by cubicle hotels led California to ban further construction of them after 1917, and most of the cubicle hotels are now gone from San Francisco (Groth 1994). The homeless shelters that have replaced them, however, are built with designs very similar to both the cubicle- and dormitory-style hotels of the first decades of the century. It is clear that accommodation of large numbers with the least financial expenditure, rather than setting minimum health standards, still characterizes urban housing policies for the poor.

The likelihood of acquiring tuberculosis in living conditions such as these was compounded by the already precarious physical condition of many South of Market residents during this period. A collection of short biographies compiled in 1928 by economists at the University of California gives testimony to the desperate poverty, debility, and hunger suffered by many migrant laborers in the district during the second and third decades of the twentieth century. For a majority of those represented in the collection, San Francisco was the endpoint of years of itinerant labor covering much of the country and several occupations, most of them semi- or unskilled. Many had labored elsewhere in California because the state's logging, mining, and agricultural industries thrived on casual or seasonal employment. According to Averbach, "exposure to the elements, the hazardous nature of mining, logging, and construction work, lack of on-the-job medical attention, insufficient diet, and the very arduous labor demanded by most [of these] jobs all determined that a high number of men would eventually find themselves incapacitated" (Averbach 1973, 207). Some simply had grown too old to sustain demanding physical labor. In either case, they ended up in South of Market looking for less-taxing work and cheap living quarters. Although it cannot be determined what percentage of the South of Market population these older, debilitated migrant workers constituted, it is clear their numbers were significant. It is also likely that their younger coresidents, though perhaps more frequently employed, were nonetheless little better off until well into the 1940s.

Howard Street, running parallel to Market, served as the place the unemployed came to find jobs for the day or for longer, if they were lucky. Known as "the slave market," it was the gathering spot for employers hiring casual laborers for odd jobs at wages hovering at or below subsistence level (Groth 1994; Olmstead et al. 1979; Averbach 1973). When even this avenue failed, men were forced to resort to the Salvation Army wood yard, where in exchange for chopping wood they received a meal and a bed if they had no room for the night. The meal, in the words of one man, was "just enough to let you get up from the table less hungry"; it was not enough to sustain physical labor or health (cited in Olmstead et al. 1979, 250). By the 1930s, the situation was worse, with employment of any kind difficult to find and even the substandard housing inadequate to accommodate everyone in need. By the late 1920s and 1930s, in addition to the cheap residential hotels and tenements, huge shelters were built in an effort to get the unemployed off the streets at night (Averbach 1973). Those shelters serving free meals were overwhelmed by the 1930s, forcing many migrants to go a day or more without food (Olmstead et al. 1979).

The Toll of Poverty and Poor Housing Policies

It is not surprising that the first extensive study of tuberculosis in San Francisco, conducted from 1912 through 1914, found tuberculosis rates of 203.2 per 100,000, significantly higher than the national average of 147.6. Also not surprisingly, the study found the highest tuberculosis rates in those districts where the poor were most prevalent (San Francisco Tuberculosis Association 1915, 6). Map 6.1 illustrates these findings, with each dot representing a death from tuberculosis during the three years from 1912 to 1914. Immediately noticeable is the fact that virtually no area of the city is unscathed;

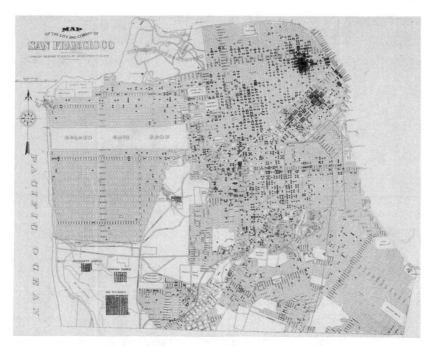

Map 6.1. Spot map of San Francisco tuberculosis cases, 1912–14. Courtesy of The Bancroft Library, University of California, Berkeley.

even the less densely populated middle- and upper-class outlying districts are not spared the ravages of the disease. Yet the greatest concentration of deaths is clearly found in the downtown and South of Market sectors of the city, where the dots are so numerous they coalesce into ominous stains covering several blocks. The most concentrated cluster of mortalities falls within the area bounded by Mason, Sansome, Sacramento, and Union, an area embracing Chinatown and the lower section of North Beach. The next highest concentration, bounded by Market, Second Street, Harrison, and Fourth, was primarily home to migrant laborers and other single men.

The city districts and their respective tuberculosis mortality rates are shown in map 6.2. Though again it is evident that every district suffered some extent of the disease, the discrepancies among districts are acute. District 33, with the highest tuberculosis mortality rate of 526.4 per 100,000, had over six times the mortality rate of district 27, a predominantly middle-class western suburb. Corresponding to geographic differences in mortality was the map of ethnic differences. Though not as widely discrepant, Asian and African American versus white mortality rates from tuberculosis

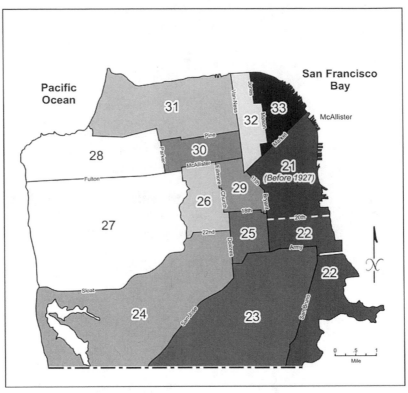

** Rate is based on 1913 district populations.
Map Source: Issel and Cherney 1986.
Data Source: San Francisco Association for the Study and Prevention of Tuberculosis, 1915.

District	Rates/ 100,000**	District	Rates/ 100,000**
27	80.8	30	160.6
28	93.1	25	183.4
32	95.4	23	197.5
26	107.2	22	200.4
31	110.0	21	339.7
24	137.1	33	526.4
29	152.6		

Map 6.2. Tuberculosis rates by city district, 1912–14. Data from San Francisco Tuberculosis Association 1915. Base map from Issel and Cherny 1986; adapted by David Cantrell.

represent a stark testament to variable economic and social opportunity in the San Francisco of the first half of the twentieth century. Whereas the white population had a composite tuberculosis mortality rate of 173.94 per 100,000 in 1914, the Chinese tallied a rate of 621.9, the Japanese 228.0, and the African American population 651.5 (San Francisco Tuberculosis Association 1915, 6–7, 20).

Given San Francisco's history of anti-Asian sentiment, perhaps the biggest surprise is the comparatively low mortality rate of the city's Japanese population. Although it is difficult to determine precisely why they fared better than most ethnic minorities, one possibility is that many of the Japanese who arrived in San Francisco were better off economically than the vast majority of immigrants to the city (Issel and Cherny 1986). Though they subsequently faced a rash of discrimination in the early twentieth century, many nonetheless found economic niches in the city and maintained them. For the most part, these niches were service industries for the growing Japanese community such as restaurants, pool halls, bars, and laundries (Takaki 1989). Other Japanese engaged in farming, usually small-scale truck farming feeding San Francisco markets (Takaki 1989). According to Takaki, the relative success of many Japanese in California was due to ethnic solidarity and "the mutual-support systems . . . [that] provided a network of social relations buttressing economic cooperation and assistance for employment, housing, and credit" (Takaki 1989, 193).

These support systems not only aided success in business but helped ensure better quality housing for many Japanese despite being forced, like the Chinese earlier, to concentrate in one area of the city (Godfrey 1988). Their later arrival also meant that Japantown was located in an outlying area, that is, the northeastern corner of the Western Addition, in contradistinction to the cramped inner-city location of Chinatown. Mutual support systems may also have provided a safety net for those Japanese finding themselves temporarily without jobs or otherwise in financial straits. Particularly during the depression years of the 1930s, such aid networks made the difference for many between provisional livelihood and a descent into poverty and disease. Finally, the involvement of so many Japanese in agriculture may also have meant access to a better diet than many of the poor had at this time. Together, these factors resulted in the Japanese having the overall lowest tuberculosis mortality rate in San Francisco by the mid-1930s (Works Progress Administration 1937).

Not so surprising is the high rate of tuberculosis suffered by the Chinese community. Outright blame of the Chinese for disease had waned after the second episode of plague in 1909. Yet hostility was replaced with the more insidious policy of neglect, while discrimination in areas of employment and housing continued. Opportunities to find work outside of Chinatown were constrained even further in the twentieth century than they were in the nineteenth, either because employers would not hire Chinese or because the growth of labor unions precluded hiring Chinese over union workers. Blue-collar whites and newer immigrants from southern and eastern Europe often replaced Chinese in service and manufacturing jobs (Takaki 1989; Daniels 1980). The rising popularity of Chinatown as a tourist attraction created more service jobs in restaurants, souvenir stores, laundries, and markets, but these generally entailed extremely long hours and little financial reward. By 1940, 61 percent of Chinese workers were in these low-paying service jobs (U.S. Census 1940). Chinese women were usually employed either in domestic service or in the garment industry. The latter occupation in particular was physically grueling, with factories opening at seven in the morning and running until ten at night (Cather 1932, 60); workrooms were cramped, often unventilated, and ill lit, and wages were minimal. Even when the owners of garment factories were themselves Chinese, the exploitation in this sector was rampant (Takaki 1989).

The depression made matters worse in Chinatown. Two of the major Chinese banks, the China Mail and the Canton Bank, failed, and with them went people's savings or the hopes of garnering loans to start or continue businesses (Cather 1932). Tourism diminished, and Chinese businesses suffered from the drop in patronage both from tourists and from Chinese within the community. In the meantime, no other employment opportunities were available to mitigate the loss, while Chinatown's population grew as Chinese released from agricultural jobs came back to the city (Cather 1932).

Added to low wages and deleterious working conditions, the Chinese occupied some of the most insalutary housing in the city. The earthquake of 1906 destroyed much of Chinatown, but the buildings that went up in the years following were some of the worst tenements in San Francisco (Scott 1959; Groth 1994). Buildings were designed with tiny cubicles and a minimum of amenities to accommodate a population still predominantly single and male in the first decade of the century due to the Chinese exclusion laws. But the 1906 fire burned the majority of municipal records, including those containing the immigration status of the city's Chinese population. Chinese men could subsequently claim to have been born in the United States, enabling them to bring their wives and families over from China (Takaki 1989). Between 1907 and 1924, when a new immigration act again prohibited Chinese immigration, some ten thousand Chinese females entered the country (Takaki 1989, 234–35). The consequence in terms of housing was a density in many buildings four times that set by the building standard (Groth 1994, 158). A Community Chest survey in 1930 showed that of the fifty-three families studied in Chinatown, thirty-two averaging five members each had only one room to live in (Cather 1932, 61). The average number of individuals per bathroom was 20.4, and several families had to share limited kitchen space (Takaki 1989, 246). Many units had no windows or had only inside windows affording no ventilation and very little light (Cather 1932, 61). It was little wonder that Chinatown's tuberculosis mortality rates were three times those for whites in the city by 1936 (Works Progress Administration 1937, 6).

Despite statistical evidence by the early twentieth century of Chinatown's high tuberculosis mortality rates, San Francisco's health department did very little to ameliorate the situation. As H. V. Cather stated, "The Chinese are no longer a problem to the city, and [instead] they have been forgotten" (Cather 1932, 62). The 1915 health survey showing high rates of tuberculosis in Chinatown did engender the opening of a tuberculosis clinic there in 1918 (Hiscock 1930). Yet a subsequent health department survey performed in 1929 showed that in contrast to the rest of San Francisco's population, tuberculosis death rates were not diminishing in Chinatown. Though the Chinese represented only 1.5 percent of the city's population in 1929, they represented 8.5 percent of total deaths from tuberculosis (Hiscock 1930, 40). They also had the lowest case-reporting rate of any other group in the city: in 1936 a full 77 percent of tuberculosis cases in Chinatown went unreported until death or one month before death (Works Progress Administration 1937, 46).

The worst rate of tuberculosis mortality in the city was found among the African American population. Alarming in itself, this statistic becomes even more disturbing when compared to the rates for African Americans outside San Francisco. In 1910, the average tuberculosis mortality rate for blacks nationally was 446 per 100,000; by 1920, it had dropped to 262 (McBride 1991, 46). In most American cities, African Americans died from tuberculosis at rates three times the white population (McBride 1991, 11); in San Francisco throughout the first three to four decades of the century, they died at rates five times the white population (Works Progress Administration 1937). The reasons behind these statistics, as always with tuberculosis, must be looked for in the social and economic conditions affecting African Americans in San Francisco during this period.

Like the Chinese and Japanese in San Francisco, African Americans faced widespread discrimination in housing and employment that in some respects worsened in the first half of the twentieth century (Daniels 1980). Because there were so few blacks in San Francisco in the nineteenth century, many were able to pursue economic opportunities without posing the threat of potential job loss to white workers. But by the early twentieth century the growth of larger-scale businesses and powerful labor unions had shut many African Americans out of jobs (Daniels 1980). An increase in white immigrant labor, as in the case of the Chinese, also provided replacements for those positions once held by blacks. One example of this was the Palace Hotel, which in the late 1870s and 1880s was the primary employer of African Americans in San Francisco (Olmstead et al. 1979). When it opened in 1875, it hired two hundred blacks as cooks, kitchen help, and waiters (Daniels 1980). By 1889, a white restaurant workers' union had forced the hotel to hire white union laborers and to dismiss its black workers (Daniels 1980; Broussard 1993). Similar layoffs of African Americans occurred elsewhere in the service and domestic sectors during the last decade of the nineteenth and first decades of the twentieth century (Broussard 1993). By the early twentieth century, the only occupations open to African American males were as elevator operators, redcaps, doormen, or railroad servicemen. Black women were overwhelmingly employed in domestic service (Broussard 1993, 40).

Although cities elsewhere in the United States discriminated against blacks, one factor affecting employment opportunities for African Americans in San Francisco was the absence of large-scale heavy industry and factories (Broussard 1993). In more industrial cities like Cleveland or Detroit, blacks were hired in large numbers to work in automobile or steel factories. Though arduous and unpleasant, these jobs paid relatively well because blacks were organized under the major trade unions (Broussard 1993). In contrast, the unions in San Francisco representing manufacturing and service industries steadfastly excluded African Americans and Asians until the middle of the century (Broussard 1993; Daniels 1980). As W. E. B. Du Bois stated in 1913, "The opportunity of the San Francisco Negro to earn a living is very difficult," and it would remain so for another three decades (cited in Daniels 1980, 34).

Finding housing presented similar obstacles for blacks, though discrimination was not legislated or organized on a large scale for the first four decades of the century. In contrast to many northeastern cities with much larger African American populations, San Francisco did not have a black ghetto, nor was there widespread agitation by white residents to keep blacks out of particular neighborhoods (Broussard 1993). Yet lower incomes and a less systematic form of housing discrimination by the 1920s and 1930s meant that African Americans frequently ended up in less desirable or substandard housing and could afford less often to buy a home rather than rent. A 1939 report on housing conditions in San Francisco noted that blacks had clustered in the poorer districts of the city such as the Western Addition and South of Market and that their households were "in poor condition and more congested than homes occupied by white families" (cited in Broussard 1993, 31). The report also stated that the Western Addition, where half the city's black population resided, contained over a third of the city's substandard housing. And yet African American families on average paid more rent than whites and spent a greater proportion of their incomes (55.5 percent) on rent than any other group in the city (Broussard 1993, 35). This, of course, left a smaller proportion of income to be spent on food and health care.

San Francisco's 1915 map of tuberculosis mortality on the surface mimicked the divide between city and country, with higher death rates in the urban core than the suburban fringe. Yet in its ethnic map of tuberculosis mortality San Francisco differed in some details from many other U.S. cities. Chinatown's location in the middle of the city, surrounded by business and financial districts, was unusual in addition to being irritating to municipal officials and businessmen. After the 1906 earthquake destroyed much of it, city planners attempted to have Chinatown rebuilt on the city's periphery, away from the main bustle of commerce and population movement (Mayne 1993). This obviously did not succeed, and the "ethnic island" (Takaki 1989) of high mortality and morbidity continued to exist adjacent to the financial zone and the wealthy residential enclave of Nob Hill. Similarly, Alvin Averbach contends that migrant laborers rarely found accommodation in the inner districts of other cities the way they did in San Francisco's South of Market. More common was for this population to establish encampments on urban fringes outside the purview of municipal tuberculosis case registration or medical assistance (Averbach 1973, 203). These factors may partially explain why San Francisco had one of the highest tuberculosis mortality rates in the country for most of the first half of the century. Yet even when the 1929 health department survey corrected San Francisco's tuberculosis death rate for "residents" only, a calculation that would have factored out the migrant labor population, it still came out ahead of other cities' death rates. Compared to Boston's rate of 81 per 100,000 population, Chicago's rate of 77, and Pittsburgh's rate of 73, San Francisco's resident tuberculosis death rate was 84.[1] Even New York, with a rate of 75, could not compare (Hiscock 1930, 40).

The scene in figure 6.1 perhaps epitomizes the image, sustained throughout the first decades of the century, of poverty and its consequences for San Francisco. A woman stands on a landing outside a very small frame house squeezed on at least two sides by other buildings and cluttered in front by

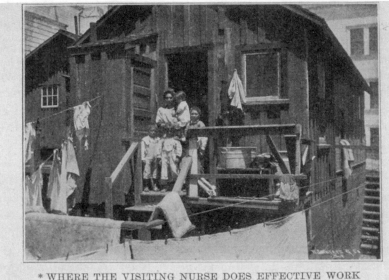

Figure 6.1. "Where the Visiting Nurse Does Effective Work." Courtesy of The Bancroft Library, University of California, Berkeley.

laundry and other household paraphernalia. The caption underneath the photograph delineates the grim outcome of poverty, overwork, congested living conditions, and poor nutrition for this woman and her family. The husband is already afflicted with advanced tuberculosis; the woman herself is showing the first signs of the disease; and all four of her children are in the liminal category of "predisposed," having physical signs that may or may not develop into active tuberculosis. For the youngest, pictured in the woman's arms, predisposition was fleeting: he died of tubercular meningitis between the time the photograph was shot and taken to press (San Francisco Tuberculosis Association 1915, 8). The caption indicates a practice common to people of all classes during this period of keeping doors and windows closed as a safeguard against colds and other respiratory ailments. This habit may not have made a significant difference in tuberculosis rates for families living in more spacious homes, but it almost certainly assisted the spread of tuberculosis in poorer houses. Spaces already cramped and airless, when closed off completely to the outside, became domestic laboratories of infection as effective as any tenement hovel.

Designing the Healthy City

The antituberculosis campaign was divided into medical and social categories, a bifurcation resulting from the shift in responsibilities of medicine and public health as a result of the bacteriological paradigm. By the turn of the century, public health had changed from focusing on the environment to focusing on individuals and those behaviors that placed them at greater risk of infection. In lieu of a vaccine or pharmaceutical cure for tuberculosis, the health department construed its responsibilities in the antituberculosis campaign as the isolation of the tuberculous in hospital facilities and, together with the San Francisco Tuberculosis Association, as the management of the tubercular at home by trained medical personnel. Besides the influence of bacteriology, this approach to tuberculosis prevention and management was guided by prevailing ontologies of poverty that implicitly recognized social causes of penury while maintaining that the poor could be helped through the avuncular guidance of the better off. Education more than structural amelioration would provide better lives for those poor individuals willing to embrace the possibilities of positive change in their lives; it would also reproduce this class as one less threatening to the remaining urban populace by diminishing their rates of tuberculosis.

Within this discourse there was room for more than one class of poor, however. As with nineteenth-century discourses of poverty, many early twentieth-century Progressives left little challenged the idea that some poor were "unworthy," beyond the hope of reeducation and control because their poverty was engendered by behavioral defects rather than structural impediments. For public health constituencies this class could not simply be neglected, however, because they posed perhaps the gravest danger for continued tuberculosis transmission. Particularly in the second and third decades of the century, the migrant laborer presented the antituberculosis campaign with its greatest challenge: how to control, reform, or isolate a highly peripatetic population.

Efforts in the Social Sphere: Reform and Restructuring

Organized in 1908, the San Francisco Tuberculosis Association coalesced when a group of physicians grew impatient with the complacency still characterizing the reaction to high rates of tuberculosis in the city, a reaction fueled in part by a lingering belief that little could be done about the disease and "the less said about it the better" (San Francisco Tuberculosis Association

1928, 8). Their organization, originally named the San Francisco Association for the Study and Prevention of Tuberculosis, embraced as its main purpose a campaign of "prevention through education" of the poor, as well as a limited restructuring of poor habitations. Education and monitoring of the poor came primarily in the form of visits from field nurses to the homes of tuberculars who either were newly discharged from sanatorium care, whose cases were not advanced enough for institutional isolation, or who were unable to gain a bed in the tuberculosis hospital. The push for structural reform on the part of the association focused upon better standards of construction for larger multiunit residential buildings, internal reconfiguration of existing homes and apartments, and the addition of outdoor sleeping porches to single-unit homes.

The idea of reducing disease rates through structural changes was not new. Sanitary engineering by the latter decades of the nineteenth century had succeeded to varying degrees in designing more efficient sewers and privy systems and in instigating better street-cleaning operations. San Francisco's public health department, though not as successful as some, had implemented ordinances for better plumbing and drainage and had rebuilt a large portion of city sewers (Municipal Reports 1880–90). The difference by the early twentieth century was public health officials' greater precision and narrower scope of spatial reference. Overarching sanitary sweeps of the city were deemphasized in favor of focusing on structural features directly impacting disease rates.

One of the earliest outcomes of this new focus nationwide was the implementation of minimum standards for houses and tenement buildings. Debates emerged over whether congestion alone caused most disease or whether restructuring should entail access to amenities such as toilets and clean water. Most cities attempted to implement some combination of the two. Housing codes regulating spatial requirements, as well as better light and ventilation, were implemented in cities like New York and Chicago, fostering the design of new tenements. In most cities the poor drainage and lack of sanitation facilities characterizing almost all impoverished districts were also addressed (Ward 1989). Zoning was another mechanism designed, among other things, to preclude the juxtapositioning of factories and noxious industries with living spaces, as well as to prevent overbuilding in lots designated for residential purposes (Klein and Kantor 1976).

San Francisco proved more reluctant to pass effective building codes. Some minor legislation was passed, such as the 1917 ordinance mandating cleanliness and good ventilation of hotel rooms (California State Board of Health Reports 1926, 99) and other ordinances requiring the installation of up-to-date plumbing and sanitation facilities in new buildings and houses (California State Board of Health Reports 1926, 99). The city proved less committed to more substantive laws. The importance accorded by the San Francisco Tuberculosis Association to this area of legislation is evident in its 1910 report:

> The record of San Francisco in the matter of health is an unenvi-able one. This fact...is due chiefly to an absence in the past of proper legal restriction and supervision in the erection of the cheaper classes of dwellings. To this condition almost exclusively is due the appalling annual mortality from tuberculosis.... The public health is closely and inseparably connected with the character of the build-ing laws, and in the details of space required for light and air. (San Francisco Tuberculosis Association 1910, 15)

This statement was made in reaction to a bill introduced that year to the board of supervisors overturning a 1909 building ordinance setting minimum sizes of lighting wells for apartment buildings and residence hotels (Groth 1994). That ordinance mandated that no building should occupy more than 90 percent of a corner lot or 70 percent of any other lot (cited in San Francisco Tuberculosis Association 1910, 15). Rather than the size of lot or building, the important precedent established by this ordinance was the ratio of empty space and light to occupied space. The bill introduced in February of 1910 would reduce the amount of space required for light and ventilation in flats and tenements, so that buildings could occupy 80 percent of any noncorner lot (San Francisco Tuberculosis Association 1910, 15, 16).

In its arguments against passing the new ordinance, the association claimed not only that reducing the required amount of space for light and air would create more slums in San Francisco but that doing so would also fly in the face of lessons learned by other cities coming to terms with their tenement sectors. While many cities were actively trying to improve their ten-ement building codes in order to ameliorate tuberculosis rates, San Francisco would be working in the opposite direction with the proposed legislation (San Francisco Tuberculosis Association 1910, 16). Despite their arguments, the ordinance passed. The contingencies faced by a city attempting to rebuild as quickly as possible after a devastating earthquake may partially explain the erosion of building standards in the midst of a local and national tuberculosis campaign. For many such as the physicians of the tuberculosis association, however, the passage of such legislation showed the limitations of a city's commitment to diminish its most costly disease.

The results of such negligence were highlighted in the same report with a description of the average lodging house for single men in San Francisco.

Claiming that no improvement had been made to these establishments over the last several years, the authors of the 1910 report went on to delineate the hazards these buildings posed, including their failure to meet even the minimum building codes still extant and their danger to public health:

> Anyone who has inspected these cheap lodging houses knows that they are not conducted in the interest of the public health. Many of them are so constructed that a large number of the rooms are entirely without sunlight, and most of them have less than the amount of cubic air space required by law. Blankets are rarely washed; sheets certainly not removed every time the bed changes its occupant. (San Francisco Tuberculosis Association 1910, 28)

To compound the capacity of these establishments to effectively transmit tuberculosis, the men who occupied them usually drifted from one such hotel to another; any who were already infected could thus spread the bacillus to a number of lodging houses, increasing exponentially the number of individuals exposed.

As with most cities in the United States, San Francisco's structural reform also focused on housing. For all classes of individuals, the agenda was to encourage more people to spend time outside their houses as well as to reconfigure their homes to allow as much air and light as possible. The porch was focused upon in the first three decades of the century as an architectural device that could be added to existing homes without radical restructuring. In its simplicity and adaptiveness, the porch could render even the most congested housing arrangement healthier and open to the outdoors. Directly inspired by the sleeping decks of sanatoriums, porches brought sanatorium care to the urban home by providing family members an open space to rest, sleep, and even eat. Those homes that did not have porches could easily add one at minimal cost. It seemed in many ways an ideal solution for combating a predominantly urban disease whose most effective antidote was fresh air and sunlight.

As part of its study published in 1915, the tuberculosis association advocated the use of porches by every household in the city as a means of preventing the onset of tuberculosis or, if tuberculosis had already been acquired by one family member, as a means of preventing its spread to other members. Figure 6.2 represents the porch as simple and purportedly universal in its application. As the caption denotes, it could benefit the wealthy as well as the poor, since all needed the benefits of fresh air. The two houses within the photograph also illustrate a porch's adaptiveness to any architectural style. It could easily be added to a lower story or an upper story, to the rear, front,

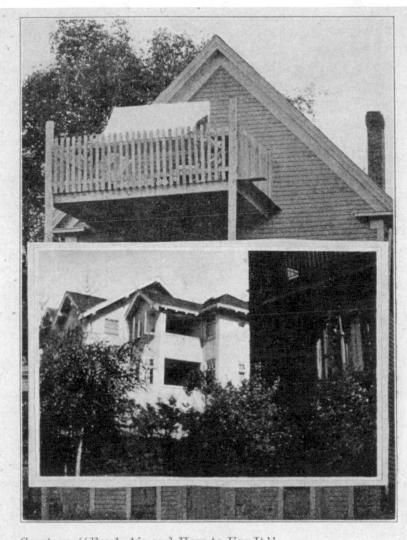

Courtesy, ''Fresh Air and How to Use It''

SLEEPING PORCHES FOR RICH AND POOR
Fresh Air Is an Essential to Health for Which There Is No Charge.

Figure 6.2. "Sleeping Porches for Rich and Poor," San Francisco, 1915.
Courtesy of The Bancroft Library, University of California, Berkeley.

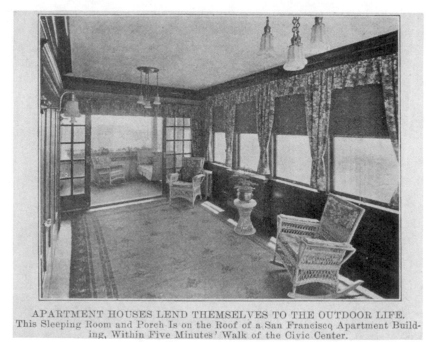

APARTMENT HOUSES LEND THEMSELVES TO THE OUTDOOR LIFE.
This Sleeping Room and Porch Is on the Roof of a San Francisco Apartment Building, Within Five Minutes' Walk of the Civic Center.

Figure 6.3. "Apartment Houses Lend Themselves to the Outdoor Life."
Courtesy of The Bancroft Library, University of California, Berkeley.

or side of a house (San Francisco Tuberculosis Association 1915, 12). Apartment living was also no impediment to the benefits of outdoor sleeping, since
porches could be rigged up on the rooftop of most apartment buildings, as
figure 6.3 illustrates. In the foreground is a comfortably outfitted room with
chairs strategically placed in front of large windows, while the room in the
background, with its even larger window, is designated for sleeping. As the
caption of the original photograph claims, apartment dwellers in the middle
of the city could "lend themselves to the outdoor life" by availing themselves
of these rooms.

The same innovation was utilized with school buildings. Open-air
schools were gaining adherents in many cities by the early twentieth century,
as public health physicians realized that preventing cases of tuberculosis early
in childhood saved money later in hospital or sanatorium fees. Using existing school buildings, large porches were built onto roofs or side buildings and
equipped with the desks for classroom instruction or cots for rest periods. Students considered vulnerable to tuberculosis because they were underweight
or had affected family members were sent to these open-air classrooms, where

they undertook their studies, meals, and rest periods fully exposed to even the severest of winter weather. By 1915, New York had fifty-three open-air schools; Chicago had twenty; and Boston had fifteen (San Francisco Tuberculosis Association 1915, 16, 23).

The first such open-air classroom to be constructed in San Francisco was the Michael Angelo school located in the Mission. It accommodated regular students in most of the building and students "predisposed" to tuberculosis in its open-air section. Another was implemented soon after in the Buena Vista school of the Mission "warm belt," a location chosen because it was less plagued by fog than some districts of the city and because it was close to the San Francisco hospital (Hiscock 1930, 49). After a 1927 state bill gave the state board of education the power to create a special education division, the Buena Vista school was made entirely open-air. Students not qualifying for this treatment were sent to schools elsewhere in the city (Hiscock 1930, 50). Only students "of normal intelligence" but of subnormal or vulnerable physical status were assigned to the open-air school, which was operated jointly by the board of education and the board of health (Hiscock 1930, 50). Whenever financing allowed, these students were sent during the summer to open-air camps designed specifically for children showing signs of early tuberculosis. There, the same philosophies of open-air living were implemented. Those with active tuberculosis, however, were barred from attending either school or camp (Hiscock 1930, 50).

It was the agenda of the tuberculosis association, as with most policy-advocating organizations, to articulate the benefits of policy recommendations rather than their limitations. There is little doubt that porches provided some reprieve from cramped living quarters, enabled urban residents to enjoy the benefits of fresh air, and brought to some extent the same structural provisions of a sanatorium to the urban residence. They had the capacity to prevent cases of tuberculosis either by isolating infected individuals from other family members or by providing families at least one space and time for being outdoors.

The limitations of the porch campaign were nevertheless significant. Who could or could not take advantage of sleeping porches was one question the association did not address. Touted as an inexpensive construction, the porch nevertheless took time, energy, and funds for building materials that some families did not possess. Nor could many afford to hire out the job. Unstated in the upbeat caption of figure 6.3 is the fact that apartment building owners had few incentives to outfit top floors as urban sanatoriums and were thus not likely to sink the necessary capital into top-floor conversions. Nor is there discussion of the logistics of access to a collection of rooms too small to accommodate an entire building's tenants. The association itself mainly provided recommendations and organized outreach campaigns; although it was able to fund some of its own recommendations, it did not have the endowment to finance all of them. There was little funding relative to need for the poorer classes to implement porch construction, and no record that the city provided any. The ability of those in greatest need of sleeping porches to obtain them was therefore in question from the start.

As figure 6.1 suggests, spatial limitations held as well. Many houses in South of Market and other congested lower-class neighborhoods had little room to add a porch. Houses were built too close together to add porches to the side; the fronts of houses abutted the streets; and the rear lot—if there was one—was frequently filled in with laundry decks and other utilitarian structures. The house in the photograph was equipped with a small porch, but the diminutive size of the house itself clearly dictated that certain domestic functions could more conveniently be undertaken outside. In this case, the porch appears to serve as the clothes-washing deck. Being able to utilize a porch for the single purpose of sleeping or outdoor relaxation, in other words, was perhaps a luxury reserved for those living in larger houses easily accommodating domestic functions internally.

Finally, the benefits of open-air classrooms and of the porch campaign were contravened by the lack of coordinated reform among living and working spaces. Children might receive the advantage of fresh air while at school, only to return every afternoon to cramped living quarters lacking ventilation and posing serious threats of tuberculosis transmission. Or families able to build porches on their houses for outdoor sleeping might return every day to workplaces posing greater health risks than their homes, risks exacerbated by the prolonged number of hours spent on the job. Admittedly more difficult to restructure, workplaces were not targeted by the tuberculosis association in its open-air campaign. It did recognize that workplace conditions were a significant impediment to improved tuberculosis rates and recommended the implementation of sick insurance for working men and women (San Francisco Tuberculosis Association 1915, 10); nevertheless, it did not actively focus upon or provide funding for workplace restructuring. Other progressive reformers campaigned for better working conditions, but these generally targeted work hours and wages rather than spatial reconfiguring. The first two were by no means irrelevant to the tuberculosis campaign, but reform in this area was slow and incomplete in San Francisco as elsewhere (Kahn 1979).[2]

A final area of housing reform was part of a much larger conglomeration of interests including but not limited to the antituberculosis campaign. As Gwendolyn Wright states in her social history of housing, "many different groups were campaigning for what they called a progressive approach to house design and upkeep." The result was what she calls the "sanitary house":

> While their social goals often were based on conflicting values, public-health nurses, arts and crafts advocates, feminists, domestic scientists, and settlement house workers favored the same simplified, standardized home to represent those values.... Architectural specifications for the sanitary house were numerous. Physicians and domestic scientists who considered dust a primary carrier of germs located dangerous "abiding-places for germs" in draperies, upholstered furniture, wall-to-wall carpets, and bric-a-brac. They urged that doorways and window casings be simpler; moldings and statuary niches disappear; cornices and other features where dust could collect be eliminated. (G. Wright 1981, 162)

The bungalow was the most exemplary sanitary house. Its interior was devoid of extraneous nooks, moldings, and architectural flourishes that could harbor bacillus-ridden dust. Bookcases, shelves, and cabinets were built in to walls to allow a greater degree of open space in the interior, and the kitchens were designed for sanitary, "germ-free food preparation" (Clark 1986, 180). Most of all, large windows and a large front porch invited the inhabitants to spend as much time as possible outside and to let nature in as much as possible when staying indoors. The general idea behind the new house design, according to one architectural journal, was to "get as close as possible to nature" (*Radford's Artistic Bungalows* [1908], cited in King 1984, 142).[3]

Economically, the bungalow was also an improvement over most previously available housing. It was inexpensive to build, with cheaper versions ranging from three hundred to twenty-two hundred dollars (King 1984). At that price, it was advocated by proponents as affordable even to those in lower-middle-class income brackets (Clark 1986). Row upon row of bungalows subsequently mushroomed in suburban communities in California and the rest of the United States (King 1984; Clark 1986; Wright 1981). San Francisco suburbs tended more toward the single-family stucco house rather than the bungalow (Walker 1995), but the latter nevertheless made its way onto the San Francisco and Easy Bay landscapes. It is difficult to determine the degree to which the new affordable housing in the Bay Area allowed those previously consigned to inner-city living a chance to own a home in a more spacious suburb. A number of upwardly mobile ethnic and white families from predominantly lower- or lower-middle-class sectors of the city undoubtedly found their escape in the relative affordability of the bungalow (Daniels 1980). Yet for San Francisco, as with most other cities in the United States, the bungalow ultimately proved beneficial to members of the middle class rather than to "all but [the] actually poor," as touted by an editor of the *Architectural Record* in the early years of the century (cited in Clark 1986, 180). For many "actually poor" and working-class persons, the ability to bring nature into the domestic sphere in the form of well-ventilated suburban housing remained an elusive prospect.

Managing the Tubercular: Nurses in the Field

Besides housing reform, the San Francisco Tuberculosis Association and the department of health recognized that any effective program of combating tuberculosis would mean locating unrecognized cases, monitoring their disease, educating them to be as responsible as possible in handling their affliction, and recommending them when necessary for institutional care. All of these were best handled by the deployment of a professional task force who would target poor neighborhoods and in effect treat them as clinical settings where the above tasks could be undertaken. Using physicians would be too expensive and somewhat inappropriate; nurses, however, would be perfect for the job because they bridged the gap between medical and social-reform facets of the antituberculosis campaign.

Rationales for monitoring poor tuberculars were located in the interrelated realms of economics, medical knowledge, and social ideology. It was assumed that the poor needed focused medical attention because their impoverished circumstances made them more vulnerable to tuberculosis while precluding them from seeking medical care. On the one hand, the status of medical knowledge made possible the greater accuracy of a tuberculosis diagnosis through the widespread deployment of medical technologies such as the X-ray machine. On the other hand, in the absence of chemotherapeutic treatment, the antituberculosis campaign was forced to rely upon environmental and behavioral therapies rather than science.

In this as with other aspects of the antituberculosis movement, space was a salient factor in both promoting and hindering the success of prevention. As always with tuberculosis it was difficult to disentangle spatial from class factors, since in attempts to discern causal relations or implement preventive measures the two were deeply interconnected. Tuberculosis was not only located in poor neighborhoods and in the bodies occupying them but needed to be discerned as well in the relationship the two had to each other. Geographic mapping of cases, in other words, was superimposed upon a map of the social body (Armstrong 1983, 8) as well as a map of the physical landscape. Yet the panoptic conditions needed to monitor the tuberculous patient were impeded by the cluttered topography of impoverished neighborhoods and the unpredictable spatial and temporal exigencies of employment. Surveillance was made difficult as well by the frequency with which many poor workers moved within the city (Olmstead et al. 1979; Broussard 1993) or in and out of the city (Averbach 1973). The task of the field nurse was not an easy one, but it was nonetheless considered one of the most important mechanisms of the antituberculosis movement.

The free tuberculosis clinic was the backbone to the field nursing endeavor, enabling the nurses to refer individuals they suspected of having tuberculosis to the clinics for a more thorough examination and subsequent confirmation or contradiction of initial diagnosis. In San Francisco the first clinic was set up in the Telegraph Hill area in 1909 by the Tuberculosis Association. Echoing current community battles over the location of services for marginalized populations,[4] the clinic's opening was met with hostility by a community clamoring to have the clinic removed or at the least to have the word "tuberculosis" removed from the entrance (San Francisco Tuberculosis Association 1928, 12). The facility and its proponents nevertheless stood firm, and by 1912 four others had opened in the North Beach, Mission, and South of Market areas (Arequipa Sanatorium Annual Reports 1912, 7). The establishment of each of these in the highest incidence areas of the city undoubtedly helped locate previously unreported cases of tuberculosis, although unreported cases in San Francisco continued to be more numerous than in many other cities (Hiscock 1930). As of 1936, 64 percent of 951 deaths from tuberculosis occurred before the first report or less than one month after (Works Progress Administration 1937, 8).

By 1915, the San Francisco Tuberculosis Association employed four nurses for the purpose of tuberculosis community work, even as it recognized that these were nowhere near the numbers needed to administer adequately to the needs of San Francisco's vulnerable population; it requested that the board of health fund sixteen more in the near future (San Francisco Tuberculosis Association 1915). By 1928, the city was funding ten nurses as well as the four still employed by the association (San Francisco Tuberculosis Association 1928, 12). In addition to social ideology, the paucity of nurses dictated that their visits to homes be "chiefly for instruction and must of necessity be so, because their time is too limited to do much actual nursing" (San Francisco Tuberculosis Association Annual Reports 1910, 28). These four women managed nevertheless to increase awareness among their clients of the existence of the free clinics and to refer a growing number of individuals over the years. Visits to the clinics increased from 1,599 in 1909 to 8,826 in 1929 (Hiscock 1930, 43).

A compilation of age and occupation statistics from those visiting the clinics provides something of a social profile of vulnerability. As figure 6.4

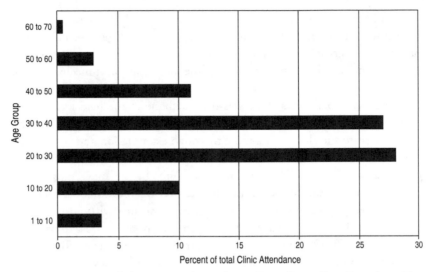

Figure 6.4. Ages of those attending clinic. Data from San Francisco Tuberculosis Association Annual Reports 1910. Courtesy of the San Francisco Archives.

suggests, tuberculosis was a disease that impacted most significantly those in their prime. Taken together, the twenty-to-thirty and thirty-to-forty age groups comprised over half of tuberculosis patients at the clinics (San Francisco Tuberculosis Association Annual Reports 1910). In the language of prevention, this was worrisome for two primary reasons: first, because this age group tended to encompass the largest spatial territory in their daily migrations between home and work, thus increasing the absolute number of contacts they had and increasing the physical area of transmission; and, second, because this was also the prime income-earning age group. Their debilitation meant a direct hit to the economy.

Figure 6.5, a graph of occupational breakdown, gives an indication by proxy of socioeconomic status. Noteworthy is the fact that housewives constituted by far the single largest occupational category of tuberculosis patients, explaining in part the reason the tuberculosis association focused so much attention in its reform campaign on the domestic arena and on the housewife herself. This disproportionate representation held for the state as a whole, with housewives heading the list of deaths from tuberculosis in 1929 at 981, and laborers constituting the next highest number of cases with 766 (California State Board of Health Reports 1930, 184). The remaining occupations on the graph are somewhat more evenly distributed over a range of blue-collar jobs. Of course this profile of vulnerability is skewed by the location of the

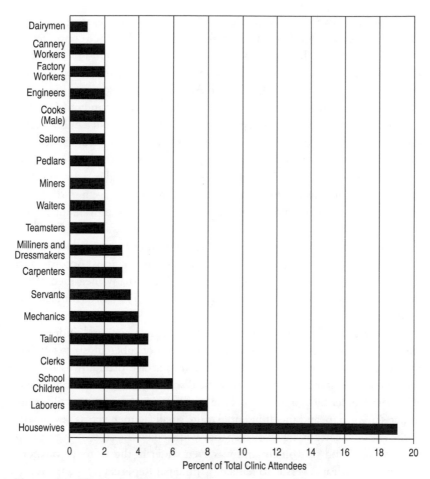

Figure 6.5. Clinic attendance by occupation. Data from San Francisco Tuberculosis Association Annual Reports 1910. Courtesy of the San Francisco Archives.

clinics in poor neighborhoods where blue-collar workers resided. Had private physicians provided similar statistics on their tuberculosis patients, a better comparison of vulnerability by class and/or occupation could have been possible. Then as now, however, those middle- and upper-class individuals able to access private physicians have had their diseases better screened from public viewing than have individuals attending public clinics where records often get published by government offices. The numbers of wealthier individuals contracting tuberculosis were small by comparison, but the mechanics of data compilation made them virtually invisible.

Despite the overwhelming representation of housewives among the clinic patients, the gender breakdown of tuberculosis in San Francisco continued to favor women despite Brown's observations to the contrary. In 1910, 175 men visited the first free tuberculosis clinic on Jackson Street versus 100 women (San Francisco Tuberculosis Association Annual Reports 1910, 24). By 1912, the total number had grown to 689 males and 242 females (San Francisco Tuberculosis Association Annual Reports 1912, 25). Attendance at a public clinic does not necessarily reflect accurately those who have active cases of tuberculosis, since a multiplicity of factors could prevent some individuals or groups from seeking medical care. Restricted mobility due to child care responsibilities, time restrictions resulting from double burdens of wage and domestic labor, and women's comparatively restricted flexibility of movement within public spaces may have combined to limit their access to a medical facility. But mortality statistics are a more accurate reflection of true prevalence, and these confirm the higher proportion of men with tuberculosis. According to the tuberculosis association's own statistics, twice as many men died of tuberculosis in San Francisco as women in 1928 (San Francisco Tuberculosis Association 1928, 6).

The reasons for this discrepancy are not clear-cut, and indeed not enough attention has been given in examinations of tuberculosis to gender-differentiated rates and their causes.[5] Looking at age breakdowns for San Francisco, for instance, it appears that the discrepancy becomes more accentuated with older age groups. In 1915 the numbers were equal (6 and 6) for the under-5 age group, and the differential quite small (19 men versus 13 women) in the 10-to-20 category. The discrepancy widened by the 20-to-30 age group with 122 men and 54 women, and was even wider in the 30-to-40 category with 176 male deaths versus 50 female (Municipal Reports 1915, 749). As figure 6.6 depicts, by 1929 more girls than boys were affected by tuberculosis in the 0-to-19 categories, but the numbers of men overtake women by the 20-to-29 category and continued to increase the gap until the 70-and-over age group (Hiscock 1930, 41). One possible explanation for higher adult male rates is if a large percentage of tuberculosis cases were contracted on job sites rather than at home. Most men and women entered the job force by the age of 20, but in the early twentieth century a much larger percentage of men than women worked at wage labor. The occupations depicted in figure 6.5 above are characterized as indoor and relatively low-paying, with the exception of carpentry work.[6] Given the significant representation of carpenters among clinic patients, though, the conditions under which laborers worked may have played a greater role in determining vulnerability to tuberculosis than did wages.

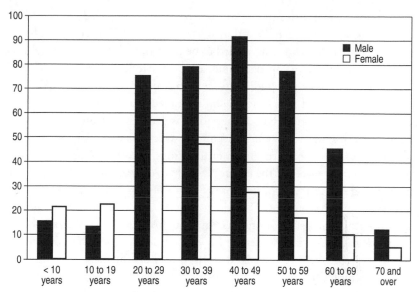

Figure 6.6. Tuberculosis (all forms) by sex and age groups, 1929. Data from Hiscock 1930.

Substandard housing was obviously the most important factor contributing to women's tuberculosis rates, but this still does not explain why more young girls contracted tuberculosis, yet fewer contracted it as adults. In addition to prolonged hours in unventilated and crowded housing, other factors influenced women's relation to the disease. For instance, there were a number of women in the labor force working under insalutary conditions and earning significantly lower wages than their male counterparts. Among the income-earning clinic attendants in 1912, the average monthly wage for males was $60.51 versus $13.05 for females (San Francisco Tuberculosis Association Annual Reports 1912, 25). Some of these women were married, but many were not, and the lower wages of the latter would only enable them to afford a very low standard of housing.[7] It is possible that tuberculosis was more often misdiagnosed among women as a cause of death, a tendency that could become more marked as perceptions grew that tuberculosis was predominantly a male disease. It is clear at any rate that the question of gender differentials in tuberculosis incidence needs further investigation.

Returning to an examination of field nursing, the majority of a nurse's time was spent not in referring patients to clinics but in helping them restructure their homes and their domestic practices to lessen the chances of transmission. Depending on the degree of poverty and condition of the home environment, the transformation of interior spaces was considered a critical component of nursing care (Robbins 1997; Bates 1992). The common habit of sleeping with windows shut needed to be broken, and the family taught to leave windows and doors open as much as possible to let in fresh air and sunlight (San Francisco Tuberculosis Association Annual Reports 1910, 28). The nurse often suggested that furniture be rearranged so that beds were nearer to windows, and the tuberculous individual isolated away from other family members in sleeping arrangements. Families were then encouraged to get rid of extraneous pieces of furniture, clothing, rugs, or other household items that could harbor dust and the tubercle bacillus. Any rags or other items used in collecting sputum were burned or otherwise eliminated (Bates 1992).

Hygiene was an area well scrutinized by the nurses in their visits to the poor tubercular, and suggestions were made to keep the house well scrubbed and whitewashed. Walls needed to be washed down, floors mopped regularly, the kitchen kept spotless, and clothing and bed linens well laundered. Nurses attempted to visit patients once a week (San Francisco Tuberculosis Association Annual Reports 1910, 28), both to see if families needed any material assistance but also to monitor the degree to which they were adhering to suggestions for domestic upkeep. Unfortunately for those tuberculous individuals with offspring, foster care was found for the children whenever possible in order to remove them from a threatening environment (Municipal Reports 1916). Whether this was done with or without parental consent is unclear from the records; it seems to have been a medically rationalized expedient for a poor population whose construction as childlike ultimately rendered them voiceless.

For San Francisco, the role of field nurse was an exhausting one. At the peak of their service in the 1920s and 1930s there were only nine tuberculosis and thirty general public health nurses hired by the city. In 1929 alone the nine tuberculosis nurses made 10,534 home visits to 1,999 cases or suspected cases of tuberculosis. According to the 1930 health department survey, this was only one-third the number of visits considered adequate for the number of cases residing in the city (Hiscock 1930, 46). Though not unique in its acute shortage of public health field nurses, San Francisco was apparently the only city of its size to not utilize more fully this "most valuable element in health work" (Emerson and Phillips 1923, 115). The seven other U.S. cities of approximately the same size had a field nursing fleet ranging from 112 for Pittsburgh to 64 for Los Angeles (Emerson and Phillips 1923, 115). The outcome of San Francisco's shortage of field nurses was a high number of tuberculosis cases that went unreported and of reported cases that received no assistance in monitoring their health or in supplementing inadequate incomes with needed material goods.

Even within the context of a serious public health campaign, San Francisco proved itself reluctant to prioritize expenditures to the poor.

The role of the public health nurse was undoubtedly beneficial in tracking previously unreported cases, tracing family contacts of tuberculars, and providing material support to families further impoverished by disease. Yet their undertakings were not entirely without controversy or shortcomings. The class difference between nurses and their clients translated at times into a patronizing attitude on the part of the nurse and a lack of understanding of the needs of a poor family and the causes of their impoverishment. Nurses were themselves working within a public health framework that never sought to remedy poverty but rather to render it less dangerous to the public. It is understandable, then, that many poor families met the public health nurse with hostility when she only suggested superficial ways to live better within the same circumstances rather than helping them solve the long-term problems of grossly inadequate incomes and an unsteady labor market (Robbins 1997). The improvements possible within these confines were of course limited. Families continued to live in the same cramped housing and continued to work under the same deleterious workplace conditions whether they received visits from a nurse or not. The main difference was that tuberculous individuals might learn the basics of not infecting those around them.

The Migrant as Public Health Menace

For the public health nurse and the antituberculosis campaign as a whole, migrants represented the most dangerous of any group of individuals. As casual laborers, they tended to be the poorest of the poor, the group of single men — and a few women — who occupied the cheapest tenements and flophouses of the city. Their employment was inconstant and variable, either because they did not want to work full-time, because age or debility limited their options, or because the only work they could find was temporary or seasonal. They tended not to stay in one place for long, migrating from one city to the next in search of jobs or for a place to rest until the next round of seasonal employment. Even within cities, they tended to migrate among the cheap lodging houses, spending nights in those hotels where they found beds available (San Francisco Tuberculosis Association Annual Reports 1910; Groth 1994).

As with homeless populations today, migrant laborers were generally seen by public health reformers from a behavioral rather than social-political perspective. They were not understood as outcomes of a changing economy where technological progress in agriculture and manufacturing had made many workers redundant or necessary only on a seasonal basis even by the early years of the century. As Paul Groth attests, "a bumper crop, a new railroad company, sudden demands for lumber, or an oil boom instantly employed thousands of new people.... Just as instantly, business downturns wiped out those positions" (Groth 1994, 134). During the first months of every year in San Francisco, an average of twenty-one thousand workers lost their jobs as industrial employers cut back their labor force (Groth 1994, 135). The inability of many, especially older men, to sustain employment was not understood as debility resulting from involvement in jobs that as yet had few accommodations to safety or the limitations of human physiology and function. Migrants were seen, in the words of Groth, not only as *down* on the socioeconomic ladder but as *out*, a highly marginalized population generally characterized as shiftless, drunken, and lazy.[8] They were thus unwelcome in most cities including San Francisco, even though they were necessary to both rural and urban economies (Groth 1994, 132). Notwithstanding their welcome, San Francisco in 1920 recorded seventeen thousand general laborers (Groth 1994, 134).[9]

From a public health standpoint, the migrant laborer was unwelcome because the conditions under which he lived generated high rates of tuberculosis but also made difficult any attempts to monitor it. Everything about the migrant lifestyle abrogated the rules of antituberculosis reform. Their peripatetic behavior made it virtually impossible for the public health nurse to pay visits since clients were not likely to be in the same place from one week to another. The rooms in which migrants could afford to stay were so ill accommodated that there was little a nurse could suggest to improve them, especially when the majority of flophouse rooms did not even have access to a window. The management, not the migrant, was responsible for keeping the rooms clean and fresh linens supplied, and they had little interest in doing so. The migrant was also single in the vast majority of cases (Groth 1994). In the eyes of the public health worker, this meant that there was little good influence at home abetting attempts to remedy unhealthy behaviors. As the 1910 tuberculosis association report stressed, the approach was to get one family member to become an ally and subsequently take over the nurse's duties by "teach[ing] their families the value and blessing" of healthy living (San Francisco Tuberculosis Association Annual Reports 1910, 28).

A second problem of migrants was the number of people they encountered in their daily movements. Flophouses might segregate their residents into cubicles, but the cheap coffee shops and restaurants patronized by migrants provided the necessary forum for greater germ transmission. Whether wandering the streets, standing in line for a job, or changing hotels every night, the migrant had numerous opportunities for close contact with the general public. And given the inevitable "promiscuous mingling" on city streets, not all of these contacts were necessarily those of their own class. For these reasons, the third annual report of the tuberculosis association concluded that "our only solution to this class of patients is to send them to the City and County Hospital." Obviously the agenda in this case was to sequester migrant tuberculars away from public access rather than to provide them with medical care. Having said this, however, the author goes on to admit that even this tactic was not especially effective, since out of forty-one cases sent to the hospital, "thirty have disappeared, which means that they are traveling about...spreading the disease among others" (San Francisco Tuberculosis Association Annual Reports 1910, 28).

For California as a whole, the definition of migrant seemed a flexible one, at the same time that the result from a public health standpoint was the same: danger to the general population. In the 1922 state board of health report, it was the ex-military migrant who threatened California's attempts to diminish its tuberculosis rates. Coming at a time when civilian migrant cases were supposedly lessening, California "found herself the vantage ground of hundreds of ex-service men suffering with tuberculosis.... [M]igration into California and migration between hospitals has created a serious public health problem. Patients can not supervise their own cure successfully,... [but] climate without the patient's desire to follow rules laid down by men wiser than they will not effect a cure" (California State Board of Health Reports 1922, 99). Encapsulated here are two assumptions: first, that even the ex-military variety of migrant was too irresponsible to be trusted with self-treatment; and, second, that physicians had superseded climate as the necessary vehicle for successful treatment of tuberculosis. Having made claim to the necessity of medical supervision, though, the author goes on to bemoan that the large number of ex-military tuberculars, together with "the great number of aliens," not only constituted a serious health problem but one in which hospitals would be taking the brunt (California State Board of Health Reports 1922, 99). The suggestion of the board was for a more careful physical examination at the port of embarkation so that tuberculous migrants would be barred from entering the state to begin with (California State Board of Health Reports 1922, 99).

The mention of aliens in the 1922 report foreshadowed a later 1920s convergence of class and nationality in characterizations of the diseased migrant in California. Sounding eerily similar to current discourses of migrants from "across the border," the 1928 state board of health report focused upon the Mexican migrant as especially threatening to public health. No doubt this newer construction of the migrant menace was in response to the number of Mexicans who came into California each year in answer to the state's huge demand for seasonal agricultural labor. Specifying the problem as more serious in southern California, the report urged the examination of every Mexican laborer entering the country and the deportation "of all aliens who have entered this country and are spreading disease wherever they go" (California State Board of Health Reports 1928, 127). The force of this statement comes with the explicit representation of the alien entering the United States as infecting the California populace rather than supporting the state's agricultural economy. Extending its analysis to the poor migrant as a whole, the report concludes with the uncharitable remark that "we need legislation to control these migratory people who may be an asset as far as the disposal of third and fourth hand automobiles are concerned, but that is all" (California State Board of Health Reports 1928, 128). Ironically, a survey of migrant health reported in the 1936 state board of health report concluded that the migrant tuberculosis situation was much worse among whites than among any foreign group, including Mexicans (California State Board of Health Reports 1936, 127).

The whole chronology of the migrant in California is relayed with weary resignation in the 1940 state board of health report. "California had first, the migration of the individual, either sent here or whose funds became exhausted, then the migratory ex-service man with tuberculosis. We have always had the migratory alien. Now we have the migratory family." Many of these families, as with all other migrant groups in the public health eye, were assumed to be riddled with tuberculosis. Every migrant incarnation was also considered a problematic element in the campaign against tuberculosis because of the specific kind of poverty and lifestyle the migrant inhabited. Deportation as an answer to the migrant menace was not always effective, however, as many had been in California long enough to gain legal residence (California State Board of Health Reports 1940, 112).

Seen from the perspective of the migrant rather than the public health worker, tuberculosis posed a grave problem. Over the course of time it debilitated individuals and incapacitated them from participating in the labor market, which in the case of the migrant meant the difference between marginal economic survival and complete penury. The absence of programs in California to help tuberculars train for jobs that could accommodate their disease and the physical limitations it imposed meant the increased likelihood that migrants could not get back on their feet (California State Board of Health Reports 1940, 117).[10] Receiving hospital care was not always easy either. Municipal hospitals generally accepted anyone, but, as will be seen below, beds were not always available, especially for tuberculars. County hospitals in and outside California often had residence requirements for admission, a step taken to defray the costs of indigent care. In some counties of California there was a minimum two-year residency requirement to qualify for county hospital treatment, which automatically disqualified most migrants (California State Board of Health Reports 1930, 128). In addition, many migrants had lost residency in their home states, meaning that they could not go back there for institutional treatment. For many of these noncitizens, the answer sometimes lay in getting care "only until the immigration authorities could deport them" (California State Board of Health Reports 1930, 128). For most others, it meant receiving no care at all.

While making it more difficult for migrant laborers to find institutional care for their disease, California also seems to have made few if any attempts to improve their living conditions. While urban flophouses more often than not were unreconstructed tuberculosis laboratories, agricultural camps were little better in terms of sanitation, dirt, and crowding. In the 1936 board of health survey of migrant health, observations were made of migrant camps in Kern, Shasta, and other agricultural counties. In one camp alone, fifty-nine people in fifty families were found to be actively tuberculous, while the sanitation of the camps was found to be "deplorable" (California State Board of Health Reports 1936, 125). Yet nowhere in the state board of health reports is there mention of systematic attention focused upon these camps to improve their conditions and to stem the transmission of tuberculosis and other communicable diseases. Even a statement of need for such an undertaking is lacking.

The public health constabulary, in other words, constructed a discourse of migrants as dangerous to the general population because of their own lifestyle choices, character defects, and unwillingness to be disciplined. In reality public health constituencies at all levels imposed structural barriers preventing migrants from seeking treatment for their tuberculosis or consciously neglected to regulate those areas of domestic and material life that contributed to the high tuberculosis rates among this group. Contrary to exhibiting a desire to diminish tuberculosis among migrants, then, the public health constabulary as a whole displayed an eagerness to maintain as impermeable the boundaries between polluted indigent bodies and everyone else. Indigents were represented as culpable, as somehow actively producing disease through the inherently defective quality of their character. Such discursive tactics served the important function of obfuscating the reality of public health neglect and rationalizing a policy of exportation rather than effective engagement.

The Limitations of Medical Purview: The Tuberculosis Hospital

The early-twentieth-century tuberculosis hospital served several functions within the urban framework. Like the sanatorium, it isolated the infectious individual from family members and other contacts, at least for the period of hospitalization. It served as a link to sanatoriums, funneling patients on the mend to a sanatorium that had an opening and receiving from sanatoriums those patients who had progressed too far in their disease to continue sanatorium treatment.[11] It was a repository for advanced cases referred by public health nurses or one of the free tuberculosis clinics. Finally, it served for the majority of tuberculars as a place to die: in 1929, 490 out of 626 tuberculosis deaths occurred in hospitals (Hiscock 1930, 47). The tuberculosis hospital generally was not, however, a place for medical treatment and the chance for recovery. As summarized by one report, the tuberculosis hospital's primary function was "segregating and caring for far-advanced and dying cases which would otherwise be a menace to public health" (Emerson and Phillips 1923, 13).

The first hospital built specifically to house tuberculosis patients in San Francisco came in 1906, during the chaotic aftermath of the earthquake. Ironically, this chaos necessitated a building design strongly resembling a sanatorium, though it was located on the edge of the city on a corner of the City and County Hospital grounds. The "tubercular colony" consisted of eleven tents — ten for patients, two to a tent, and one for a doctor and nurse. In addition it had a kitchen, bath, laboratory, toilet, linen closet, and open-air dining tables. The object was to try the open-air treatment run along the same lines as the German-style closed sanatorium that had yet to be instituted outside the city. Barbed wire ringed the tent colony, and no one was allowed in or out except by permission of a warden (Municipal Reports 1907, 563).

Though the urban sanatorium seemed successful at least in achieving weight gain in most patients, it was abandoned when money and means became available to build a more conventional hospital structure. The intermediate stage came in the form of seven wooden buildings and six lean-tos erected on the grounds of the City and County Hospital to accommodate tuberculosis patients while the more permanent tuberculosis hospital was being built (Municipal Reports 1911, 289). The final product, though of the latest design and most modern standard of efficiency (Emerson and Phillips 1923, 11), was inadequate before it even opened its doors. According to the 1915 assessment of the tuberculosis situation in San Francisco, the city needed a minimum of 600 beds for advanced cases of tuberculosis (San Francisco Tuberculosis Association 1915); the new San Francisco Hospital provided a mere 240 (San Francisco Tuberculosis Association 1928). It was inevitably inadequate as a curative institution as well. Touting the hospital as modern meant essentially that it had incorporated relatively recent interior design innovations enabling better isolation and more efficient management of each patient. Without concomitant advances in therapy, the new hospital did not necessarily improve patients' chances for survival. For the advanced tubercular of any socioeconomic class, the prognosis remained grim until the use of streptomycin in the 1940s (Bates 1992).

The location of the new hospital, at least, was less criticized. Positioned on the boundaries of the Mission and Potrero, the hospital was far enough from downtown, and amply far away from wealthier suburbs, to avoid outcry over the presence of contagious disease. Except for the poorer sections of North Beach, it was closer to those districts of the city most clearly needing the services of a free tuberculosis hospital. According to a 1923 survey of health care in San Francisco, the Mission accounted for 28 percent of admissions to the San Francisco Hospital, South of Market for 21 percent, and the Western Addition for 19 percent. More hospital patients came from these three districts than all other districts combined (Emerson and Phillips 1923, 69).[12]

One problem plaguing the tuberculosis hospital was its enormous expense. The disproportionate representation of the poor among tuberculars meant that a disproportionate number of tuberculous patients could not pay for their institutional care. The lengthy stay required for most patients, an average of 112 days (Hiscock 1930, 48), increased exponentially the financial output needed to maintain these hospitals. In 1920, San Francisco Hospital provided 122,748 free days of bed care for its tuberculosis patients, compared to 60,129 for general medical treatment (San Francisco Tuberculosis Association 1928, 5); by 1929, the number had increased to 142,134 (Hiscock 1930, 47). Using what the author of a 1930 health department survey considered a conservative estimate of three dollars and fifty cents per patient per day, San Francisco expended in one year approximately five hundred thousand dollars for the institutional maintenance of its tuberculous population (Hiscock 1930, 48). Starting in 1917 the state funded one hundred beds in the San Francisco Hospital for three dollars per day, but this sum did not begin to cover the costs expended by the city (San Francisco Tuberculosis Association 1928, 17).

According to the 1922 report of the Tuberculosis Bureau of the California State Board of Health, however, it does seem that the added funds allowed county tuberculosis institutions to raise their standards of care and to better follow the bureau's guidelines for a tuberculosis hospital. Issued in 1916, these guidelines included the separation of tuberculosis buildings from other hospital wards; the segregation of advanced tuberculosis patients from less advanced within the tuberculosis wing; locating the hospital with priority given to accessibility to the patient; the sufficient provision of isolation rooms, kitchens, and bathrooms; and the allowance of at least three feet six inches of space between beds (California State Board of Health Reports 1916, 166). Such standardization established minimum criteria for care of the tuberculous but also provided better assurances of reaching target populations and of better managing them once access had been gained.

Ironically, the improvement of facilities brought out the class biases of some hospital administrators, a reflection of the degree to which migrants and other indigent were considered undesirable even within medical institutions built to confront a disease primarily afflicting the poor. In the 1922 Bureau of Tuberculosis report, the authors state that the largest change in care over the last few years was in the type of patient receiving care. "From the old miserable lodging provided before the subsidy, when only the tuberculous tramp would accept such a place for a hospital, we find now what the director has reiterated over and over again, that once decent places were provided our sanatorium population would change" (California State Board of Health Reports 1922, 97). The continued availability of free beds makes this statement a little mystifying, though the sentiment is clear. For some hospital directors, maintenance of boundaries between themselves and the poorest of the poor, and between hospitals and the poor, had higher priority than reaching those in greatest need of care.

The financial drain of tuberculosis hospitals was one reason for the chronic shortage of institutional beds for the tubercular in San Francisco. The number of beds provided for tuberculosis patients eventually increased to 350 (Hiscock 1930, 46), but the simultaneous increase of San Francisco's population and number of tuberculous individuals eroded any progress this increase of beds might have made in reaching more patients in need of care. A 1930 appraisal of San Francisco's public health program determined that its tuberculosis services were approximately 72 percent of what they needed to be (Hiscock 1930, 20). Besides the acute shortage of public health nurses, one of the most critical shortcomings was the inadequacy of beds for women (Hiscock 1930, 48). More facilities were slated for construction at the time of the 1930 report, but San Francisco never provided the number of beds needed by its tuberculous population.

A chronic shortage of beds undermined the antituberculosis initiative in several ways. First, the most obvious result was to leave infectious cases unisolated in the community. Second, a less obvious result was the implementation of a triage system within the San Francisco Hospital that designated some as more in need than others based on stage of illness. The highest priority in admissions was given those with the most advanced cases of tuberculosis. As the 1928 report of the San Francisco Tuberculosis Association conceded, these patients were the least likely to improve; it was for "humane reasons," that is, primarily to give these individuals a place to die, that they were given first consideration. This prioritization meant that others whose tuberculosis warranted institutional care, who were infectious to others, and who might stand a chance of at least arresting their disease in a hospital setting had to stay on a waiting list until a bed opened up. Third, persistent demand for beds made it necessary to discharge some patients before their cases were sufficiently arrested. With a grim irony, chances were high that these individuals would eventually return to the hospital since they likely would "again break down with the disease and again become dependent upon the community" (San Francisco Tuberculosis Association 1928, 18–19).

While understandable in light of circumstances, the practice of admitting only the most advanced cases of tuberculosis eroded seriously the benefits hospital care might have provided poor communities and the rest of San Francisco. The sustained refusal of the board of supervisors to provide funding for hospital beds commensurate with city needs meant the perpetuation of the tuberculosis problem. Though public health nurses and care in free clinics may have helped ease the burden of disease for those unable to gain institutional care, their lack of isolation from the community and the unchanging conditions of their domestic and work conditions meant a sustained legacy of disease.

Conclusion

As the public health historian George Rosen eloquently puts it, by 1900 the relationship between tuberculosis and the structures of poverty had attained a wider symbolic sense. It had made tuberculosis "the epitome of urban maladies, the mirror of a community's mode of life and the milieu in which that life was passed, revealing the deprivation, dirt, and disease which pervaded the existence of so many people" (Rosen 1975, 10). But tuberculosis was mirroring not just a mode of life but also the political policies and social ideologies that maintained it. In its wider symbolic sense, tuberculosis brought to the forefront how society felt about the poor and the lengths it was willing to go to assist them. Older discourses blaming poverty on moral character defects competed with newer discourses located in the Progressive Movement that saw poverty as a product of industrial imperative and municipal neglect. Within the public health domain, lip service was paid to the structural impediments reproducing poverty while the privileged discourse remained the older focus on deviant behavior. Addressing tuberculosis meant essentially treating the pathologies of character. This particular interpretation of poverty had a profound influence on the course of the antituberculosis campaign.

From this discursive foundation, education inevitably followed as the keystone of public health initiative. Field nurses thus educated tuberculosis cases in hygiene, nutrition, and fresh air as part of a process of allocating full responsibility for health upkeep to the poor themselves. The key to success in this process was a focus on the home and home life, implicitly visioned as constituting a family in a single-family structure. If the locus of tuberculosis diminution resided in behavioral changes, then the family and their domestic arena proffered the most important single location of antituberculosis efforts. The home was the primary site of social reproduction and thus of behavioral engineering, and in this respect if the public health agent could impact the behavior of one family member, the rest would inevitably be reformed in turn. As the secretary of the California State Board of Health claimed in his 1904 report, there were many spaces in which tuberculosis bred and disseminated including schools, theaters, churches, and assembly halls. All of these places needed thorough and regular disinfection, yet in the end these measures were peripheral:

> But important as are all these things, consumption can not be stamped out or very materially lessened until the people find out that their home life has more to do with it than their public life.... [I]f they persist in living and sleeping in overheated rooms, often without the possibility of a change of air, the clean school and theater will not save them.... [T]he eradication of consumption is more a matter of education than anything else. (California State Board of Health Reports 1904, 15)

And the first agenda of education, before behavioral reform could even be initiated, was recognition by the tubercular that he "is a danger and a menace to others only as he makes himself so" (California State Board of Health Reports 1904, 15).

The particular construction of this rhetorical shift meant an almost inevitable classification of the poor into those who were educable and those who were not. During the first decades of the century, the primary constituents of the latter category were migrant laborers and other indigents, a hobo class created by changing industrial structures and concomitant shifts in the demand for labor. Regardless of the causal factors of their poverty, migrants were often characterized by the public health constabulary as irresponsible, shiftless, and unpredictable. From a public health standpoint, migrant laborers were indeed a population needing attention because their extreme poverty and peripatetic lifestyle meant a combination of high tuberculosis rates and greater opportunities for infecting others. But the issue of migrants and other truly impoverished went deeper. Much of the characterization of this group was a social fictioning reflecting a profound distrust of those who did not easily fit into the "normal" categories constituting society — the family, the steadily employed, the spatially immobile — even when such abrogations were largely dictated by economic expediency. As understood by public health and medical authorities, the socially marginal behaviors of the migrant laborer were as dangerous for their failure to adhere to disciplinary reform as for their potential to spread disease.

Later in the 1920s and 1930s, outside San Francisco the body of the migratory indigent was made even more ominously deviant by being racialized. In southern California, Mexicans, Filipinos, and other "aliens" who seasonally entered California to meet the demands of a huge agricultural industry were represented by state public health officials as the most dangerous element lurking in California, the diseased and peripatetic alien who not only spread infection wherever he went but ultimately ended up in a state- or county-supported institution draining the state of resources. For these undesirables, the answer was quick deportation and legislation that would mandate physical examinations for all Mexicans and other more indigent foreigners entering the state. This legislation did not pass, but the rhetoric behind it provided strong precedent for current discursive representations of poor migrants as having a deleterious impact on the economic and physical health of states.

Though tuberculosis rates were undoubtedly high among the most impoverished populations of the state, the threat of disease along with character-fictioning became an effective political tool for expropriating these populations either out of the state or away from population nodes. Yet hiding behind the rhetorical veil of irresponsibility lay the true impediments faced by migrants if and when they tried to seek medical assistance for their tuberculosis. Many county hospitals would not take them, and others did not want them; public health nurses generally did not target them or the flophouses in which they resided; and economic assistance during months of unemployment was scarce or unavailable. The signs all pointed in one direction: a hasty exit by the migrant away from the city and out of the state so that they would no longer constitute a menace to mainstream society or a drain on government coffers. If that failed, there was always the recommendation of the secretary of the California State Board of Health in 1940, one that revealed an enduring synonymity between disease and deviance and the willingness to deploy carceral tactics for the worst offenders: "A state camp is recommended for all...who have made trouble in the unemployed camps, the group who are inebriate and suffering with venereal disease, the group who make life miserable for the patients who are trying to take the cure properly, the group who insist upon using the hospital as a lodging house" (California State Board of Health Reports 1940, 105). A virtual prison camp was what this public health official seemed to be suggesting, a method of isolating undesirables from mainstream populations but also from public health purview. Those refusing to come under the control of "men wiser than they" clearly deserved corrective measures of a more punitive kind.

One of the results of the ascendancy of medical science in public health policy was a shift in purview. Where the nineteenth-century sanitary movement had taken the larger environment as its responsibility in improving the public's health, post–germ theory public health policy focused upon the individual and the types of behaviors that could make the individual vulnerable to the transmission of germs. Absent from this policy shift were those contingent factors that were acknowledged to have some impact upon health but were nonetheless deemed the responsibility of other constituencies. Housing, workplace conditions, length of workday, and wage levels were consciously left out of the fold of medical or public health authority even though they were known to play roles in tuberculosis rates. The 1930 recommendations of the committee surveying San Francisco's public health program reflect what in effect have become institutionalized standards of public health policy: continued efforts at case tracing and reporting; more funds to extend nursing personnel; better methods of record-keeping for comparative statistical data; and the development of educational outreach to vulnerable populations (Hiscock 1930, 54). While these recommendations were commendable in their own right, their positive effect was necessarily jaundiced by the sustained impact of those social factors equally significant in the production of disease.

San Francisco fit the norm in constructing its antituberculosis campaign within this framework, but in carrying it out it proved more parsimonious than many cities. In short, San Francisco was never willing to adequately fund the two most important medical institutions in the antituberculosis efforts: hospital beds and field nurses. From their inception both remained insufficient to meet the needs of the tuberculous, and they remained so despite repeated efforts on the part of the tuberculosis association and the board of health to acquire more funding. San Francisco was certainly not unique in this, but its parsimony in addressing its most deadly disease was less than commendable. As shown by two health care reviews conducted in the 1920s, San Francisco ranked somewhere in the middle of larger U.S. cities in their institutional provision for the tuberculous poor (Emerson and Phillips

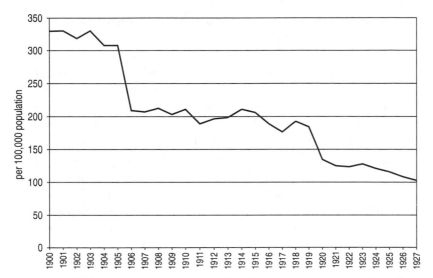

Figure 6.7. Tuberculosis death rate for San Francisco, 1900–1927. Data from the San Francisco Tuberculosis Association 1928.

1923; Hiscock 1930). There were worse places to be when impoverished and diseased, but there more far more humane places as well.

Outside the United States, France and Germany were two countries that proffered more humanitarian views on treating the tuberculous poor. In Germany, these views were operationalized through a tax law dictating that each laborer and employer pay a small sum to the state. The money subsequently went toward treating the tuberculous indigents who could not pay for their own care. In 1899, there were already fifty sanatoriums in Germany constructed expressly for the poor and laboring classes (Schweimitz 1899). In France, municipal societies existed to help the tuberculous poor through dispensaries. These were much like the free tuberculosis clinics of San Francisco, but offered more extensive material assistance and medical care. They also functioned as a "priceless agent of popular education and propaganda against consumption" (Calmette 1902). Material benefits usually included coal, beef, bread, and milk, as well as amenities like washbasins and laundry facilities that the poor were not likely to have in their homes (Calmette 1902).

Despite the limitations of the campaign, tuberculosis rates steadily declined throughout the first decades of the century in San Francisco as elsewhere. As seen in figure 6.7, the decline was dramatic, from well over 300 per 100,000 in 1900 to just above 100 by 1927 (San Francisco Tuberculosis Association 1928). The reasons for the drop are unclear, but by the 1930s the urgency had to some extent gone from the antituberculosis campaign as tuberculosis rates dipped well below those of cancer and heart disease (Bates 1992; Rothman 1992; Works Progress Administration 1937). Some analysts maintain that a significant role was played by sanatoriums and hospitals in declining tuberculosis rates for the United States and Britain (L. Wilson 1990). While not invalidating the overall benefits of these institutions to the tuberculous individual, it seems probable that their role in the decline was not preeminent. As Linda Bryder asserts (Bryder 1991), in only taking advanced cases the hospitals shielded tuberculars from society for a very short proportion of their contagious period. More likely is the suggestion made by Bates of a synergistic effect of slowly improving nutrition levels brought about by refrigeration technology and lower food prices; increased ventilation in factories, homes, and schools; and the institution of such devices as exhaust fans that diminished levels of dust (Bates 1992, 322–25). Contemporary explanations included a decrease in the 1920s of desperately poor people, shorter work hours, better homes, better wages, and cheaper transportation enabling better access to fresh air and sunshine outside the city (San Francisco Tuberculosis Association 1928, 21).

Marring this show of progress was the recognition by the San Francisco Tuberculosis Association and other public health overseers that improvements were more remarkable for some than for others. Rates for African Americans and Chinese continued to be significantly higher, showing no signs of narrowing the gap with rates for whites. In fact, the 1930 public health overview of San Francisco noted that rates for the Chinese population had not dropped proportional to overall rates (Hiscock 1930, 40); African American rates of tuberculosis meanwhile remained five times the rate for white San Franciscans (Works Progress Administration 1937). Incidence among migrants and other indigent groups was not offset, making a comparison over time impossible. Unfortunately, San Francisco's antituberculosis campaign was typical in engineering a movement that benefited least those whose mortality rates were highest (Bates 1992, 287).

Another mar on San Francisco's success was its standing among other cities (see figures 6.8 and 6.9). By 1912, its tuberculosis rates were higher than the majority of large cities, including heavily industrialized cities such as Pittsburgh and Detroit. By 1929 even New York and Boston had lower tuberculosis death rates (Hiscock 1930). Determining reasons for this poor showing would require a more detailed examination of each city than is possible here. Tentative explanations would include the sustained neglect of housing conditions in San Francisco and a higher proportion of large fourth-class hotels housing the poor (Groth 1983). Many of these latter were built as temporary barracks

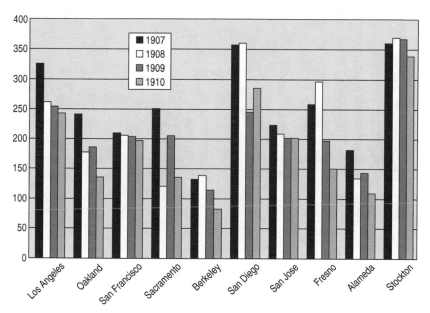

Figure 6.8. Death rate from tuberculosis per 100,000 population for selected major California cities. Data from San Francisco Tuberculosis Association Annual Reports 1912.

for the influx of workers helping to reconstruct the postearthquake city. As Paul Erling Groth puts it, reformers thought that "like packing crates, the single people and their temporary workers' housing would go away just a few years after the shining city was conveyed into reality" (Groth 1983, 276). They were obviously wrong. Increased crowding and medical neglect in Chinatown must certainly have played a role in sustaining San Francisco's high tuberculosis rates as well. After their intrusive approaches to infectious diseases at the turn of the century, public health officials adopted a "benign neglect" policy toward tuberculosis, rationalizing that the Chinese Six Companies were probably in a better position to help their own people than was the board of health (Trauner 1978, 85). Not until 1933 was a tuberculosis clinic established in Chinatown.

Finally, tuberculosis and responses to it raised a number of questions that remained largely unanswered and that have regained trenchancy in the resurgence of tuberculosis and the rise of HIV in the 1980s and 1990s. One of these questions involved the registration of cases. Control over knowledge of who has what disease historically has been a tricky issue contested among physicians, public health institutions, and the general public. At stake is not only

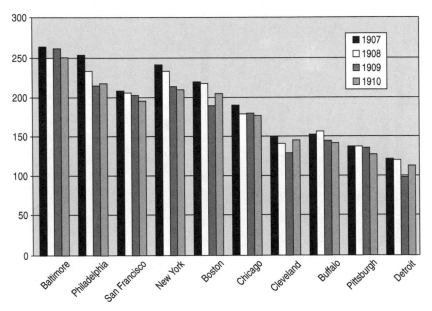

Figure 6.9. Death rate from tuberculosis per 100,000 population for selected major U.S. cities. Data from San Francisco Tuberculosis Association Annual Reports 1912.

who has access to knowledge of individual cases but how that knowledge will be handled and for what purposes. For many physicians at issue is the confidentiality of the doctor-patient relationship and whether this is betrayed even through anonymous case-reporting. The outcome of this debate for tuberculosis in the early twentieth century remains typical today for tuberculosis and HIV: public clinics and hospitals report cases to the department of health, whereas private physicians and hospitals do not (Hiscock 1930).

The exact purpose for case registration itself was, and still is, a contentious point. The public safety argument is easily countered by the instruction private physicians are able to give their infectious patients concerning minimization of risks to themselves and others with whom they come in contact. Contact-tracing can also be accomplished through interviews between the physician and patient. Monitoring changes over time of the incidence and prevalence of disease has value in determining whether prevention programs are effective or what diseases need intensified targeting. Yet the suspicion remains that information gained through case registration could be used for surveillance of the diseased rather than for monitoring the public health (Patton 1990). In the case of tuberculosis in San Francisco, knowledge of who had the disease was often signaled by the visit of a public health nurse or other official, and the knowledge impinged significantly upon the infected individual's rights. As one San Francisco Tuberculosis Association report conceded, many patients did not want public health nurses visiting them because it could mean eviction from housing when landlords found out they were tuberculous (San Francisco Tuberculosis Association Annual Reports 1910). Parallel issues have arisen for tuberculars and persons living with AIDS today.

A second question involved management of recalcitrant cases. Occasionally tuberculars continued life uninfluenced by the guidelines dictated for minimizing risk of infection to others. The points of transgression could be one or several, but in most cases they did not come under any existing laws (San Francisco Tuberculosis Association Annual Reports 1910). It was legal, for example, for a tubercular to work at any job even when some occupations, such as food handling or hospital service, posed particular threats to the public health. In 1909 the tuberculosis association got an ordinance passed in San Francisco declaring tuberculosis a communicable disease dangerous to the public health (San Francisco Tuberculosis Association 1928, 8), but little real power came with this. In 1908 a bill entered the state legislature requiring registration of all cases of tuberculosis, protection of records, approval of occupation by a health officer, prohibition of carelessness of persons with tuberculosis, and penalty for failure of physicians to report tuberculosis cases to the department of health. The bill passed the legislature but was subsequently vetoed by then Governor Gillett (San Francisco Tuberculosis Association Annual Reports 1910, 18). State and city health officials had the authority under the state quarantine laws to detain recalcitrant cases of tuberculosis, but the authority was rarely used (California State Board of Health Reports 1930, 183).

Before these debates could play themselves out they became largely irrelevant in the opinion of public health officials. General economic prosperity in the United States after World War II and the advent of streptomycin in the late 1940s together brought tuberculosis down to negligible levels. In the eyes of the medical constabulary, another victory had been scored for scientific medicine in vanquishing a ravaging disease through the advances of "magic bullet" pharmaceuticals. For public health agencies, surveillance of cases could be relaxed and education programs ended because tuberculosis was no longer a threat; the epitome of urban maladies was considered history.

7

ENVISIONING AN EPILOGUE
TO URBAN MALADIES

The collective outcome of disease in San Francisco was dualistic and in some respects contradictory. On the one hand, response to epidemic benefited the general population because it entailed piping water to every district, paving streets, rebuilding sewers, improving privy connections, and instituting regular municipal garbage collection. Domestic architectures incorporated better ventilation and sunlight, and hospitals were rebuilt along a "pavilion" model to more effectively isolate infectious patients. Public health laws forbade businesses such as dairies and slaughterhouses from practicing within city limits, while the idea of healthy spaces for public use influenced the establishment of a park system. Disease was not solely responsible for all of these new urban characteristics, but the fight against infection and the need to prevent further epidemics informed a city at once more "modern" in appearance and in the efficiency of its public services. Advances in bacteriology not only brought about the elucidation of disease etiologies, but eventually brought vaccines for prevention and effective drugs for treatment. The benefits of these cannot be overestimated.

On the other hand, a more ominous legacy of disease circulated through less visible arteries. The keystone of public health response to epidemic was the inscriptive practice of representing some bodies as diseased and as culpable for being so. Simultaneously evident in these practices were the social forces informing official action and the naturalizing thrust of medical authority. These discursive campaigns reinforced, redefined, or reproduced the fault lines of race, class, and gender in San Francisco, forcefully — and forcibly — pushing the physiognomically different, the sexually threatening, and the economically burdensome further into the political margins. Where "the margins" are often depicted as an undifferentiated peripheral location, however, the case of nineteenth- and twentieth-century San Francisco illustrates the degree to which social category and disease ascription determine the qualitative nature of marginalization. Ascribing smallpox or plague to the Chinese not only placed them further into peripheral territory but also rendered their particular brand of marginality as pathological, highly contagious, and intensely threatening. The poor tubercular, in contrast, experienced marginal inscriptions of disdain, childish irresponsibility, and a less-threatening form of infectivity. Disease acted both as an optic for seeing the degree to which even the social margins are hierarchized and as a powerful determinant of that hierarchy.

Of course it followed that as the nature of marginalization differed, so too did its consequences. If disease more firmly appropriated each group into hierarchies of marginality, it authorized corollary degrees of intervention at the same time. The diseased Chinese body required far more aggressive tactics to render it less threatening than did the diseased poor body. And always these tactics achieved material violence through spatial operations. First through pathologizations of place and then through interventions into those pathologies, public health policies responding to epidemic pivoted around spatial strategies that ascribed meaning; ordered bodies; and isolated, stigmatized, reconfigured, reordered, and defined parameters of social behavior in particular districts. In other words, responses to epidemic produced place, and conversely a very particular production of place was critical to public health policy.

In the case of Chinatown, public health sanctions combined with legal restrictions on external employment or housing built a white space around the district delimiting how the Chinese could behave, where they could go, and how they could support themselves. Representational tactics penetrated Chinatown through the inevitable internalization of difference and the endurance of overt social aggression. Chinatown became in turn a reactive space, a place to hide from white hostility, escape police surveillance, defend against the intrusion of public health officials, and reappropriate social practices inscribed as pathological even after the ascendancy of germ theory. Physical interventions disrupted employment and business, destroyed living spaces, and effectively isolated the Chinese from the rest of the city. Chinatown existed before the first smallpox epidemic, but it was subsequently reproduced through a combination of symbolic iconographies, physical intervention, bodily inscription, and institutional oversight.

The neglect of poor neighborhoods and later the minimal rearrangement of suboptimal housing in response to tuberculosis reflect in turn attitudes about poverty in the nineteenth and twentieth centuries. Public health officials as usual activated these policies, but the political anatomy of the poor as shiftless, puerile, and worthy at best of benign patrimony was common currency throughout the nineteenth and early twentieth centuries, if not now. The relationship was a reciprocal one, as the crowding, filth, and squalor characterizing the poorest neighborhoods confirmed professional opinions that the poor were irremediable and thus unworthy of anything but the most parsimonious portion of the municipal budget. The resulting lack of better housing, tenement legislation, workplace improvements, hospital expansions, or sanatorium subsidies ensured that squalor and disease continued to characterize the poorest neighborhoods. Neglect in this case was as violent as the sanitary assaults upon Chinatown if viewed via the number of lives that might have been saved with more humane public health action that could have addressed direct precipitates of disease as well as the more insidious inequities of turn-of-the-century capitalism. Ultimately, explanations of poverty rooted in cultural determinism proved more enduring than theories of environmental influence or the Progressive focus on structural cause. The public health responses emerging from cultural explanations consequently had more to do with taming the underclass threat and less to do with social justice or amelioration of the urban penalty.

Without denying the liberatory potential of marginal locations (hooks 1990; Soja and Hooper 1993),[1] it is important to note here that ascriptions of epidemic disease left little room for counterhegemonic cultural production or political action. The Chinese fought successfully for a repeal of discriminatory public health policies targeting their community, but these legal battles did little to throw off the mantle of pathological deviance. Nor did they disrupt detrimental political outcomes of disease ascription such as restrictive immigration laws. White working-class women chose to contest the suffocating discipline of the sanatorium regimen, but doing so returned them to impoverished homes, oppressive jobs, and the debilitation of untreated tuberculosis. Imbricating with low wages, long work hours, language barriers, and narrow channels of legal representation, disease ascriptions ensured that spaces of resistance were relatively constrained. Through its various material and discursive ruptures of social identity, disease also made difficult a "cultural politics of difference and identity" (Soja and Hooper 1993, 189) that could successfully contest, much less reappropriate, highly negative representations of difference. The obloquy of contagion proved relatively resistant to reinscription.

Disease, however, did not reify social relations in space, nor are the preceding discussions meant to suggest a static rendering of spatial production. Every spatialized policy of public health officials generated some kind of response among the public that also informed a meaningful production of space and the social identities it enabled or constrained. Whether it was the contestation by other physicians of discourses of Chinese infectivity, circumvention of smallpox quarantine laws, white missionary "rescue" of Chinese prostitutes, or Progressive agitation for equitable work and housing mandates, a multiplicity of competing discourses and political actions disrupted to some extent the pervasive workings of public health policy. Such policies or their contestation also obviously did not work alone in informing the production of place. Factors including tourism, industrial location, shifting sectoral employment, and suburban growth intersected with public health policies and ensured that the production of Chinatown, South of Market, North Beach, and other neighborhoods was always dynamic if not conflictual. The pathologization of Chinatown in the late nineteenth century did not preclude, for instance, its appeal as a tourist destination in the early twentieth.

The overall legacy of disease was nevertheless significant in San Francisco and predominantly negative. Where public health policies might have helped mend the fractures of race and poverty highlighted by disease, they widened the rupture. Where they might have overturned social inequities resulting in disease, they reinscribed them. Where the devastation of disease might have created for public health authorities, in other words, a new enunciative site for articulating "culturally hybrid social identities" (Bhabha 1991, 211) and their attendant spaces, it created instead the opportunity to reimpose a socially fragmented status quo and to augment its underlying hierarchies.

The return of tuberculosis and the advent of HIV in the 1980s have often been represented as disjunctures from the previous four decades of relative disease quiescence (Fee and Fox 1992). The introduction of antibiotics in the 1940s and other new pharmaceuticals signaled an era of unprecedented medical capacity to keep infectious diseases at bay, even if chronic diseases continued their ascent. Looked at another way, however, tuberculosis and HIV represent more continuity than discontinuity with the past, and it is the links to previous disease episodes and institutional histories that prove more instructive for a current history of these epidemics.

"Many arguments have been made...that the tuberculosis death rate, in spite of economic conditions, will continue to decline. It is doubtful if this is true." These words by a California State Board of Health secretary in 1936 (California State Board of Health Reports 1936, 123) might well have been heeded in the past four decades. For one thing, rhetoric of the demise of tuberculosis belies the extent to which public health agencies and the state still incorporate, and in turn reproduce, often racialized definitions of citizenship. Tuberculosis never did go away in the United States; it merely receded into urban pockets of predominantly black poverty such as Harlem, but these communities were not considered worthy of continued funding for tuberculosis prevention programs (Lerner 1998). Nor were they mentioned in the narratives of biomedical victory over a long-standing contagious disease. The resurgence of tuberculosis by the mid-1980s should also have been predictable, and perhaps would have been, had the field of public health been defined a different way or had other public agencies incorporated disease outcomes into their institutional purview. As seen in the previous chapter, the advent of germ theory caused a shift in public health at the turn of the century from a largely environmental approach to one dominated by a focus on individual behavior (Fee and Porter 1992; Lerner 1993). This trajectory has continued relatively unchanged today.[2] As a result, the same conditions of deepening poverty such as homelessness and unemployment that generated tuberculosis in the nineteenth and early twentieth century did not signal to a public health constabulary in the 1970s a warning that tuberculosis would ascend again within the next decade (Joseph 1993). The signal was not read in part because the location of public health precluded it from reading signs inscribed on the social and economic landscape; even now, tuberculosis is not seen as a social problem. Municipal and state public health departments accordingly continue to address tuberculosis along lines similar to the early twentieth century, with a focus on particular populations and greater control over their behaviors.[3] The one difference today is the administration of drug therapy, but this solution has become partially ineffective in cities such as New York where multi-drug-resistant strains of tuberculosis have developed (Lerner 1993). As Barron Lerner summarizes it, the rise of bacillus strains resistant to known drug therapies could create a preantibiotic scenario with the majority of tuberculosis cases untreatable and therefore fatal (Lerner 1993).

In this most recent resurgence of tuberculosis, the homeless have replaced the migrant workers of the early twentieth century as a population posing overwhelming difficulties for treatment. Like itinerant laborers, homeless often do not stay long in one place. While in one city, they might move among different districts in search of services, available shelters, solitude, or employment. Movement among cities is also generated by the vicissitudes of regional employment patterns or by climate. The long treatment period for tuberculosis, up to a year of daily drug therapy, makes this itinerant pattern problematic, as does the inability of the homeless to pay for medical care. The disproportionate time spent by many homeless in public spaces has raised again the specter of "promiscuous mingling of classes in close proximity on the street" (E. Wilson 1991, 29), a situation made dangerous as well as uncomfortable by a contagious disease.

As with the tuberculous migrant of the 1930s and 1940s, several solutions have been invoked by urban municipalities to deal with homeless populations seen as annoying and, increasingly, as diseased. One of them is the planned spatial barriers described in the introduction. Given the virtual impossibility of closing off borders to the homeless, an alternative solution is found in dispersing barriers of access throughout a city. The message of desired expulsion is still clear: if homeless individuals cannot find a park to camp in, a bench to rest on, or a doorway to find shelter in, eventually they will move on to urban arenas more hospitable to their dereliction. But not all homeless respond as directed to the spatial lexicon of undesirability confronting them, and other approaches are necessary for those among them known to be tuberculous. Directly observed therapy (DOT) has been the solution in many large cities in the United States, and it is not without promise. With this program, social workers are hired to track down the homeless known to be tuberculous, provide them with their medications, and ensure compliance by watching them take their drugs (*Los Angeles Times,* October 24, 1993; *San Francisco Chronicle,* September 27, 1992). Despite some degree of success the problems with this approach are numerous, including difficulty in tracking down peripatetic individuals, the expense of intense and prolonged surveillance, and the contestation of those who resent being policed. It also does little to prevent the disease, except among contacts of observed cases.

But the recurrence of tuberculosis and the persistence in seeing it as solely a medical problem are not just by-products of the developmental trajectories of medicine and public health. They are reflections as well on social and state attitudes toward the poor that have not changed noticeably from the nineteenth century. San Francisco in the early twentieth century may have been worse than many cities, but it was not exceptional in its categorization of most poor as "unworthy," in its lack of institutional provisions for tuberculosis, and its refusal to address those material conditions spawning the disease. The rest of the United States developed similar codifications, and similar blinders, to the social components of tuberculosis in the first half of the twentieth century (Bates 1992; Rothman 1994; Lerner 1993). Likewise, during the resurgence of tuberculosis in the late 1970s and 1980s, the same ambivalence if not disdain toward the impoverished remained. Reagan administration cutbacks of social programs including Aid to Families with Dependent Children (AFDC), Unemployment Insurance, and the Comprehensive Employment Training Act

(CETA) succeeded in launching an estimated half-million people into poverty[4] and made poverty worse for thousands more (Danziger and Gottschalk 1995). Economic growth was supposed to compensate for diminished government assistance, but the result instead was augmented income inequality, increased homelessness, decline in the standard of living of the poor, and rising tuberculosis rates (Danziger and Gottschalk 1995). More than a failed experiment in trickle down, 1980s legislation is a testament to recurrent blame of the poor that emerges out of, but also finds substantiation in, their discursive fictioning as indolent and dishonest. Like the nineteenth-century discourses on poverty, today's dominant characterization of the poor "compounds various forms of dependence and deviance into one convenient and derogatory category defined more by behavior than poverty" (Katz 1986, 277).

Tuberculosis plateaued in most states by the mid-1990s.[5] It will likely continue its pattern of recurrence, however, as long as public and congressional opinion persist in seeing poverty as a deviant behavior rather than as deeply entrenched in the economic restructuring of postindustrial society. With the exception of a modest rise in the minimum wage, few policies designed to ensure a minimum standard of living for the poor have been legislated in recent years. The most recent welfare restructuring places time limits on assistance, yet concomitant programs such as job training, child care assistance, or housing subsidies are not widely implemented to ensure that those moving off welfare are actually moving into jobs with viable wages and benefits. Tuberculosis will also recur as long as the institution of public health continues to produce itself as apolitical and the issues it addresses as divorced from economic contexts or the broader agenda of social justice. A departure from historical trajectory might see public health lending its institutional weight to advocating for decent and affordable housing, child care subsidies, job tracking, or wages that are sufficient to allow the working poor to remain housed and adequately fed. Such measures would provide far more effective means of tuberculosis prevention than free clinics or case surveillance.

As with previous eras of public health efforts, the inappropriateness of current policies is reflected most vividly in the landscape, with inscriptions of poverty most visibly evident in the inner city. Housing in poor urban districts is characterized by a proliferation of housing projects, single-residency occupation (SRO) and other fourth-class hotels, and homeless shelters (Groth 1994) — all designed to hide the poorest of the poor behind walls, segregated from mainstream urban districts. The insalubrity of the homeless shelter has already been described, but the SRO and housing project are equally conducive to transmitting tuberculosis and other infectious diseases. Even the minimal legislation of the early twentieth century integrating better light and ventilation into architectural design of multiple-residency structures seemingly has been forgotten. If recent welfare restructuring proves to intensify poverty for some, these landscapes will only multiply.

Affirming the reciprocity of spatial production and social practice, the structures of poverty blighting urban landscapes in turn inform discourses on the poor and policies toward them. Housing projects have become symbols of everything that is negative about inner cities: material degradation, crime, prostitution, drug abuse, and disease. The embarrassment of unsightly SROs, homeless shelters, and homeless encampments has caused a shift in many American cities in the direction of even greater intolerance toward the homeless or the precariously housed. Businesses don't want them hanging around, and no one wants them in their residential neighborhoods. The resulting locational politics means a highly restricted area in which the homeless may find residence or other social services (Dear and Wolch 1987). In the meantime, homeless encampments are being forcibly dismantled even in socially tolerant cities such as San Francisco. Housing projects are being slowly dismantled as well, yet former residents are all too often relocated within other impoverished inner-city neighborhoods (*New York Times,* September 28, 1998). This conscious ghettoization of undesirable constituencies into inner cities suggests the inability of society and a medical constabulary to separate ideologies of difference from epidemiologies of disease.

But tuberculosis is no longer just a disease of poverty. Its dissemination into prison and AIDS populations has added the taint of deviancy to the slur of poverty, making it more than ever a behavioral disease from both social and public health perspectives. Unlike the early-twentieth-century tubercular, however, the late-twentieth-century tubercular's disease is a product of social practices born of degradation rather than ignorance, and as such AIDS and tuberculous bodies are converging in public health and social taxonomies. They are also actually converging in the same bodies, since tuberculosis is an increasingly common opportunistic infection of the person with AIDS. Like smallpox before them, these diseases are now serving in part as codifiers of normality, a discursive categorization driven largely by medical discourse and embraced by a society wanting to believe itself outside the boundaries of the pathological. As Waldby suggests, "biomedical knowledge is always a discourse about social order, worked out in bodily terms" (Waldby 1996, 32). In this case, AIDS and tuberculosis mark the socially pathological through discourses locating the diseases in hedonistic pleasures of sex and drugs that are perceived as voluntary as well as deviant (Epstein 1995). One purpose of these "stigmatizing narratives" is "largely to reassure the artificially invented "general population" that they are "safe" from taint as long as they resist such chosen pleasures" (Epstein 1995, 169). Social order is thus maintained by making visible the dire consequences of deviance, while fear is assuaged by creating supposedly clear-cut boundaries between the normal and the diseased.

The perceived concentration of HIV and tuberculosis among particular populations means that these diseases also serve to shape definitions of sexuality, class, gender, and race in urban America. Like syphilis and the Chinese prostitute, AIDS and tuberculosis have been added to the long list of social pathologies defining not only the homosexual male but more recently the African American and Latino / Latina. Though both diseases are present in other populations, it is the white gay male and the underclass ethnic minority who bear the brunt of representational politics wielding disease as an affirmation of marginality (Wilton 1997; Hammonds 1997). This inscription finds substantiation in official numbers showing the fastest rise of AIDS cases over the past several years among African Americans and Latinos, but the numbers are often taken as confirmation of degradation rather than examined for causal factors. Indeed, the causes of HIV are increasingly rooted in "inequitable economies of health care, and the relations between poverty, unemployment, educational ghettoization, urban despair, and family dispersement" (Epstein 1995, 169). Yet these epidemiologies are largely ignored by public policy and health constituencies refusing to see AIDS, like tuberculosis, as a social and economic problem (Patton 1990; Singer 1998).

This is not to suggest that public health constituencies are failing to target lower income and largely ethnic neighborhoods. The problem is that they target them with tactics such as educational outreach and free condoms, approaches that are needed but that by themselves are inadequate. A tiny clinic located in one of San Francisco's poorest districts exemplified the shortsightedness of public health policies focused upon such epidemiological mainstays as contact-tracing and "behavioral modification." Posters on the walls educated the viewer to practice safe sex, a message supported by the basket of free condoms on the receptionist's counter. The clinic offered testing and counseling, two services that while needed in this neighborhood did nothing in the way of prevention. The largely homeless population accessing this clinic were, by their own assessments (anonymous 1991), more concerned with getting their lives back on track, getting off drugs, getting their children back, and getting jobs than with getting AIDS. Knowledge does not always lead to an ability to change behavior, and behavior is too inextricably embedded in social economies to be treated in isolation. Thus rather than seeing drug or alcohol abuse and homelessness as irremediable behaviors, these issues need to be recognized as consequences of poverty and addressed as part of inner-city HIV-prevention programs.

The representation of women in AIDS discourse is problematic as much for what is left out as for what is represented and how. Women are gaining ground quickly in percentage of new AIDS cases (Stine 1995), yet their treatment in epidemiological literature largely remains relational — that is, what their seropositive status means in relation to childbearing or to the uninfected male (Treichler 1992b). Even though it is easier for women to become HIV positive from men than the reverse, it is the woman, and more specifically the prostitute, who has been represented as a "reservoir" of infection threatening to victimize the unsuspecting client (Gilman 1985). That prostitutes themselves are infected and not just infectious is rarely the focus of analysis (Treichler 1992b; Waldby 1996). As Waldby suggests, the pathologization of female bodies results from biomedicine's designation "as an origin and cause those identity categories that are in fact the effects of institutions, practices, discourses" (Butler 1990, xi, cited in Waldby 1996, 22).

Other discursive representations portray women as threatening their unborn children with HIV. One public health poster (figure 7.1) depicts a baby with the message "She has her father's eyes and her mother's AIDS." The representational tactics of this poster are unequivocal in the assignment of culpability. Whereas the father is responsible only for passing on positive biological traits, the mother is guilty not only of acquiring HIV but of ultimately killing her child with it. The scenario leaves conveniently absent any indication that the father might have been the one to infect the mother during the process of impregnation. Having assigned blame, the poster sends an underlying message concerning the ignorance and irresponsibility of women, characteristics that in other circumstances might be unfortunate but in this case are deadly. It is a throwback to the turn of the century and the discourse of women as endangering their families through class-coded ignorance, except that this time the uninformed woman threatens to give her family AIDS rather than tuberculosis. The targeting of women as responsible for HIV is particularly egregious given that sexual politics still find women largely at the subordinate end of inequitable power dynamics dictating the conditions of sexual exchange.

Though not made explicit by the public health poster, the message of mothers with AIDS is a class and racially coded one. The disproportionate number of African American and Hispanic cases of HIV seropositivity, combined with the tendency to seek associations of AIDS with social categories rather than social context, has resulted in a tendency to see ethnicity itself as a risk factor (Hammonds 1997). It is not primarily the middle-class white woman who is at risk, but the lower-class ethnic woman because she is more likely to belong to at least one "risk" category of prostitute, intravenous drug

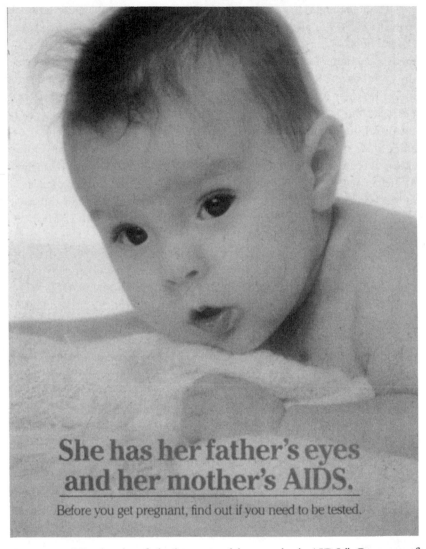

She has her father's eyes
and her mother's AIDS.

Before you get pregnant, find out if you need to be tested.

Figure 7.1. "She has her father's eyes and her mother's AIDS." Courtesy of the National Library of Medicine.

user, or the partner of a drug user. The African American and Hispanic versions of this public health poster in particular send the message that like the Chinese prostitute, the African American and Hispanic woman is increasingly seen not only as poor and deviant but as possessing the capability of tainting a new generation with a debilitating disease.

Critiquing these representational tactics is all the more trenchant because they are a part of, but also help reproduce, policies that miss the mark. In placing the onus of responsibility for HIV on women, the public health message elides the gendered economies and inequitable politics that place many women at risk for HIV. It ignores the fact that an economy based increasingly on employing women in low-paying service jobs produces a class with few resources, limited access to medical care, and a higher risk of HIV. It fails to recognize that welfare cuts hit women harder because of unmet child care responsibilities and because of continued gender inequities in the labor force. It ignores the fact that preventing HIV among women will mean addressing these problems. In portraying women as irresponsible in their sexual and reproductive lives, it provides a rationale for placing blame on the individual rather than on the detritus of racism, poverty, and inequitable gender politics underlying risk. That a national AIDS prevention campaign could produce such a poster speaks volumes about the problematic politics and institutional myopia characterizing public health. Unfortunately, the continued rise in HIV cases among low-income African American and Hispanic women speaks louder to the ineffectiveness of current prevention efforts.

The continued bifurcation of medical and social-economic purviews will result in the persistence of tuberculosis and AIDS for both men and women, especially when the undercurrent of blame for these diseases dictates a focus on control rather than prevention.[6] It will also mean a continued production of inner cities, gay neighborhoods, and other "marginal" zones not only as socially disdained but as pathological. Recognition that public health is very much about politics, and should be as much about social equity as it is about behavior, could finally disrupt the long cycle of epidemics and their more unfortunate material and spatial taxonomies. Perhaps then more urban communities will have another chance, at least, for life.

Introduction

1. Personal communication with Dr. Andrew Moss, December 1991. Infection rates for homeless populations living in shelters in other U.S. cities can be even higher. For example, a 1990 study came up with a stunning 79 percent positive test rate among homeless men living in the Fort Washington Men's Shelter in New York City (see Paul et al. 1993). Other estimates of asymptomatic tuberculosis among homeless populations range from 20 to 50 percent (Schieffelbein and Snider 1988; Slutkin 1986).

2. Most of this literature focuses on AIDS and is too voluminous to cite. A few examples are Waldby 1996; Treichler 1992a, 1992b; Wilton 1997.

3. This was especially true when it was not clear through just what actions, or through what bodily medium, the virus could be passed on. Thus drinking from the same cup, hugging, touching, or any other bodily contact was suspect for its potential for viral transmission (Doka 1997; Oppenheimer 1992).

4. In his book *AIDS and Accusation* (1992), Paul Farmer documents the discrimination faced by Haitians living in U.S. cities after the CDC's claim of a Haitian origin of AIDS. The fallout included many Haitians losing their jobs, public admonitions to employers not to hire Haitians, and the general characterization of Haitian immigrants as not only dirty and illiterate but now diseased as well. In his astute observations of international economies, Farmer notes that the repercussions of these discriminations in the United States affected individual welfare within Haiti as remittances ceased to flow into the country from family members in the United States who had lost their jobs and the claim of a well-established epidemic on the island caused tourism to take a drastic plunge.

5. With some notable exceptions (Urla and Terry 1995; Arnold 1993; Brandt 1987; Fee and Fox 1988), analyses of deviant bodies and their implications tend toward the ahistorical, leaving the impression that discursive pathologizations did not occur before the advent of AIDS and overlooking the analytical depth gained from historical comparison and institutional precedent.

6. Though I have changed his categories to some degree, I thank Chris Philo for disaggregating the different body types that are usually the subject of normalizing discourses — besides the diseased body, Philo includes those with visual marks of stigma, functional disability, out-of-placeness, and smell (personal communication, January 1998).

7. These transgressions include the blatant display of what is usually termed promiscuity — in terms of both the number of partners and the chosen sites of sexual undertaking — and of course the same-sex, nonprocreative, and "aberrant" nature of sexual exchanges.

8. Specifically, according to the authors of the *Journal of the American Medical Association* article, the CDC "defines heterosexual transmission as sexual contact with a partner who has a primary risk factor (e.g., IDU or male-male sex) or is known to have HIV or AIDS" (Wortley and Fleming 1998, 356). Heterosexuals might be at risk, in other words, but only because they have crossed boundaries — social and body — in dangerous ways. Sexual contact with someone known to have AIDS is a seeming afterthought, a vague description of those not falling into the "primary risk" categories and not numerous enough to represent more specifically.

9. When 292 students at a middle-class southern California high school tested positive for tuberculosis, an extensive part of the coverage in the *New York Times* centered upon the double trajectory of tracing the original case back to a Vietnamese girl who contracted tuberculosis in her home country, thus, on the one hand, confirming the "outsider" status of the case but, on the other hand, informing the public that tuberculosis is no longer "the disease of the impoverished, the immigrant, and the homeless," but rather "has come home to roost...among those in places that have always been considered safe havens, such as sunny, open-air California high schools" (quote from Dr. Richard Jackson, chief of the California State Division of Communicable Disease Control, *New York Times,* July 18, 1994, A6).

10. Even with the Americans with Disability Act, the question of whether asymptomatic seropositive individuals are covered, and thus whether or not they can be fired from their jobs, is up to state interpretation (*New York Times,* January 20, 1998).

11. Of course tuberculosis never really went away after the 1950s. Its containment within small pockets of poverty such as Harlem rationalized the neglect of the disease, and the poor (Lerner 1998). The federal government subsequently cut budget allocations toward tuberculosis clinics during the 1970s despite the warnings of public health practitioners, yet the (declined) requests for funding primarily were for more research projects and clinics, not for measures that would address poverty itself (*New York Times,* October 11, 1992).

12. I want to make the distinction here that public health *practitioners* who work with tuberculous and/or HIV-positive constituencies are often the

first to see the interrelatedness of disease and social economy. It is public health as an institution that defines its purview so narrowly as to restrict the parameters of public health practice.

13. My thanks to Dereka Rushbrook for bringing this example to my attention.

14. Joan B. Trauner (1978) does an admirable job of this for Chinatown, but not for San Francisco as a whole.

15. Currently, for example, poorer populations tend to be overrepresented in disease reporting because they receive medical care through public clinics or clinics receiving federal funding, making these institutions more likely to report communicable diseases to state departments of health. Private physicians, though held to the same laws of reporting, are more notorious in refusing to report the diseases of their private patients because it abrogates their Hippocratic oath.

1. Tuberculosis, Tenements, and the Epistemology of Neglect

1. "Consumption" was the term in common parlance in the nineteenth century, until the discovery of the tubercle bacillus by Robert Koch in 1882. The term referred to the tuberculous body's propensity to waste away, as if being quite literally consumed by disease.

2. I am following David Barnes (1995) here in my use of "spatial relations" to mean how the individual body's relations with the environment — including climate, food and alcohol intake, and eventually area of residence within the city — impacted health. It also refers to the epistemologies of control in the fight against the diseased body.

3. Just how much the consumptive — or anyone else — was supposed to emulate the healthy primitive was left vague given the ambivalent attitude exhibited by the physicians writing about these consumptive-free societies. On the one hand, these peoples managed to remain unscathed by a disease that ravaged so much of the rest of the world, especially the Western world. On the other hand, they were simple primitives. And though tuberculosis might be a bane of European and American society, it was a disease "peculiarly the product of civilized society," the prevalence of which "might be a sufficient index in determining the degree of culture in any given community" (Abrams 1886–87, 3).

4. It should be noted that Kober wrote this after Koch's discovery of the tubercle bacillus. While acknowledging the infectious nature of tuberculosis, Kober nonetheless maintains older theories of tuberculosis susceptibility and causation.

5. According to Feldberg, observations of regional differentiation in tuberculosis rates came early in American history, with eighteenth-century physicians such as Philadelphia's Benjamin Rush writing on the topic. Not only did particular regions of the United States suffer less tuberculosis, ac-

cording to Rush, but the disease was also less common among Indians; in the country (rather than the city); in active, temperate, nonsedentary modes of life; and among men as opposed to women (Feldberg 1995).

6. While medical theories of environmental therapeutics backed these physicians, just how therapeutic San Francisco's climate was did not go undebated. Several accounts, some by physicians, claim that in fact the climate of San Francisco itself was unhealthy for the consumptive because of its high winds and cold fog. Other areas in the vicinity are recommended instead. See Saxon 1861, 10; Hatch 1871, 24; and Bancroft, n.d., 708.

7. It should not be inferred from this that tuberculosis at this time, especially in San Francisco, was associated directly with industrialization. This is why the body was an important signifier, since — as will be discussed further — the penury caused by the shifting employment needs of capitalist production and the structural extensions of this penury (in the form of substandard housing and other factors) were not emphasized at this time in discussions of consumption's epidemiology.

8. See especially Limerick, Milner, and Rankin 1991.

9. See also Municipal Reports 1867, 1871, and 1881.

10. As for the first factor, the developers of the Central Pacific worked with the eastern rails as well and charged less to bring freight cars full of East Coast products to San Francisco than the other way around. Consequently, California products were not selling well in the East, while eastern products were cheap and plentiful.

11. According to Issel and Cherny (1986, 25), the typical workshop in San Francisco hired "fewer than five hands" as late as 1880, though some enterprises hired between twenty-five and fifty workers.

12. One is reminded, for example, of the decisions by some major scientific journals not to publish the viewpoints of Peter Duesberg, the University of California, Berkeley, virologist who, contrary to majority scientific opinion, does not believe that AIDS is caused by a virus or that it is a separate disease at all.

13. Feldberg 1995; Lerner 1993, 759; Hardy 1993.

14. See Hardy 1993, 211–19, for analysis of the debate; cf. McKeown 1976; Cronje 1984; Smith 1988; L. Wilson 1990; and Bryder 1991.

15. See also Municipal Reports 1881, 1884, 1897, 1891.

16. Not all practices were gender- or class-coded. Other bodily practices as preventive tactics were recommended in various medical journal editorials. One physician, for example, suggests the tuberculous individual sponge with cold water, rub his or her body, wrap it in linen cloth, and recline for an hour; the rationale of the suggestion is that this procedure would strengthen the skin and make the body less susceptible to "atmospheric variations" (*Western Lancet* 3, no. 2, April 1879, 92).

17. On the topic of the "cult of true womanhood," see Baker 1984; Welter 1966; Sklar 1973; Smith-Rosenberg 1985.

18. See Limerick 1987, 100–106, for a discussion of the numerous difficulties and frequent failures facing those rushing for riches in the Sierra foothills.

2. Sewers and Scapegoats

1. There are many good accounts of the anti-Chinese movement in San Francisco, including Saxton 1971; Cross 1935; Issel and Cherny 1986.

2. That is, it was the most deadly epidemic to hit San Francisco as a mature city, since several waves of smallpox had traversed California before San Francisco's first major growth in the 1840s. According to Sherburne Cook, one of the most devastating swept through in 1828, with another hitting in 1837. The collective damage of these epidemics was the virtual decimation of the Indian population, thousands of Mexicans dead, and the few remaining whites either vaccinated or immune (Cook 1940). According to J. Saunders, the 1828 smallpox epidemic struck California because of the relaxation of vaccination and quarantine laws implemented by the Spanish government in the late eighteenth century and strictly enforced until 1820 or so. He also credits the epidemic of the 1830s, and consequently the decimation of the Indian population of California, to malaria rather than smallpox (Saunders 1967). The paucity of surviving descriptions of this epidemic makes it difficult to prove either assertion. That smallpox wiped out much of the native population of the rest of the country, however, is not in question (cf. Hopkins 1983; Tremble 1986).

3. That is, when looking just at the continental United States. Yellow fever also thrived in Central and South America and other warm, wet climates where the *Aedes egypti* mosquito could thrive.

4. Cholera was prevalent on the California-Oregon Trail in the 1840s, though, which probably indicates its common presence in California before 1850; higher population density by 1850 might have been the key to epidemicity versus isolated cases. Thanks to Richard Walker for pointing this out.

5. The concept of the "Other," as will be seen further below, is taken from Stallybrass and White 1983, and indirectly from Edward Said.

6. Many argue that Chinese workers also took only or primarily those jobs that whites did not want. Cross (1935, 315n. 8) holds that this argument is not valid, given the list of jobs performed and wages received by Chinese and white laborers. As noted in chapter 2, before the arrival of Chinese immigrants the Irish were the ones at the bottom of the social totem pole who took the jobs spurned by others. Thus, as Robert A. Burchell notes, the Chinese were ironically of great importance to the Irish by providing them with an automatic means of social elevation in relative, if not real, terms (Burchell 1980, 181).

7. In retrospect, many scholars agree that white male laborers generally were not displaced by the hiring of Chinese workers. Olmstead, for instance, points out that in reality the Chinese did not contribute that extensively to white unemployment rates since there was high unemployment in trades that never employed Chinese workers and since "there was no great boom in those businesses that did benefit from low Chinese wages" (Olmstead et al. 1979, 123–24). Also see Shumsky 1972.

8. In part this might result from the tendency throughout the century for San Francisco to look toward Asia rather than eastward, especially with increasing commerce after the opening of Japan. This does not go far in explaining the direction of medical rhetoric, however.

9. If the Chinese were indeed "unassimilable" into white American culture, the reason for this may in part derive from the fact that most hoped to keep their stay in San Francisco as short as possible. As Ronald Takaki points out, the numbers of Chinese returning to China exceeded those immigrating to San Francisco for almost every year until the Exclusion Act of 1882, a fact ignored by municipal officials of the time (Takaki 1989, 116).

10. In his book *Silent Travelers* (1994, 78–82), Alan Kraut discusses the importance of the growing Chinese population in San Francisco to the increasing tendency to impute origins of epidemic diseases to the Chinese community.

11. The inclusion of malaria as one of the three most feared diseases in San Francisco in the 1880s is rather mystifying, given that malaria felled very few people by this time. An almost complete lack of reference to it in municipal and medical reports would also indicate that not much concern was generated over it by the latter part of the century. The fact that tuberculosis and even diphtheria are not included among these ghouls indicates once more the lack of fear inspired by these diseases at this time.

12. By fabrication and pathologization I do not mean that there was no material basis for suggesting that Chinese prostitutes had syphilis; many of them did. The point is that all female Chinese bodies, no matter what the status of the individual body, were inscribed as lewd, beastly, full of malicious intent toward the white male, and diseased.

13. It does appear that many Chinese prostitutes practiced their trade in conditions worse than their white counterparts. Some arrived in San Francisco contracted to brothel owners who kept them as virtual slaves, controlling the money they earned, keeping them in the basest of conditions, sometimes physically abusing them, and often leaving them on the streets if they did become diseased (Issel and Cherny 1986; Pascoe 1990). Peggy Pascoe has an interesting account of white missionary women's attempts in the late nineteenth and early twentieth centuries to rescue these women and give them new, and newly Christianized, lives in San Francisco (Pascoe 1990).

14. See Judith Walzer Leavitt's similar account of smallpox's role in spurring Milwaukee's sanitary movement (Leavitt 1985).

15. Debate over "soil or seed," or contagion versus miasmatic origins of disease, continued throughout the nineteenth century in the United States and Europe, constituting the focal point of national and international sanitary science meetings (see Feldberg 1995).

16. This obsession had actually spilled over, or at least was known, to others outside the public health constabulary. As Anthony Wohl cites in his examination of public health in nineteenth-century Britain, the poet John Ruskin once proclaimed "a good sewer" to be "a far nobler and a far holier thing... than the most admired Madonna" (Wohl 1983, 101).

17. Mention of London sewers is made upon occasion in the Municipal Reports of San Francisco in the later nineteenth century. For London as an example of sanitary order outside San Francisco, see Barnes 1995.

18. In fact there are times in Meares's accounts of smallpox epidemics when he seems implicitly to acknowledge that defective sanitary conditions in the city might be *equally culpable* with Chinatown in producing zymotic diseases, rather than simply being Chinatown's susceptible vessel for these diseases (cf. Municipal Reports 1877, 1881).

3. Negotiating the Boundaries, Policing the Borders of Disease

1. The plague has been especially well documented in the ways people contested and negotiated public health mandate. See Calvi 1989; Carmichael 1986; Cipolla 1979.

2. Only the composite statistics were divided into categories such as gender and ethnicity; statistics by ward were not.

3. For all hospitalizations other than smallpox, the reports of the City and County Hospital also show a higher proportion of male patient loads even taking into account the imbalance in population for San Francisco. Rates for the year 1888, for example, were 2,326 male versus 588 female admissions (Municipal Reports 1888, 546).

4. It was very common during this period in San Francisco to live in a hotel, rather than in a domestic residence. Hundreds of such live-in lodging houses existed until late in the century.

5. See Leavitt 1985; Hopkins 1983; Duffy 1990.

6. One physician claimed that after the Vaccination Act of 1867 in London instituting compulsory vaccination, mortality rates from smallpox plummeted to only 12 percent in the 1867–68 London epidemic; mortality rates for San Francisco's 1868 epidemic, in contrast, hovered at 30 to 40 percent (*California Medical Gazette,* October 1868, 90).

7. Most of this regulation was a result of the realization that tuberculous cows could pass their disease on to milk consumers, and not the result of recent smallpox or other disease epidemics. To this effect, the Milk Im-

provement Association was formed in 1908 to make tuberculosis-free milk (Municipal Reports 1909, 675).

4. Structures of Susceptibility

1. Plague hit Europe in the sixth century as well, but why it did not more frequently cross Asia Minor, for example, is not known definitively but almost certainly has to do with trade configurations among countries and the routes by land and sea that this trade took. See McNeill 1976 for an account of how plague reached Europe.

2. There were two unconfirmed cases in 1898 referred to by the editor of the *Sacramento Bee* in a letter to the editor of the *Washington Post* (Freuch 1901), but there is no other information about these cases.

3. These methods follow Koch's basic principles of verifying disease. Presence of a disease cannot be proven if blood or other body fluid samples do not produce the disease in animals. It also cannot be verified if there is no pathogenic evidence of it—that is, if the specific virus, bacteria, or spirochete that produces the disease cannot be found in the body fluid of the patient.

4. The U.S. Marine Hospital Service was instituted primarily to keep in check infectious diseases entering the country from outside sources via ships coming through various ports — hence its name. It subsequently established hospitals at the major ports of entry in the country, including San Francisco. The U.S. Marine Hospital Service was the predecessor to the U.S. Public Health Service.

5. Unless otherwise indicated, the following description of the 1900 plague epidemic is taken from McClain 1988.

6. These included the discovery of pathogens for anthrax, tuberculosis, diphtheria, cholera, and yellow fever.

7. The Chinese Six Companies, or the Chinese Consolidated Benevolent Association, was a council of merchants and other associations representing the Chinese districts from which immigrants came. It acted, among other things, as an interlocutor between the Chinese and white communities and possessed the financial means and authority to contest those policies it deemed detrimental to Chinese business and social functioning (McClain 1988, 455).

8. As McClain explains, the truthfulness of this statement on the part of Kinyoun is dubious, given that it was made a month after the incident and after much criticism had been launched at the actions of the collective health constabulary in San Francisco. See McClain 1988, 469.

9. Of course to iterate that susceptibility seemed to show itself by family or ethnic grouping also raises the important question of what public health authorities were looking for, that is, what questions they were using to inform their examination of the evidence. With "the immigrant question" looming large, there were definitely tendencies to want to see higher disease rates

among, for instance, eastern European Jews or southern Italians or Asians than among Anglo-Americans. The heredity question of course either precluded or made secondary any discussion of socioeconomic factors in the spread of disease. See Kraut 1994 for a good history of blaming immigrants in the United States for various diseases.

10. In the case of New Orleans the embargo was on travelers, not goods, and it was not just Chinese and Japanese being barred from entering the city, but poor whites as well. Evident here was the association of plague with dirt and the continued association of the poor with filth in the early years of the century. See McClain 1988, 483.

11. Schrady himself, after assuring whites that they had nothing to fear, also supported the idea of removing the Chinese from Chinatown, burning the district to the ground, rebuilding it, then reestablishing the Chinese and compensating them for property loss. Obviously there was something disturbing about the prospect of plague smoldering in the middle of the city, whatever its risks to those outside the real and constructed physiological boundaries of the disease. See McClain 1988, 490.

12. On May 11, 1903, for example, the state board of health unanimously adopted a resolution calling for the removal of Chinatown from its present site in San Francisco to an "outlying and isolated district," and that pending such a measure the Chinese be removed from all underground and other tenements (California State Board of Health Reports 1903, 5). Like all the other calls for Chinatown's removal, this one was never realized.

13. The majority of analyses of the first plague in San Francisco focus attention on the political aspects of it, including the refusal of Governor Gage to recognize it, his mandate to the state board of health to not recognize it and to hereafter impede as much as possible the progress of the San Francisco Board of Health and the U.S. Marine Hospital Service to combat the epidemic, and the consequent confirmation of the presence of plague by the federally appointed committee of three. The battle went all the way to the president of the United States, although McKinley's intercessions were of less import than those of Judge Morrow of the federal circuit court. See in particular McClain 1988; and also Haas 1959; Lipson 1972; Risse 1992; Kraut 1994.

14. These are Hannah's descriptions of a panoptic setting taken from Foucault's three instruments of disciplinary power: "hierarchical observation, normalizing judgment and their combination in a procedure that is specific to it, the examination" (Foucault 1977, 170). My definition of an imperfect panopticon is not precisely what Hannah had in mind or what he elaborates upon in his article; for the purpose of this analysis, then, the idea is derivative of, not parallel to, Hannah's original idea.

15. The mention of fleas departing from a body dead from plague should not be used to infer that Blue knew the precise role of fleas in the

transmission of plague. He did not, and the statement is more a commentary on hygiene than on epidemiology.

16. This is of course not a new point to make. A burgeoning literature in cultural studies and medical history analyzes from various angles and using various case studies the reciprocal relationship between medicine and culture. A very selective sample of this literature includes Waldby 1996; Epstein 1995; Sontag 1977; Cartwright 1992; Treichler 1992a, 1992b; Urla and Terry 1995; Wilton 1997.

17. The list of such commentators has grown voluminous, but includes Poirier 1991; Shilts 1987; Patton 1990; Watney 1987; Waldby 1996.

18. Risse (1992) offers details on the funding of the plague cleanup efforts. Politically the plague epidemic showed up at a bad time; the city was rocked with scandal involving the shady financial dealings of Abe Reuf, a political "boss" of the city, and various members of the city government. The president of the city board of health was found to be involved in the financial misdealings and resigned, as did the city mayor. The city board of supervisors thus found an excuse (as it always did) to decrease the board of health's budget subsequent to its involvement in political scandal. Needless to say, the city found itself short of funds to wage a large antiplague campaign and welcomed federal support. The expenses of the sanitation campaign were not entirely taken over by the U.S. Public Health Service and U.S. Marine Hospital Service until 1908, but subsidization occurred by the latter part of 1907.

5. Reforming Bodies

1. Rural areas suffered as well, but cities had on average 50 percent higher tuberculosis rates at the beginning of the century. See Shryock 1957, 64.

2. Statistics were kept before the turn of the century, but their accuracy improved around 1900 in part due to an increased emphasis on the importance of statistical information in divulging social patterns and in part due to better reporting by local departments of public health. Better diagnostic capabilities included the increasing use of X-rays and a recognized presence of the bacillus in sputum. See Shryock 1957.

3. San Francisco Tuberculosis Association 1912, 23. This rate includes death from all forms of tuberculosis, although pulmonary tuberculosis accounted for the significant majority of all cases. See also Shryock 1957, 62–63.

4. Ward actually states that interpretations of moral causes of poverty were giving way to social causes, but in light of discourses concerning tuberculosis that will be elaborated upon in this chapter, I cannot agree with Ward's claim. Other discourses came into being and existed alongside the moral discourse, but did not supersede it.

5. Take, for example, the public health nurse from Philadelphia who in 1909 wondered whether or not a fellow nurse had become "impressed primarily with the squalor, shiftlessness, and lack of intelligence and fortitude" among the poor to whom she ministered (cited in Bates 1992, 245).

6. This figure included natural increase and any other increases such as migration from rural communities. Population figures from *War against Tuberculosis* 1928.

7. It is interesting to note that there was something of a regional pattern corresponding to physicians' acceptance of Dettweiler's ideas. Physicians in the West, noting the more independent-mindedness and aversion to authority of their patients, rejected the notion of the closed sanatorium more than their eastern counterparts (see Rothman 1994, 197).

8. Edward L. Trudeau is considered something of a father of tuberculosis treatment in the United States. He pioneered the use of the sanatorium for treating the tuberculous, even if Kretzschmer pioneered the idea of it. Trudeau was himself tuberculous, and at the brink of death he found physical reprieve in the Adirondacks. Consequently, location as well as architectural style were important to Trudeau, and he purposely located his own sanatorium in the same mountains where he himself regained health (Trudeau 1916).

9. Whether influenced by the antituberculosis campaign or not, camping and the great outdoors became popular activities and popular tropes for architects working in San Francisco and Berkeley at the time. Willis Polk, Bernard Maybeck, and Ernest Coxhead incorporated views, an abundance of wood, and a sense of outdoor rusticity into the designs of their homes at the turn of the century (see Longstreth 1983). Needless to say, these homes were for the healthy benefit of the upper classes.

10. See, for example, Chris Philo's article on the tendencies in the nineteenth and early twentieth centuries to house the mad in institutions utilizing the panopticon as designed by Bentham, or variations of panoptic architecture (Philo 1989).

11. For another example of Foucault's schemata used in the analysis of a medical(ized) phenomenon, see Dear and Wolch's discussion of twentieth-century deinstitutionalization of the mentally ill (Dear and Wolch 1987).

12. The even higher mortality rate in Stockton is due primarily to the fact that the state hospital was located there.

13. California State Board of Health Reports 1906; San Francisco Tuberculosis Association 1928; Municipal Reports 1915.

14. The evidence for this last statement is contradictory. The precipitous drop in tuberculosis rates in San Francisco between 1905 and 1907 (from approximately 309 deaths per 100,000 to 209) suggests what other public health physicians claimed, that is, that the earthquake actually made urban

conditions better in terms of tuberculosis transmission (see San Francisco Tuberculosis Association 1928). This will be discussed further in chapter 6.

15. It is interesting to note in apparent contradiction to Brown's perspective that F. B. Smith, in his examination of tuberculosis in the United States and the United Kingdom, cites the role of the pub in causing higher tuberculosis rates among urban males in the United Kingdom in the early decades of the twentieth century (F. B. Smith 1988, 18). Men may not have been obliged to go home after work, but they ended up in equally unhealthy, if more convivial, environments.

16. Brown's findings are intriguing, since they seem to find no resonance in other gender-based tuberculosis statistics for the city. In 1910, for example, out of a total of 859 deaths from tuberculosis for the city, 614 were male and only 245 female (San Francisco Tuberculosis Association Annual Reports 1910, 19). Although Brown chose to concentrate his attention on working women, the San Francisco Tuberculosis Association also found that over half the women attending its free tuberculosis clinic (this was a different clinic from Brown's, set up specifically for tuberculosis monitoring) were housewives, not working women (San Francisco Tuberculosis Association Annual Reports 1910, 25). As stated in the report, this statistic exemplified the problems of poor housing in the city. F. B. Smith (1988), however, backs up the claim of higher mortality rates for adolescent girls in most of the United States and Britain, but not for women and men in the twenty-to-forty age group. Whatever the comparative rates, though, the waiting list at Arequipa was long throughout its operation, attesting to the small capacity of the facility combined with high numbers of poorer women suffering from tuberculosis and unable to find alternative sanatorium treatment.

17. The companies that apparently thought that Arequipa was a good investment, and that subsequently paid for their employees to "take the cure" there, included Emporium Retail, Pacific States Telephone Company, and United Airlines. It seems that Pacific Telephone was the only company that continued paying salaries to employees while they were residents at Arequipa (Arequipa Sanatorium Annual Reports 1912, 6).

18. The issue of dividing the poor between the worthy and the unworthy will be taken up in more detail in the next chapter.

19. In a newspaper editorial written in 1912, a Dr. Richard Cabot states that "the great curse of tuberculosis to all but the rich (in whom it is relatively rare) is not the physical suffering it entails, but the serious expense of so long and wearing an illness stretching over months and years and the ravage which long idleness makes in the patient's character. Despondency pulls down some patients as seriously as the disease itself. Restlessness drives others into every sort of vice and folly which sanatoria endeavor in many ways to conceal and control" ("Arequipa Sanatorium" 1912, 1).

20. Thomas Mann's book *The Magic Mountain* gives some indication

of the forms of entertainment, including speakers, music, and the occasional film, that were possible for the sanatorium of means.

21. See especially Rothman 1994 for poignant excerpts from diaries and letters depicting the intense loneliness and boredom plaguing women at various sanatoriums. The number who left before their full prescribed time at the sanatorium was not large, but Rothman does give some indication, through these firsthand accounts, that monotony caused enough discontent in some to drive them to abort their attempts at institutional cure.

22. For instance a letter from a Violette Fitz Gerald says that she arrived at Arequipa on July 17, 1934, and "am very happy to be here. . . . I hope I shall be able to stay at Arequipa until I am well. It is a very cheerful and homelike place and so perfectly supervised. I had no idea I would be so contented away from home, especially in an institution" (Fitz Gerald, Correspondence dated July 23, 1934).

23. This is rather ironic given that the fitness of workers for the expansion of industrial production was in part a motivation of the antituberculosis campaign. David Rosen also makes the very plausible connection between, on the one hand, the antituberculosis campaign and, on the other, increased "mercantilist ideas" and the acquisition of colonies and markets and sources of raw materials in the pursuit of these ideas. A growing nation, thus, needed fit and productive workers, not tuberculous ones (Rosen 1975, 15).

24. Ellen Richards was the most prolific proponent of scientific housekeeping, publishing a number of books at the turn of the century and into the first decades of the twentieth century.

25. The original comment was "You work through, not the marginal position or some kind of point of resistance that's outside domination, but many kinds of not fitting" (Haraway 1995, 515). The context was an exploration of "cracks in the system of domination" and the suggestion that this is explored not so much from points of resistance but from looking at points of incommensurability within a system designed to be commensurate for the majority.

26. The importance of behavioral reform as an aspect of the antituberculosis campaign is even more clearly seen in the implementation of open-air camps for children in 1921. According to the *Trail Blazer,* the newsletter of the California Tuberculosis Association, California was the only state as of 1920 to initiate these camps. They were designed for children who were underweight or who had a family history of tuberculosis (*Trail Blazer,* April 1921). The fundamental rationale for the camps was the same as for sanatoriums: that is, to give less healthy (i.e., primarily underclass) children the opportunity to get out of the detrimental environment of the city and into the countryside for an extended period of time. Good-quality and abundant food, medical examinations, and plenty of outdoor sports constituted the basic regimen.

At the same time, however, the physical isolation of the camps and the separation of parent and child presented the opportunity to instill at both ends the coda of healthy and orderly living. While the children were at camp, field nurses visited the parents and educated them on sanitation and hygiene so that "each child returned from camp to improved home conditions." Likewise, the camp regimen was supplemented with "valuable educational work" on similar health and sanitation issues so that the child, in turn, "brought back a vibrant health message to the other members of his family" (*Trail Blazer*, April 1921, 8). Inextricably woven into the health message was "civic training in community life." Such training constituted almost military-style discipline at the camps, with roll call every morning, the supervision of every aspect of behavior down to tooth brushing, and inspections for cleanliness and neatness. As one camp staff person commented, "One can scarcely overestimate the value of the impetus given in this way to a taste for cleanliness, order and regularity" (*Trail Blazer*, April 1921, 8).

27. Like so many current public health recommendations geared toward improving health through individual behavior, these suggestions were easier to teach than to follow. It was not always possible for discharged patients to sustain better diets if they could not afford it; nor was it always possible to rest if the rigors of waged plus domestic labors did not allow for it.

28. Cf. Bryder 1991; L. Wilson 1990; Szreter 1988; McFarlane 1989; Conje 1984.

6. Reforming the City

1. The nonadjusted rate for San Francisco was 103 per 100,000 (Hiscock 1930, 40).

2. Judd Kahn (1979) gives a good history of the ups and downs of unionization in San Francisco, for example, and the general victory in the early part of the century of open-shop policies even in a relatively well-unionized town. This and the depressions of the 1890s and 1930s obviously had a downward force on wages, not to mention an impact on the availability of jobs of any kind. As Kahn's appendix (p. 308) also shows, wages for women at this time were a mere fraction of the wages earned by men. Some workers had won forty-four-hour workdays by 1920, while others, still in the majority, were working forty-eight-hour weeks (Kahn 1979, 308).

3. The back-to-nature ideology behind bungalows and other architectural movements around this time was not necessarily connected directly to the antituberculosis campaign. The general disgruntlement with urbanism, of being "crowded and hustled and irritated to the point of physical desperation in our thoroughfares and markets, our tenements and tiny apartments, our shops and street cars" (cited in King 1984, 135), found the inevitable correlate in romanticizing rusticity and the bucolic. These were predominant forces behind housing reform, although in question is to what degree those architectural

historians and geographers writing about these movements simply have not bothered to acknowledge the influence of public health campaigns on architectural reforms (cf. Walker 1995; King 1984; Longstreth 1983). For an exception to this concerning late-nineteenth-century England, see Adams 1996.

4. Dear and Wolch 1987 is the classic account of locational battles over services for the homeless. Other current battles involve the location of clinics for AIDS and other communicable diseases.

5. Rothman 1994 focuses some attention on women, but Rothman's agenda is to portray the experiences of women in sanatoriums rather than to determine the reasons for different rates among men and women. Most examinations of tuberculosis in the United States, Britain, and Europe touch briefly upon gender-differentiated incidences but do not include detailed or exhaustive analyses of why these differences existed (cf. F. B. Smith 1979; Bates 1992; Barnes 1995; Rothman 1994).

6. According to Kahn (1979), in 1920 unionized carpenters were making $40–45 per week, the highest paid occupation listed. The lowest paid were laundry workers ($15/week), waiters and waitresses ($21 and $18/week, respectively), and food and tobacco workers ($18–25/week for men and $9–13/week for women). The 1920 wages can obviously not be applied to the 1910 occupations graph, but wage differentials were probably similar for the same trades.

7. Paul Erling Groth mentions that women were a "discernible" group in the cheap hotels and flophouses of San Francisco and the United States. For the country as a whole, women represented one out of ten migrant workers during the depression, and in most cities there were cheap lodging houses specifically for women. Other hotels and flophouses took both men and women. According to one San Francisco hotel clerk, if women could not afford their own rooms in these establishments, "they ha[d] to take their chances with the rest" (cited in Groth 1994, 138).

8. Hobos themselves apparently had a tripartite system of categorization — namely, hobos who worked, tramps who generally did not, and drunkards (Groth 1994, 133). As with homeless populations today, there was always some attempt to accurately characterize the character of the hobo, for instance, the degree to which alcoholism was a factor in their lifestyle. See Works Progress Administration reports cited in Olmstead et al. 1979.

9. The category "general laborer" could mean many things, and some within this category were not necessarily temporary or seasonal workers. The category itself shows the difficulty in specifying the different types of casual labor existing at this time, much less pinpointing differences in individuals undertaking such labor. Nevertheless, the category is the best estimate of the number of "hobos" residing in San Francisco at any one time. This number though, as Groth points out, was itself highly fluctuating as laborers exited the city during the summer for agricultural jobs and came back into the city during the winter looking for urban work on the agricultural off-season (Groth 1994).

10. A bill to assist the convalescing patient did not pass in California (California State Board of Health Reports 1940, 117). Only Wisconsin and New York had passed such bills by 1940.

11. In 1929, seventy-six patients were admitted into Arequipa Sanatorium from San Francisco hospitals. Several patients came from Arequipa to the San Francisco hospital for surgical procedures (California State Board of Health Reports 1940, 48).

12. These statistics include all patients of the San Francisco Hospital, including but not singling out tuberculosis patients. The percentages just for tuberculosis, however, closely approximated the statistics listed here.

7. Envisioning an Epilogue to Urban Maladies

1. Hooks states that "as a radical standpoint, perspective, position, 'the politics of location' necessarily calls those of us who would participate in the formation of counter-hegemonic cultural practice to identify the spaces where we begin the process of re-vision. . . . For me this space of radical openness is a margin — a profound edge." (hooks 1990, 145–49, cited in Soja and Hooper 1993, 189).

2. Witness, for example, public health focus on "behavioral" problems such as smoking, alcohol consumption, and diet and the general absence of attention to such public health threats as environmental toxins.

3. More specifically, New York instituted screening of at-risk populations, the administration of drug therapy, and detention of recalcitrant tuberculars not adhering to dictated therapeutic regimens (Lerner 1993). San Francisco has instituted similar measures (Lown, personal communication, 1991).

4. An estimate calculated by the House Ways and Means Committee (U.S. House of Representatives 1984).

5. The reason behind a halt in the rise of cases is as difficult to ascertain as the reason behind tuberculosis's decline earlier in the century. It can probably, however, be attributed to a stronger economy (diminished unemployment and rising real wages for some) combined with case observance and contact-tracing.

6. The *New York Times* on September 25, 1998, reported a "wave" of new public health reporting laws that signals a shift to greater surveillance of persons with HIV. The article quotes Lawrence Gostin, director of the Georgetown University–Johns Hopkins University Program on Law and Public Health, as saying that the "legislative trend is that we've moved from a period where civil rights and civil liberties for a person with H.I.V. prevailed to a compulsory and punitive approach" (*New York Times,* September 28, 1998, A1).

BIBLIOGRAPHY

Primary Sources

Abrams, Albert. 1886–87. *Pulmonary Phthisis: Report of the Committee on Microscopy and Histology.* California Medical Association Committee on Microscopy and Histology. Reprinted from the *Transactions of the Medical Society of the State of California.*

Act to Establish a Quarantine and Sanitary Laws for the City and County of San Francisco. 1870. San Francisco: City Printing Office.

Alta of San Francisco (newspaper). 1868–87. Bancroft Library, the University of California, Berkeley.

Alta Sanatorium for Early Tuberculosis Reports. 1909, 1912. Bancroft Library, the University of California, Berkeley.

An Appeal from the California Club for a State Sanatorium for the Treatment and Cure of Consumption. 1906. Sacramento: California State Printing Office (December).

"Arequipa Sanatorium." 1912. *The Survey,* December 7.

Arequipa Sanatorium: An Appeal. 1938. Pamphlet.

Arequipa Sanatorium, correspondence of patients. 1929–34. Bancroft Library, the University of California, Berkeley.

Arequipa Sanatorium, correspondence of staff and physicians. 1912–54. Bancroft Library, the University of California, Berkeley.

Arequipa Sanatorium Annual Reports. 1912–24. Fairfax, Calif.: Arequipa Sanatorium Printing.

Ashby, Ruth. N.d. "Life in a Lung Resort." *The Hi-Life.* (Newsletter of the Arequipa Sanatorium, Arequipa, California.)

Aubert, Dr. 1868. "The Smallpox Scare: Wholesale Vaccination, Is Smallpox Contagious, Etc." *Alta of San Francisco,* July 29 and August 6.

Bancroft, H. H. 1891. *History of California.* Vol 7. San Francisco: History Company.

Barney, Edward. 1899. *Truth Unveiled.* Bancroft Library, the University of California, Berkeley.

Benetes, General José. N.d. *California's First Medical Survey.* Translated by Sherburne Cook. Bancroft Library, the University of California, Berkeley.

Bersford, Thomas. 1908. *Theories and Facts for Students of Longevity and Health.* San Francisco: City Printing Office.

Blue, Rupert. Correspondence with H. H. Glennan, Surgeon of Public Health and U.S. Marine Hospital Service, San Francisco. Bethesda, Md.: National Archives.

———. Correspondence with Walter Wyman, Surgeon General, Washington, D.C. Bethesda, Md.: National Archives.

Boone, Dr. H. W., and A. T. Prescott. 1872. "The Sanitary Situation in San Francisco." *Western Lancet* 1, no. 4 (April).

Brown, Dr. Philip King, 1909–10. *The San Francisco Polyclinic Tuberculosis Class.* Unpublished pamphlets.

———. 1910–31. Correspondence with patients, Arequipa Sanatorium. Bancroft Library, the University of California, Berkeley.

———. 1911a. Correspondence with Edward Trudeau. Bancroft Library, the University of California, Berkeley.

———. 1911b. "The Opening of Arequipa Sanatorium." *San Francisco Chronicle,* April 6.

———. 1938. *Arequipa Sanatorium: An Appeal.* Fairfax, Calif.: Arequipa Sanatorium Printing.

———. n.d.[a]. "The Opening of a Sanatorium for Early Cases of Tuberculosis in Wage-Earning Women." N.p.

———. n.d.[b]. "Tuberculosis Case Work in the San Francisco Polyclinic." N.p.

Bureau of Tuberculosis, Department of Public Health, State of California. 1922. *Status of Tuberculosis.* Sacramento: California State Printing Office.

———. 1927. *Report of the High School Clinics.* Sacramento: California State Printing Office.

Cabot, Robert. 1912. "Arequipa Sanatorium: Where a Tuberculosis Patient Can Be Cured without Expense to Himself or Anyone Else." *Survey,* December 7.

California Department of Public Health. 1934. *Tuberculosis in California: The Development of a State Policy.* Sacramento: California State Printing Office.

California Interagency Council on TB and California Department of Public Health. 1964. *A Program for the Eradication of Tuberculosis in California.* Sacramento: California State Printing Office.

California Medical Gazette. July 1868; August 1868; October 1868; March 1869; November 1869.

California State Board of Health. 1903. "Resolution Passed May 11, 1903 to Remove Chinatown." Sacramento: California State Printing Office.

———. N.d. "Consumption: Its Restriction and Prevention." Extract from the Fourteenth Biennial Report.

California State Board of Health Reports. 1870–1940. Sacramento: California State Printing Office.

Call of San Francisco. 1882–88. Bancroft Library, the University of California, Berkeley.

Calmette, A. 1902. "Social Crusade against Consumption in the French Working Classes: The Émile Roux Dispensary at Lille." Berlin.

Cather, H. V. 1932. *The History of San Francisco's Chinatown.* Sacramento: California State Printing Office.

Chipman, J. 1880. Editorial in *San Francisco Chronicle,* March 6.

Cole, Beverly. 1873. "Our Lying-in Hospital and Foundling Asylum." *Western Lancet* 2, no. 9 (September).

Committee to Investigate Chinatown. 1880. "Chinatown Declared a Nuisance!" San Francisco.

Commonwealth Club. 1911. *Report on Syphilis and Gonorrhoea.* San Francisco.

Currie, Donald. 1901–5. Journal recording plague operations.

Emerson, L., and E. Phillips. 1923. *Hospitals and Health Agencies of San Francisco.* Report prepared for the Municipal Health Agency of San Francisco.

Fitz Gerald, Violette. 1934. Correspondence dated July 23.

Freuch, H. A. 1901. Letter to the editor, *Washington Post,* March 10.

Geiger, J. C., et al. 1939. *The Health of the Chinese in an American City.* San Francisco Department of Public Health, San Francisco.

Glennan, H. H., Surgeon of Public Health and U.S. Marine Hospital Service, San Francisco. 1903. Correspondence with Surgeon General Wyman, Washington, D.C., January 30.

Goodman, T. H. 1900. Correspondence with D. A. Chambers, Attorney, Washington, D.C., June 23.

Grancher, Dr. 1883. "Early Diagnosis of the Various Forms of Phthisis Pulmonalis." *Western Lancet* 12, no. 12 (December).

Hatch, Dr. F. W. 1871. *Report on Epidemics and Climatology of California with Remarks on the Relation of the Climate to Consumption.* Philadelphia: Collins Printing.

Hewston, George. 1878. Editorial on yellow fever in *Western Lancet* 7, no. 5 (July).

Hi-Life. 1912–32. (Publication of Arequipa Sanatorium.) Bancroft Library, the University of California, Berkeley.

Hiscock, R. 1930. *An Appraisal of the Public Health Program, 1929–1930.* Sacramento: California State Printing Office.

Hittell, John S. 1878. *A History of San Francisco, and Incidentally of the State of California.* San Francisco: A. L. Bancroft.

———. 1882. *Commerce and Industries of the Pacific Coast.* San Francisco: A. L. Bancroft.

"A Home for Consumptives." 1869. *California Medical Gazette* (June).

"About Hospitals." 1869. Editorial in *California Medical Gazette* (September).

Keating, J. M. 1879. *History of the Yellow Fever Epidemic of 1878.* Memphis: Howard Association.

Kober, George Martin. N.d. "The Etiology and Prevention of Tuberculosis." *Modoc County Correspondent.*

Langley's City Directory. 1869. San Francisco.

Lebert, H. 1873. "Tuberculosis in the Female Generative Organs." *Western Lancet* 2, no. 5 (May).

MacCormac, Henry. 1869. "The Crucial Test in Regard to the Origin of Phthisis and Tubercle." *California Medical Gazette* (April).

Mack, Mary. 1920. *Outwitting the 'TB Bugs': A Little Message of Hope, Help, and Common Sense for Those Who Seek Better Health.* San Francisco: Cahill Publishing.

McNutt, W. F. 1879. "Valedictory Address to the Graduating Class of the Medical Department of the University of California." *Western Lancet* 8, no. 10 (December).

Medico-Literary Journal of San Francisco. 1878–80.

Minnesota State Board of Health. 1911. *Report of Division of Epidemiology.* Minneapolis.

Morse, E. Malcolm. 1869. "Something about the Smallpox Epidemic." *California Medical Gazette* (January).

Municipal Reports of San Francisco. 1866–1915. Bancroft Library, the University of California, Berkeley.

National Board of Health. 1881. *Annual Report for 1880.* Washington, D.C.: Government Printing Office.

National Board of Health. 1881–82. *Bulletin.* Washington, D.C.: Government Printing Office.

Nordhoff, Charles. 1872. *California: For Health, Pleasure, and Residence.* New York: Harper.

Northern, W. F. 1908. "Report on Tuberculosis among Negroes." In U.S. Census for 1900. Washington, D.C.: Government Printing Office.

Ordinances of the City and County of San Francisco. 1909. San Francisco.

Ordinance 369 of the City and County of San Francisco: Providing Sanitary Regulations for the Protection of the Public Health in the City and County of San Francisco, and particularly to Prevent the Propagation and Spread of Bubonic Plague. 1909. San Francisco: City Printing Office.

Oswald, Dr. Felix. 1882. "The Fresh-Air Habit." *Western Lancet* 11, no. 3 (March).

Pacific Dispensary for Women and Children. 1875. *First Report.* March 24.

"People's Open Illustrated Letter." 1886. San Francisco (May 1).

Regulations of the Arequipa Sanatorium. N.d. Fairfax, Calif.: Arequipa Sanatorium Printing.

Remondino, Dr. P. C. 1890a. "Empyema and Pulmonary Abscess." *Journal of the American Medical Association,* December 17.

———. 1890b. "Ventilation and Impure Air as Prophylactic or Causative of Disease." Paper presented before the American Public Health Association.

———. 1893. *The Modern Climatic Treatment of Invalids with Pulmonary Consumption in Southern California.* N.p.

Report of the Special Health Commissioners Appointed by the Governor to Confer with the Federal Authorities at Washington respecting the Alleged Existence of Bubonic Plague in California. 1901. Sacramento: California State Printing Office.

Richardon, B. W. 1879. Editorial in *Western Lancet* 1, no. 5 (January).

Roosevelt, President Theodore. 1907. Correspondence with Surgeon General Wyman, Washington, D.C., September 5.

Saint Helena Sanitarium News. 1940–41. St. Helena, California.

San Francisco Association for the Study and Prevention of Tuberculosis (San Francisco Tuberculosis Association). 1908–24. Annual Reports. San Francisco.

———. 1915. *A Report of the Tuberculosis Situation in San Francisco.* San Francisco (July).

———. 1928. "The War against Tuberculosis in San Francisco." San Francisco.

Saxon, Isabelle. 1861. *Five Years within the Golden Gate.* San Francisco: Bancroft.

Schweimitz, E. A., Chief Biochemistry Director, Agricultural Department. 1899. Correspondence to John Hay, Secretary of State, June 2.

Shorb, J. Campbell. 1868. "The Public Health — the Public Responsible for the Diffusion of Small Pox." *California Medical Gazette* (September).

Smith, F. 1912. Correspondence with the Surgeon General of the United States, August 22.

Smith, Mary Roberts. 1895. *Notes on Almshouse Women.* Boston: n.p.

Stallard, J., et al. 1876. *Female Health and Hygiene on the Pacific Coast.* San Francisco: City Printing Office.

Stanley, Dr. Leo. 1938–39. "TB in San Quentin." *California and Western Medicine* 49, no. 6 (December 1938) and 50, no. 1 (January 1939).

Stout, Arthur B. 1868. "Hygiene as Regards the Sewage of San Francisco." *California Medical Gazette* (October).

Symms, Frank, Chair of Merchants' Association of San Francisco. 1903. Correspondence with Francis Loomis, Assistant Secretary of State, June 5.

Todd, Frank Morton. 1909. *Eradicating Plague from San Francisco: Report of the Citizens' Health Committee.* San Francisco: City Printing Office.

Trail Blazer. 1920–21. (Newsletter of the California Tuberculosis Association.) San Francisco.

Trudeau, Edward Livingston. 1916. *An Autobiography.* New York: Doubleday.

U.S. Census. 1860, 1900, 1910, 1940, 1960. Washington, D.C.: Government Printing Office.

The War against Tuberculosis in San Francisco. 1928. San Francisco: San Francisco Publishing.

The Wasp. May 26, 1882.

Western Lancet (medical journal). 1872–83. San Francisco.

White (no initial), Assistant Surgeon of U.S. Marine Hospital Service. 1901. Correspondence to Surgeon General Wyman, Washington, D.C., September 27.

Whitney, Jessamine, Statistician of the United States Public Health Service. 1922. Correspondence to Frank Balderrey, Department of Public Safety, Perrysburg, New York, February 2.

Whittaker, Dr. 1880. "The Resemblances between Tuberculosis and Syphilis." *Western Lancet* 9, no. 8 (October).

Williams, C. J. B. 1869. "Nature and Treatment of Pulmonary Consumption as Exemplified in Private Practice." *California Medical Gazette* (January).

Works Progress Administration. 1937. *A Study of 2739 Cases of TB Reported to the San Francisco Department of Public Health during 1934, 1935, and 1936.* San Francisco.

Secondary Sources

Adams, Annmarie. 1996. *Architecture in the Family Way: Doctors, Houses, and Women 1870–1900.* Kingston, Canada: McGill-Queen's University Press.

Anderson, Kay. 1992. *Vancouver's Chinatown: Racial Discourse in Canada, 1874–1980.* Kingston, Canada: McGill-Queen's University Press.

Anonymous. 1991. *Personal Communications with Homeless Individuals Accessing Clinic.* San Francisco, September–December.

Armstrong, David. 1983. *Political Anatomy of the Body: Medical Knowledge in Britain in the Twentieth Century.* Cambridge: Cambridge University Press.

Arnold, David. 1993. *Colonizing the Body: State Medicine and Epidemic Disease in Nineteenth Century India.* Berkeley: University of California Press.

Arnstein, Lawrence. 1972. "Earl Warren and the State Department of Public Health." Interviews conducted by Gabrielle Morris. California State Department of Public Health.

Averbach, Alvin. 1973. "San Francisco's South of Market District, 1850–1950: The Emergence of Skid Row." *California Historical Quarterly* 3, no. 3 (fall): 196–223.

Baker, Paula. 1984. "The Domestication of Politics: Women and American Political Society, 1780–1920." *American Historical Review* 89, no. 3 (June): 620–47.

Barnes, David. 1995. *The Making of a Social Disease: Tuberculosis in Nineteenth-Century France.* Berkeley: University of California Press.

Bates, Barbara. 1992. *Bargaining for Life: A Social History of Tuberculosis, 1876–1938.* Philadelphia: University of Pennsylvania Press.

Bauer, John. 1959. *The Health Seekers of Southern California, 1870–1900.* San Marino, Calif.: Huntington Library.

Bell, David, et al. 1994. "All Hyped Up and No Place to Go." *Gender, Place, and Culture* 1, no. 1:31–48.

Benjamin, Walter. 1978. *Reflections: Essays, Aphorisms, and Autobiographical Writings.* Edited by Peter Demetz. Translated by Edmund Jephcott. New York: Schocken Books.

Bhabha, Homi K. 1991. "'Race,' Time, and the Revision of Modernity." *Oxford Literary Review* 13, nos. 1–2:193–219.

Bondi, Liz. 1992. "Gender Symbols and Urban Landscapes." *Progress in Human Geography* 16:157–70.

Bordo, Susan. 1993. *Unbearable Weight: Feminism, Western Culture, and the Body.* Berkeley: University of California Press.

Boyer, Paul. 1978. *Urban Masses and Moral Order in America, 1820–1920.* Cambridge, Mass.: Harvard University Press.

Brandt, Allan M. 1987. *No Magic Bullet: A Social History of Venereal Disease in the United States since 1880.* Oxford: Oxford University Press.

———. 1991. "AIDS and Metaphor: Toward the Social Meaning of Epidemic Disease." In *In Time of Plague: The History and Social Consequences of Lethal Epidemic Disease,* edited by Arien Mack. New York: New York University Press.

Broussard, Albert S. 1993. *Black San Francisco: The Struggle for Racial Equality in the West, 1900–1954.* Lawrence: University Press of Kansas.

Brown, Michael. 1997. *Replacing Citizenship: AIDS and Activism in Vancouver.* New York: Guilford.

Bryder, Linda. 1988. *Below the Magic Mountain: A Social History of Tuberculosis in Twentieth-Century Britain.* Oxford: Clarendon Press.

———. 1991. "Comments on 'The Historical Decline of Tuberculosis in Europe and America: Its Causes and Significance.'" *Journal of the History of Medicine* 46 (July): 358–62.

Burchell, Robert A. 1980. *The San Francisco Irish 1848–1880.* Berkeley: University of California Press.

Butler, Judith. 1990. *Gender Trouble.* London: Routledge.

Caldwell, Mark. 1988. *The Last Crusade: The War on Consumption 1862–1954.* New York: Atheneum.

Calvi, Giulia. 1989. *Histories of a Plague Year: The Social and the Imaginary in Baroque Florence.* Berkeley: University of California Press.

Canguilhem, Georges. 1991. *The Normal and the Pathological.* New York: Zone Books.

Carmichael, Ann G. 1986. *Plague and the Poor in Renaissance Florence.* Cambridge: Cambridge University Press.

Cartwright, Lisa. 1992. "Women, X-rays, and the Public Culture of Prophylactic Imaging." *Camera Obscura* 29:19–56.

Choay, Françoise. 1969. *The Modern City: Planning in the 19th Century.* Translated by Marguerite Hugo and George R. Collins. New York: George Braziller.

Cinel, Dino. 1982. *From Italy to San Francisco: The Immigrant Experience.* Stanford, Calif.: Stanford University Press.

Cipolla, Carlo M. 1979. *Faith, Reason, and the Plague in Seventeenth-Century Tuscany.* Ithaca, N.Y.: Cornell University Press.

———. 1981. *Fighting the Plagues in Seventeenth-Century Italy.* Madison: University of Wisconsin Press.

Clark, Clifford Edward, Jr. 1986. *The American Family Home 1800–1960.* Chapel Hill: University of North Carolina Press.

Coleman, William. 1982. *Death Is a Social Disease: Public Health and Political Economy in Early Industrial France.* Madison: University of Wisconsin Press.

Condran, Gretchen, and Eileen Crimmins. 1980. "Mortality Differentials between Rural and Urban Areas of States in the Northeastern United States 1890–1900." *Journal of Historical Geography* 6, no. 2:179–202.

Conje, G. 1984. "Tuberculosis and Mortality Decline in England and Wales, 1851–1900." In *Urban Disease and Mortality*, edited by R. I. Woods and J. Woodward. New York: St. Martin's Press.

Cook, Sherburne. 1940. *Population Trends among the California Mission Indians*. Berkeley: University of California Press.

Craffey, Brynn. 1992. "Death in the Air: The Shocking Return of a 19th-Century Killer." *San Francisco Examiner (Image)*, June 14, 6–15.

Cresswell, Tim. 1996. *In Place/Out of Place: Geography, Ideology, and Transgression*. Minneapolis: University of Minnesota Press.

Crimp, Douglas. 1992. "Portraits of People with AIDS." In *Cultural Studies*, edited by Lawrence Grossberg, Cary Nelson, and Paula Treichler. New York: Routledge.

Cronje, G. 1984. "Tuberculosis and Mortality Decline in England and Wales, 1851–1900." In *Urban Disease and Mortality*, edited by R. I. Woods and J. Woodward. New York: St. Martin's Press.

Cross, Ira B. 1935. *A History of the Labor Movement in California*. Berkeley: University of California Press.

Daniels, Douglas Henry. 1980. *Pioneer Urbanites: A Social and Cultural History of Black San Francisco*. Philadelphia: Temple University Press.

Danziger, Sheldon, and Peter Gottschalk. 1995. *America Unequal*. Cambridge, Mass.: Harvard University Press.

Dear, Michael J. 1981. "Social and Spatial Reproduction of the Mentally Ill." In *Urbanization and Urban Planning in Capitalist Society*, edited by M. Dear and A. J. Scott. London: Methuen.

Dear, Michael J., and Jennifer Wolch. 1987. *Landscapes of Despair: From Deinstitutionalization to Homelessness*. Oxford: Polity Press.

Delaporte, François. 1986. *Disease and Civilization: The Cholera in Paris, 1832*. Cambridge, Mass.: MIT Press.

Dennis, Richard. 1984. *English Industrial Cities of the 19th Century: A Social Geography*. Cambridge: Cambridge University Press.

Dicker, Laverne Mau. 1979. *The Chinese in San Francisco: A Pictorial History*. New York: Dover.

Doka, Kenneth J. 1997. *AIDS, Fear, and Society: Challenging the Dreaded Disease*. London: Taylor and Francis.

Douglas, Mary. 1966. *Purity and Danger: An Analysis of the Concepts of Pollution and Taboo*. New York: Routledge.

———. 1991. "Witchcraft and Leprosy: Two Strategies of Exclusion." *Man* 26:723–36.

Dubos, Rene, and Jean Dubos. 1987. *The White Plague: Tuberculosis, Man, and Society*. 1952. Reprint, New Brunswick, N.J.: Rutgers University Press.

Duffy, John. 1974. *A History of Public Health in New York City 1866–1966*. New York: Russell Sage Foundation.

———. 1985. "Social Impact of Disease in the Late 19th Century." In *Sickness and Health in America: Readings in the History of Medicine and Public Health*, edited by J. Walzer Leavitt and R. Numbers. Madison: University of Wisconsin Press.

———. 1990. *The Sanitarians: A History of American Public Health.* Champaign: University of Illinois Press.

Economist. September 12, 1998, 93–94.

Ellis, John. 1992. *Yellow Fever and Public Health in the New South.* Lexington: University Press of Kentucky.

Epstein, Julia. 1995. *Altered Conditions: Disease, Medicine, and Storytelling.* New York: Routledge.

Evans, D. M. 1978. "Alienation, Mental Illness, and the Partitioning of Space." *Antipode* 10:10–23.

Evans, Richard J. 1992. "Epidemics and Revolutions: Cholera in Nineteenth-Century Europe." In *Epidemics and Ideas: Essays on the Historical Perception of Pestilence,* edited by T. Ranger and P. Slack. Cambridge: Cambridge University Press.

Eyler, John M. 1992. "The Sick Poor and the State: Arthur Newsholme on Poverty, Disease, and Responsibility." In *Framing Disease: Studies in Cultural History,* edited by C. Rosenberg and J. Golden. New Brunswick, N.J.: Rutgers University Press.

Eyles, J., and K. J. Woods. 1983. *The Social Geography of Medicine and Health.* London: Croom Helm.

Farmer, Paul. 1992. *AIDS and Accusation: Haiti and the Geography of Blame.* Berkeley: University of California Press.

Fee, Elizabeth, and Roy M. Acheson. 1991. *A History of Education in Public Health: Health That Mocks the Doctor's Rules.* New York: Oxford University Press.

Fee, Elizabeth, and Daniel M. Fox, eds. 1988. *AIDS: The Burdens of History.* Berkeley: University of California Press.

———, eds. 1992. *AIDS: The Making of a Chronic Disease.* Berkeley: University of California Press.

Fee, Elizabeth, and Dorothy Porter. 1992. "Public Health, Preventive Medicine and Professionalization: England and America in the Nineteenth Century." In *Medicine in Society: Historical Essays,* edited by Andrew Wear. Cambridge: Cambridge University Press.

Feldberg, Georgina D. 1995. *Disease and Class: Tuberculosis and the Shaping of Modern North American Society.* New Brunswick, N.J.: Rutgers University Press.

Figlio, Karl. 1978. "Chlorosis and Chronic Disease in 19th Century Britain: The Social Constitution of Somatic Illness in a Capitalist Society." *Social History* 3:167–97.

Foucault, Michel. 1965. *Madness and Civilization: A History of Insanity in the Age of Reason.* Translated by Richard Howard. New York: Random House.

———. 1975. *The Birth of the Clinic: An Archaeology of Medical Perception.* New York: Vintage Books.

———. 1977. *Discipline and Punish: The Birth of the Prison.* Translated by Alan Sheridan. New York: Vintage Books.

Galishoff, Stuart. 1975. *Safeguarding the Public Health: Newark, 1895–1918.* Westport, Conn.: Greenwood Press.

Gilman, Sander. 1985. *Difference and Pathology: Stereotypes of Sexuality, Race, and Madness.* Ithaca, N.Y.: Cornell University Press.

———. 1988. *Disease and Representation: Images of Illness from Madness to AIDS.* Ithaca, N.Y.: Cornell University Press.

———. 1995. *Picturing Health and Illness.* Baltimore: Johns Hopkins University Press.

Godfrey, Brian J. 1988. *Neighborhoods in Transition: The Making of San Francisco's Ethnic and Nonconformist Communities.* Berkeley: University of California Press.

Grosz, Elizabeth. 1994. *Volatile Bodies: Toward a Corporeal Feminism.* Bloomington: Indiana University Press.

———. 1995. *Space, Time, and Perversion.* New York: Routledge.

Groth, Paul Erling. 1983. "Forbidden Housing: The Evolution and Exclusion of Hotels, Boarding Houses, Rooming Houses, and Lodging Houses in American Cities." Ph.D. diss., University of California, Berkeley.

———. 1994. *Living Downtown: The History of Residential Hotels in the United States.* Berkeley: University of California Press.

Haas, Victor H. 1959. "When Bubonic Plague Came to Chinatown." *American Journal of Tropical Medicine* 8:141–47.

Hammonds, Evelynn. 1997. "Seeing AIDS: Race, Gender, and Representation." In *The Gender Politics of HIV/AIDS in Women: Perspectives on the Pandemic in the United States,* edited by Nancy Goldstein and Jennifer Manlowe. New York: New York University Press.

Hannah, Matt. 1997. "Imperfect Panopticism: Envisioning the Construction of Normal Lives." In *Space and Social Theory: Interpreting Modernity and Postmodernity,* edited by Georges Benko and Ulf Strohmayer. Cambridge, Mass.: Blackwell.

Hansen, Gladys, ed. 1973. *San Francisco: The Bay and Its Cities.* New York: Hastings House.

Haraway, Donna. 1995. "Nature, Politics, and Possibilities: A Debate and Discussion with David Harvey and Donna Haraway." *Environment and Planning D: Society and Space* 13:507–27.

Hardy, Anne. 1993. *The Epidemic Streets: Infectious Disease and the Rise of Preventive Medicine 1856–1900.* Oxford: Clarendon Press.

Harris, Henry. 1932. *California's Medical Story.* Baltimore: Grabhorn Press.

Harvey, David. 1989. *The Condition of Postmodernity: An Enquiry into the Origins of Social Change.* Cambridge: Basil Blackwell.

———. 1995. "Nature, Politics, and Possibilities: A Debate and Discussion with David Harvey and Donna Haraway." *Environment and Planning D: Society and Space* 13:507–27.

———. 1997. "The Body as an Accumulation Strategy." Paper given at the University of Arizona, fall.

Henderson, George. 1999. *California and the Fictions of Capital.* New York: Oxford University Press.

Himmelfarb, Gertrude. 1984. *Idea of Poverty: England in the Early Industrial Age.* New York: Knopf.

hooks, bell. 1990. *Yearnings: Race, Gender, and Cultural Politics.* Boston: South End Press.

Hopkins, Donald R. 1983. *Princes and Peasants: Smallpox in History*. Chicago: University of Chicago Press.

Howard, Ebenezer. 1962. "The Garden City." 1898. Reprinted in *City and Country in America*. New York: Appleton-Century-Crofts.

Hubbard, Phil. 1998. "Sexuality, Immorality, and the City: Red-light Districts and the Marginalization of Female Street Prostitutes." *Gender, Place, and Culture* 5, no. 1:55–72.

Humphreys, Margaret. 1992. *Yellow Fever and the South*. New Brunswick, N.J.: Rutgers University Press.

Issel, William, and Robert W. Cherny. 1986. *San Francisco 1865–1932: Politics, Power, and Urban Development*. Berkeley: University of California Press.

Jones, J. R. 1964. *History of the Medical Society of the State of California*. Sacramento: Historical Committee of the Sacramento Society for Medical Improvement.

Joseph, Stephen. 1993. "Editorial: Tuberculosis, Again." *American Journal of Public Health* 83, no. 5:647–48.

Kahn, Judd. 1979. *Imperial San Francisco: Politics and Planning in an American City, 1897–1906*. Lincoln: University of Nebraska Press.

Katz, Michael. 1986. *In the Shadow of the Poorhouse: A Social History of Welfare in America*. New York: Basic Books.

Kearns, Gerry. 1985. *Urban Epidemics and Historical Geography: Cholera in London 1848–49*. Norwich, England.

———. 1989. "Zivilis or Hygaeia: Urban Public Health and the Epidemiologic Transition." In *The Rise and Fall of Great Cities*, edited by R. Lawton. London: Bellhaven.

———. 1991. "Biology, Class, and the Urban Penalty." In *Urbanising Britain: Essays on Class and Community in the Nineteenth Century*, edited by Gerry Kearns and Charles Withers. Cambridge: Cambridge University Press.

Kern, Stephen. 1983. *The Culture of Time and Space 1880–1918*. Cambridge, Mass.: Harvard University Press.

King, Anthony. 1984. *The Bungalow: The Production of a Global Culture*. London: Routledge and Kegan Paul.

Klein, Maury, and Harvey Kantor. 1976. *Prisoners of Progress: American Industrial Cities 1850–1920*. New York: Macmillan.

Kraut, Alan M. 1994. *Silent Travelers: Germs, Genes, and the "Immigrant Menace."* New York: Basic Books.

Kristeva, Julia. 1982. *Powers of Horror: An Essay on Abjection*. Translated by Leon S. Roudiez. New York: Columbia University Press.

La Berge, Ann. 1992. *Mission and Method: The Early Nineteenth Century French Public Health Movement*. Cambridge: Cambridge University Press.

Lavender, David. 1972. *California: Land of New Beginnings*. Lincoln: University of Nebraska Press.

Leavitt, Judith Walzer. 1982. *The Healthiest City: Milwaukee and the Politics of Health Reform*. Princeton, N.J.: Princeton University Press.

———. 1985. "Politics and Public Health: Smallpox in Milwaukee, 1894–1895." In *Sickness and Health in America: Readings in the History of Medicine and Public Health,* edited by J. Walzer Leavitt and R. Numbers. Madison: University of Wisconsin Press.

Leavitt, Judith Walzer, and R. Numbers, eds. 1985. *Sickness and Health in America: Readings in the History of Medicine and Public Health.* Madison: University of Wisconsin Press.

Lefebvre, Henri. 1991. *The Production of Space.* Cambridge: Basil Blackwell.

Lerner, Barron. 1993. "New York City's Tuberculosis Control Efforts: The Historical Limitations of the 'War on Consumption.'" *American Journal of Public Health* 83, no. 5:758–66.

———. 1998. *Contagion and Confinement: Controlling Tuberculosis along the Skid Road.* Baltimore: Johns Hopkins University Press.

Lert, France. 1982. "Emergence and devenir du systeme de prise en charge de la tuberculose en France entre 1900 et 1940." *Social Science and Medicine* 16:2073–82.

Limerick, Patricia. 1987. *Legacy of Conquest.* New York: W. W. Norton.

Limerick, Patricia, Clyde Milner, and Charles Rankin, eds. 1991. *Trails: Toward a New Western History.* Lawrence: University Press of Kansas.

Lipson, Loren G. 1972. "Plague in San Francisco in 1900." *Annals of Internal Medicine* 77:303–10.

Lockwood, Charles. 1979. "Rincon Hill Was San Francisco's Most Genteel Neighborhood." *California History* 58 (spring): 47–62.

Longstreth, Richard. 1983. *On the Edge of the World: Four Architects in San Francisco at the Turn of the Century.* New York: Architectural History Foundation; Cambridge, Mass.: MIT Press.

Los Angeles Times. October 24, 1993.

Los Angeles Times Magazine. October 24, 1993.

Lown, Ann. 1991. Personal communication. September.

Mack, Arien, ed. 1991. *In Time of Plague: The History and Social Consequences of Lethal Epidemic Disease.* New York: New York University Press.

Martin, Emily. 1994. *Flexible Bodies: The Role of Immunity in American Culture from the Days of Polio to the Age of AIDS.* Boston: Beacon Press.

Marx, Karl. 1976. *Capital.* Vol. 1. New York: Vintage.

Matthaei, Julie. 1982. *An Economic History of Women in America: Women's Work, the Sexual Division of Labor, and the Development of Capitalism.* New York: Schocken Books.

Mayne, Alan. 1993. *The Imagined Slum: Newspaper Representation in Three Cities, 1870–1914.* Leicester: Leicester University Press.

McBride, David. 1991. *From TB to AIDS: Epidemics among Urban Blacks since 1900.* Albany: State University of New York Press.

McClain, Charles. 1988. "Of Medicine, Race, and American Law: The Bubonic Plague Outbreak of 1900." *Law and Social Inquiry* 13:447–70.

McClintock, Ann. 1995. *Imperial Leather: Race, Gender, and Sexuality in the Colonial Conquest.* New York: Routledge.

Mcfarlane, Neil. 1989. "Hospitals, Housing, and Tuberculosis in Glasgow." *Social History of Medicine* 2.

McGrath, Roberta. 1990. "Dangerous Liaisons: Health, Disease, and Representation." In *Ecstatic Antibodies: Resisting the AIDS Mythology*, edited by Tessa Boffin and Sunil Gupta. London: Rivers Oram Press.

McKeown, T. 1976. *The Modern Rise of Population*. New York: Academic Press.

McNeill, William H. 1976. *Plagues and Peoples*. New York: Doubleday.

Merrill, Malcolm. 1972. "A Director Reminisces." Interview by Gabrielle Morriss. California State Department of Public Health.

Mitchell, Don. 1996. *The Lie of the Land: Migrant Workers and the California Landscape*. Minneapolis: University of Minnesota Press.

Musto, David. 1988. "Quarantine and the Problem of AIDS." In *AIDS: The Burdens of History*, edited by Elizabeth Fee and Donald M. Fox. Berkeley: University of California Press.

Nelkin, Dorothy, and Sander Gilman. 1991. "Placing Blame for Devastating Disease." In *In Time of Plague: The History and Social Consequences of Lethal Epidemic Disease*, edited by Arien Mack. New York: New York University Press.

New York Times. October 11, 1992; October 12, 1992; October 13, 1992; July 18, 1994; January 20, 1998; September 28, 1998.

Olmstead, Roger, et al. 1979. "The Yerba Buena Center: Report on Historical Cultural Resources." Prepared for the San Francisco Redevelopment Agency (August).

Oppenheimer, Gerald. 1992. "Causes, Cases, and Cohorts: The Role of Epidemiology in the Historical Construction of AIDS." In *AIDS: The Making of a Chronic Disease*, edited by Elizabeth Fee and Daniel M. Fox. Berkeley: University of California Press.

Pascoe, Peggy. 1990. *Relations of Rescue: The Search for Female Moral Authority in the American West, 1874–1939*. New York: Oxford University Press.

Patton, Cindy. 1990. *Inventing AIDS*. New York: Routledge.

———. 1995. "Between Innocence and Safety: Epidemiologic and Popular Constructions of Young People's Need for Safe Sex." In *Deviant Bodies*, edited by Jacqueline Urla and Jennifer Terry. Bloomington: Indiana University Press.

Paul, Eugene, et al. 1993. "Nemesis Revisited: Tuberculosis Infection in a New York City Men's Shelter." *American Journal of Public Health* 83, no. 12:1743–45.

Pelling, Margaret. 1978. *Cholera, Fever, and English Medicine 1825–1865*. Oxford: Oxford University Press.

Philo, Chris. 1987. "Fit Localities for an Asylum: The Historical Geography of the Nineteenth-Century 'Mad-Business' in England as Viewed through the Pages of the *Asylum Journal*." *Journal of Historical Geography* 13:398–415.

———. 1989. " 'Enough to Drive One Mad': The Organization of Space in 19th-Century Lunatic Asylums." In *The Power of Geography: How Territory Shapes Social Life*, edited by Jennifer Wolch and Michael Dear. Boston: Unwin Hyman.

Poirier, Richard. 1991. "AIDS and Traditions of Homophobia." In *In Time of Plague: The History and Social Consequences of Lethal Epidemic Disease*, edited by Arien Mack. New York: New York University Press.

Pooley, M., and C. Pooley. 1984. "Health, Society, and Environment in Victorian Manchester." In *Urban Disease and Mortality,* edited by R. I. Woods and J. Woodward. New York: St. Martin's Press.

Poovey, Mary. 1993. "Anatomical Realism and Social Investigation in Early Nineteenth-Century Manchester." *Differences: A Journal of Feminist Cultural Studies* 5, no. 3:1–30.

Porter, Roy. 1994. "Gout: Framing and Fantasizing Disease." *Bulletin of the History of Medicine* 68, no. 1 (spring): 1–28.

Pratt, Geraldine, and Susan Hanson. 1994. "Geography and the Construction of Difference." *Gender, Place, and Culture* 1, no. 1:5–30.

Pred, Allan. 1984. "Place As Historically Contingent Process: Structuration and the Time-Geography of Becoming Places." *Annals of the Association of American Geographers* 74, no. 2:279–97.

———. 1990. *Making Histories and Constructing Human Geographies.* Boulder, Colo.: Westview Press.

Reichman, Lee. 1993. "Fear, Embarrassment, and Relief: The Tuberculosis Epidemic and Public Health." *American Journal of Public Health* 83, no. 5:639–41.

Riis, Jacob A. 1971 [1901]. *How the Other Half Lives: Studies among the Tenements of New York.* New York: Dover.

Risse, Guenter B. 1988. "Epidemics and History: Ecological Perspectives and Social Responses." In *AIDS: The Burdens of History,* edited by Elizabeth Fee and Daniel M. Fox. Berkeley: University of California Press.

———. 1992. "'A Long Pull, a Strong Pull, and All Together': San Francisco and Bubonic Plague, 1907–1908." *Bulletin of the History of Medicine* 66:260–82.

Robbins, Jessica. 1997. "Class Struggles in the Tubercular World: Nurses, Patients, and Physicans, 1903–1915." *Bulletin of the History of Medicine* 2, no. 3 (fall): 412–34.

Rogers, Naomi. 1992. *Dirt and Disease: Polio before FDR.* New Brunswick, N.J.: Rutgers University Press.

Rosen, George. 1975. *Preventive Medicine in the U.S. 1900–1975: Trends and Interpretations.* New York: Science History Publications.

Rosenberg, Charles. 1962. *The Cholera Years: The United States in 1832, 1849, and 1866.* Chicago: University of Chicago Press.

———. 1992a. *Explaining Epidemics and Other Studies in the History of Medicine.* Cambridge: Cambridge University Press.

———. 1992b. "Framing Disease: Illness, Society, and History." In *Framing Disease: Studies in Cultural History,* edited by Charles Rosenberg and Janet Golden. New Brunswick, N.J.: Rutgers University Press.

Rosenberg, Charles, and Carroll Smith-Rosenberg. 1985. "Pietism and the Origins of the American Public Health Movement: A Note on John H. Griscom and Robert M. Hartley." In *Sickness and Health in America: Readings in the History of Medicine and Public Health,* edited by Judith Walzer Leavitt and R. Numbers. Madison: University of Wisconsin Press.

Rosenberg, Charles, and Janet Golden. 1992. *Framing Disease: Studies in Cultural History.* New Brunswick, N.J.: Rutgers University Press.

Rosenkrantz, Barbara Gutmann. 1972. *Public Health and the State: Changing Views in Massachusetts, 1842–1936.* Cambridge, Mass.: Harvard University Press.

———. 1991. "Case Histories — an Introduction." In *In Time of Plague: The History and Social Consequences of Lethal Epidemic Disease,* edited by Arien Mack. New York: New York University Press.

Rosner, David, ed. 1995. *Hives of Sickness: Public Health and Epidemics in New York City.* New Brunswick, N.J.: Rutgers University Press.

Rothman, Sheila M. 1978. *Women's Proper Place: A History of Changing Ideals and Practices, 1870 to the Present.* New York: Basic Books.

———. 1994. *Living in the Shadow of Death: Tuberculosis and the Social Experience of Illness in American History.* New York: Basic Books.

Ruskin, John. 1962. "The Stones of Venice, Vol. I." 1851. Reprinted in *City and Country in America,* edited by David Weimer. New York: Appleton-Century-Crofts.

San Francisco Chronicle. 1868–1992.

Saunders, J. D. de C. M. 1967. "Geography and Geopolitics in California Medicine." Reprinted from the *Bulletin of the History of Medicine* 41, no. 4 (July-August): 296–324.

Saxton, Alexander. 1971. *Indispensable Enemy: Labor and the Anti-Chinese Movement in California.* Berkeley: University of California Press.

Schilling, Chris. 1995. *The Body and Social Theory.* Thousand Oaks, Calif.: Sage Press.

Scott, Mel. 1959. *The San Francisco Bay Area: A Metropolis in Perspective.* Berkeley: University of California Press.

Shilts, Randy. 1987. *And the Band Played On: Politics, People, and the AIDS Epidemic.* New York: St. Martin's Press.

Shryock, Richard. 1957. *National Tuberculosis Association 1904–1954.* New York: National Tuberculosis Association.

Shumsky, Neil Larry. 1972. "Tar Flat and Nob Hill: A Social History of Industrial San Francisco during the 1870s." Ph.D. diss., University of California, Berkeley.

Shumsky, Neil Larry, and Larry Springer. 1981. "San Francisco's Zone of Prostitution, 1880–1934." *Journal of Historical Geography* 7 no. 1:71–89.

Sibley, David. 1995. *Geographies of Exclusion.* New York: Routledge.

Singer, Merrill. 1998. *The Political Economy of AIDS.* Amityville, N.Y.: Baywood.

Sklar, Katherine. 1973. *Catherine Beecher: A Study in American Domesticity.* New Haven, Conn.: Yale University Press.

Smith, F. B. 1979. *The People's Health 1830–1910.* New York: Holmes and Meier.

———. 1988. *The Retreat of Tuberculosis 1850–1950.* London: Croom Helm.

Smith-Rosenberg, Carroll. 1985. *Disorderly Conduct: Visions of Gender in Victorian America.* New York: Knopf.

Soja, Edward. 1989. *Postmodern Geographies: The Reassertion of Space in Critical Social Theory.* New York: Verso Press.

Soja, Edward, and Barbara Hooper. 1993. "The Spaces That Difference Makes: Some Notes on the Geographical Margins of the New Cultural Politics." In *Place and the Politics of Identity,* edited by Michael Keith and Steve Pile. New York: Routledge.

Sontag, Susan. 1977. *Illness As Metaphor.* New York: Farrar, Straus and Giroux.

———. 1989. *Aids and Its Metaphors.* London: Allen Lane.

Stallybrass, Peter, and Allon White. 1986. *The Politics and Poetics of Transgression.* Ithaca, N.Y.: Cornell University Press.

Stine, Gerlad. 1995. *AIDS Update 1994–1995.* Englewood Cliffs, N.J.: Prentice Hall.

Sullivan, Andrew. 1996. "When Plagues End: Notes on the Twilight of an Epidemic." *New York Times Magazine,* November 10, 52–62.

Szreter, Simon. 1988. "The Importance of Social Intervention in Britain's Mortality Decline, c. 1850–1914: A Reinterpretation of the Role of Public Health." *Social History of Medicine* 1.

Takaki, Ronald. 1989. *Strangers from a Different Shore: A History of Asian Americans.* New York: Penguin Books.

Thrift, Nigel. 1985. "Flies and Germs: A Geography of Knowledge." In *Social Relations and Spatial Structures,* edited by Derek Gregory and John Urry. London: Macmillan.

Tilly, Charles. 1984. "Notes on Urban Images of Historians." In *Cities of the Mind: Images and Themes of the City in the Social Sciences,* edited by Lloyd Rodwin and Robert Hollister. New York: Plenum Press.

Tindall, George Brown, and David E. Shi. 1992. *America: A Narrative History.* New York: W. W. Norton.

Trauner, Joan B. 1978. "The Chinese as Medical Scapegoats in San Francisco 1870–1905." *California History* (spring): 70–87.

Treichler, Paula. 1992a. "AIDS and HIV Infection in the Third World: A First World Chronicle." In *AIDS: The Making of a Chronic Disease,* edited by Elizabeth Fee and Daniel M. Fox. Berkeley: University of California Press.

———. 1992b. "Beyond *Cosmo:* AIDS, Identity, and Inscriptions of Gender." *Camera Obscura: A Journal of Feminism and Film Theory* 28:21–78.

Urla, Jacqueline, and Jennifer Terry. 1995. "Introduction: Mapping Embodied Deviance." In *Deviant Bodies,* edited by Jacqueline Urla and Jennifer Terry. Bloomington: Indiana University Press.

U.S. House. 1984. Committee on Ways and Means. *Effects of the Omnibus Budget Reconciliation Act of 1981 (OBRA), Welfare Changes, and the Recession on Poverty.* Washington, D.C.: Government Printing Office.

Valentine, Gill. 1993. "(Hetero)sexing Space: Lesbian Perceptions and Experiences of Everyday Spaces." *Environment and Planning D: Society and Space* 11:395–413.

Waldby, Catherine. 1996. *AIDS and the Body Politic: Biomedicine and Sexual Difference.* New York: Routledge.

Walker, Richard. 1995. "Landscape and City Life: Four Ecologies of Residence in the San Francisco Bay Area." *Ecumene* 2, no. 1:1–35.

———. 1996. "Another Round of Globalization in San Francisco." *Urban Geography* 17, no. 1:60–94.

Wallace, Roderick. 1990. "Urban Desertification, Public Health and Public Order: 'Planned Shrinkage,' Violent Death, Substance Abuse, and AIDS in the Bronx." *Social Science and Medicine* 31, no. 7:801–13.

Wallace, Roderick, and Deborah Wallace. 1995. "U.S. Apartheid and the Spread of AIDS to the Suburbs: A Multi-city Analysis of the Political Economy of Spatial Epidemic Threshold." *Social Science and Medicine* 41, no. 3:333–45.

Ward, David. 1984. "The Progressives and the Urban Question: British and American Responses to the Inner City Slums 1880–1920." *Transactions of the Institute of British Geographers* n.s. 9:299–314.

———. 1989. *Poverty, Ethnicity, and the American City 1840–1925: Changing Conceptions of the Slum and the Ghetto.* Cambridge: Cambridge University Press.

Watney, Simon. 1997. *Policing Desire: Pornography, AIDS, and the Media.* London: Methuen.

Weimer, David R., ed. 1962. *City and Country in America.* New York: Appleton-Century-Crofts.

Weitz, Rose. 1991. *Life with AIDS.* New Brunswick, N.J.: Rutgers University Press.

Welter, B. 1966. "The Cult of True Womanhood, 1820–1860." *American Quarterly* 18:151–74.

White, Morton, and Lucia White. 1962. *The Intellectual versus the City: From Thomas Jefferson to Frank Lloyd Wright.* Oxford: Oxford University Press.

Williams, Raymond. 1980. *Problems in Materialism and Culture.* London: Verso Press.

Wilson, Elizabeth. 1991. *The Sphinx in the City: Urban Life, the Control of Disorder, and Women.* Berkeley: University of California Press.

Wilson, Leonard. 1990. "The Historical Decline of Tuberculosis in Europe and America: Its Causes and Significance." *Journal of the History of Medicine* 45 (July):366–96.

Wilton, Tamsin. 1997. *Engendering AIDS: Deconstructing Sex, Text, and Epidemic.* London: Sage Press.

Wohl, Anthony S. 1983. *Endangered Lives: Public Health in Victorian Britain.* Cambridge, Mass.: Harvard University Press.

Wollenberg, Charles. 1975. *Golden Gate Metropolis: Perspectives on Bay Area History.* Berkeley: Institute of Governmental Studies, University of California.

Woods, Robert, and John Woodward, eds. 1984. *Urban Disease and Mortality in Nineteenth-Century England.* New York: St. Martin's Press.

Wortley, Pascale, and Patricia L. Fleming. 1998. "Increasing Incidence of AIDS among Women." (Letter.) *Journal of the American Medical Association* 279, no. 5:356.

Wright, Gwendolyn. 1981. *Building the Dream: A Social History of Housing in America.* Cambridge, Mass.: MIT Press.

Wright, P., and A. Treacher, eds. 1982. *The Problem of Medical Knowledge.* Edinburgh: Edinburgh University Press.

Young, Iris Marion. 1990. *Justice and the Politics of Difference.* Princeton, N.J.: Princeton University Press.

Yung, Judy. 1995. *Unbound Feet: A Social History of Chinese Women in San Francisco.* Berkeley: University of California Press.

INDEX

SUSAN CRADDOCK is assistant professor of women's studies at the University of Arizona. She is also associated with the Southwest Institute for Research on Women at the University of Arizona.